In Vivo Perfusion and Release of Neuroactive Substances

Methods and Strategies

Contributors

CHRISTOPHER D. ANDREWS
BENITO ANTÓN
ALEJANDRO BAYÓN
CLAES-HENRIC BERTHOLD
IRENE CASTAÑO
ANDRÉ CHÉRAMY
JOSÉ M. R. DELGADO
DAVID DÍAZ-PONTONES
RENÉ DRUCKER-COLÍN
FRANCISCO ESTRADA-VILLANUEVA
JACQUES GLOWINSKI
ANDERS HAMBERGER
DEAN R. HAUBRICH
TOSHIHIKO IIJIMA
INGEMAR JACOBSON
BIRGITTA KARLSSON
NORMAN W. KASTING
PETER J. KNOTT
JAKOB KORF
K. LEDERIS
ANDERS LEHMANN
JUAN LERMA
GREGORY E. MARTIN
KENNETH E. MOORE
KATHYRNE J. MUELLER
JANN A. NIELSEN
KAZUO NUNOKI
BRITTA NYSTRÖM
MARÍA TRINIDAD PACHECO
ATHINEOS PHILIPPU
QUENTIN J. PITTMAN
VICTOR D. RAMÍREZ
PETER REDGRAVE
RAFAEL MARTÍN DEL RÍO
RANULFO ROMO
WILLIAM D. RUWE
MATS SANDBERG
EUGENE P. SCHOENER
SARA SOLANO
JOSÉ M. SOLÍS
H. S. SWARTZWELDER
JAN A. M. VAN DER HEYDEN
WARREN L. VEALE
FRANCISCO VELASCO
MARCOS VELASCO
KOR VENEMA

IN VIVO PERFUSION AND RELEASE OF NEUROACTIVE SUBSTANCES

Methods and Strategies

Edited by

ALEJANDRO BAYÓN
Departamento de Biología Molecular
Instituto de Investigaciones Biomédicas
Universidad Nacional Autónoma de México
Mexico City, Mexico

RENÉ DRUCKER-COLÍN
Centro de Investigaciones en Fisiología Celular
Universidad Nacional Autónoma de México
Mexico City, Mexico

1985

ACADEMIC PRESS, INC.
(Harcourt Brace Jovanovich, Publishers)

Orlando San Diego New York London
Toronto Montreal Sydney Tokyo

ACADEMIC PRESS, INC.
Orlando, Florida 32887

United Kingdom Edition published by
ACADEMIC PRESS INC. (LONDON) LTD.
24–28 Oval Road, London NW1 7DX

Library of Congress Cataloging in Publication Data
Main entry under title:

In vivo perfusion and release of neuroactive substances.

Includes index.
1. Neurotransmitters. 2. Brain chemistry. 3. Perfusion (Physiology). I. Bayón, Alejandro. II. Drucker-Colín, René Raúl. [DNLM: 1. Neurochemistry. 2. Brain Chemistry. 3. Neuroregulators–physiology. 4. Perfusion. QV 126 I35]
QP364.7.I5 1985 599.01'88 84-21541
ISBN 0–12–083350–6 (alk. paper)

PRINTED IN THE UNITED STATES OF AMERICA

85 86 87 88 9 8 7 6 5 4 3 2 1

Contents

Contributors

Numbers in parentheses indicate the pages on which the authors' contributions begin.

Christopher D. Andrews (141), Department of Pharmacology, Marshall University School of Medicine, Huntington, West Virginia 25704

Benito Antón (69), Departamento de Biología Molecular, Instituto de Investigaciones Biomédicas, Universidad Nacional Autónoma de México, 04510 Mexico City, Mexico

Alejandro Bayón (1, 69), Departamento de Biología Molecular, Instituto de Investigaciones Biomédicas, Universidad Nacional Autónoma de México, 04510 Mexico City, Mexico

Claes-Henric Berthold (119), Department of Anatomy, University of Göteborg, S-400 33 Göteborg, Sweden

Irene Castaño (69), Departamento de Biología Molecular, Instituto de Investigaciones Biomédicas, Universidad Nacional Autónoma de México, 04510 Mexico City, Mexico

André Chéramy (161), Chaire de Neuropharmacologie, Groupe NB, Collège de France, 75231 Paris 05, France

José M. R. Delgado (95), Departamento de Investigación, Centro Ramón y Cajal, Madrid 28034, Spain

David Díaz-Pontones (69), Departamento de Biología Molecular, Instituto de Investigaciones Biomédicas, Universidad Nacional Autónoma de México, 04510 Mexico City, Mexico

René Drucker-Colín (1), Centro de Investigaciones en Fisiología Celular, Universidad Nacional Autónoma de México, 20 Mexico City, Mexico

Francisco Estrada-Villanueva (271), Division of Neurophysiology, Scientific Research Department, National Medical Center, Instituto Mexicano del Seguro Social, 03020 Mexico City, Mexico

Jacques Glowinski (161), Chaire de Neuropharmacologie, Groupe NB, Collège de France, 75231 Paris 05, France

Anders Hamberger (119), Institute of Neurobiology, University of Göteborg, S-400 33 Göteborg, Sweden

*Dean R. Haubrich** (293), Department of Pharmacology, Merck Sharp & Dohme Research Laboratories, West Point, Pennsylvania 19486

Toshihiko Iijima (41), Department of Pharmacology, Tohoku University School of Medicine, Sendai 980, Japan

Ingemar Jacobson (119), Institute of Neurobiology, University of Göteborg, S-400 33 Göteborg, Sweden

Birgitta Karlsson (119), Institute of Neurobiology, University of Göteborg, S-400 33 Göteborg, Sweden

Norman W. Kasting (233), Department of Physiology, University of British Columbia, Vancouver, British Columbia, Canada

Peter J. Knott† (141), Department of Pharmacology, Marshall University School of Medicine, Huntington, West Virginia 25704

Jakob Korf (51), Department of Biological Psychiatry, University Psychiatric Clinic, 9713 EZ Groningen, The Netherlands

K. Lederis (233), Department of Medical Physiology, Faculty of Medicine, University of Calgary, Calgary, Alberta T2N 4N1, Canada

Anders Lehmann (119), Institute of Neurobiology, University of Göteborg, S-400 33 Göteborg, Sweden

Juan Lerma (95), Departamento de Investigación, Centro Ramón y Cajal, Madrid 28034, Spain

Gregory E. Martin‡ (293), Department of Pharmacology, Merck Sharp & Dohme Research Laboratories, West Point, Pennsylvania 19486

Kenneth E. Moore (177), Department of Pharmacology and Toxicology, Michigan State University, East Lansing, Michigan 48824

Kathyrne J. Mueller (141), Department of Pharmacology, Marshall University School of Medicine, Huntington, West Virginia 25704

Jann A. Nielsen§ (177), Department of Pharmacology and Toxicology, Michigan State University, East Lansing, Michigan 48824

Kazuo Nunoki (41), Department of Pharmacology, Tohoku University School of Medicine, Sendai 980, Japan

Britta Nyström (119), Institute of Neurobiology, University of Göteborg, S-400 33 Göteborg, Sweden

María Trinidad Pacheco (271), Division of Neurophysiology, Scientific Research Department, National Medical Center, Instituto Mexicano del Seguro Social, 03020 Mexico City, Mexico

Athineos Philippu (221), Department of Pharmacodynamics and Toxicology, University of Innsbruck, A-6020 Innsbruck, Austria

*Present address: Sterling-Winthrop Research Institute, Rensselaer, New York 12144.

†Present address: Departments of Psychiatry and Pharmacology, The Mount Sinai Medical Center, One Gustave L. Levy Place, New York, New York 10029.

‡Present address: McNeil Pharmaceutical, Department of Biological Research, Spring House, Pennsylvania 19477.

§Present address: Program of Pharmacology, Northeastern Ohio University, College of Medicine, Rootstown, Ohio 44272.

Quentin J. Pittman (233), Department of Medical Physiology, Faculty of Medicine, University of Calgary, Calgary, Alberta T2N 4N1, Canada

Victor D. Ramírez (249), Department of Physiology and Biophysics, University of Illinois, Urbana, Illinois 61801

Peter Redgrave (11), Department of Psychology, University of Sheffield, Sheffield S10 2TN, England

Rafael Martín del Río, (95), Departamento de Investigación, Centro Ramón y Cajal, Madrid 28034, Spain

Ranulfo Romo (161), Chaire de Neuropharmacologie, Groupe NB, Collège de France, 75231 Paris 05, France

William D. Ruwe (233), Department of Medical Physiology, Faculty of Medicine, University of Calgary, Calgary, Alberta T2N 4N1, Canada

Mats Sandberg (119), Institute of Neurobiology, University of Göteborg, S-400 33 Göteborg, Sweden

Eugene P. Schoener (25), Department of Pharmacology, Wayne State University, School of Medicine, Detroit, Michigan 48201

Sara Solano (69), Departamento de Biología Molecular, Instituto de Investigaciones Biomédicas, Universidad Nacional Autónoma de México, 04510 Mexico City, Mexico

José M. Solís (95), Departamento de Investigación, Centro Ramón y Cajal, Madrid 28034, Spain

H. S. Swartzwelder (201), Department of Medicine, Division of Neurology, Duke University Medical Center, Durham, North Carolina 27705

Jan A. M. van der Heyden (51), Department of Pharmacology, Duphar B. V., 1380 AA Weesp, The Netherlands

Warren L. Veale (233), Department of Medical Physiology, Faculty of Medicine, University of Calgary, Calgary, Alberta T2N 4N1, Canada

Francisco Velasco (271), Division of Neurophysiology, Scientific Research Department, National Medical Center, Instituto Mexicano del Seguro Social, 03020 Mexico City, Mexico

Marcos Velasco (271), Division of Neurophysiology, Scientific Research Department, National Medical Center, Instituto Mexicano del Seguro Social, 03020 Mexico City, Mexico

Kor Venema (51), Department of Biological Psychiatry, University Psychiatric Clinic, 9713 EZ Groningen, The Netherlands

Preface

The birth of neuroscience as an interdisciplinary subject largely originated from the necessity of unifying the conceptual maps produced within the different traditional disciplines studying the nervous system. The *in vivo* techniques that allow the concerted study of neurochemical, pharmacological, electrophysiological, and behavioral aspects of brain function have played a paramount role in this endeavor. In spite of the fact that these techniques—the subject matter of this book—have for two decades been our main window for the direct observation of these correlations, their use within the scientific community has been limited by misinformation, misconceptions, and/or inexperience. Only recently has this panorama begun to change. As a result of improved procedures, probes, and detectors, and due to the availability of more specific and sensitive neurochemical assays, these techniques have provided new strategies for the study of brain function, and their success has resulted in the recognition of their unique value.

The feeling that these developments are opening a new epoch for the *in vivo* study of the brain has stimulated several scientific events on this topic, including a symposium in the Annual Meeting of the Society for Neuroscience (1981), a workshop at the European Society for Neuroscience (1981), and recently a symposium entitled "*In Vivo* Release of Neuroactive Substances in the CNS," held in 1983 in Mexico City. From these meetings it was clear that in this changing scientific atmosphere it is necessary not just to analyze the emerging possibilities and alternatives, but also to evaluate the state of the art and the depth of its accomplishments.

Our main concern in editing this book is to provide the reader with sound criteria to engage with, use, and improve on the methods and strategies utilized to study *in vivo* neurochemistry, in order to correlate it with electrophysiological and behavioral events. We do not intend to give the best of recipes for *in vivo* perfusion and release techniques. This is possible only by careful consideration of current knowledge and personal experience, along with practical tests of the suitability of the methods for one's own necessities. Nonetheless, in the Introduction we present an overview of methodological alternatives and experimental strategies that we think are critical for the outcome of this type of research. The chapters that follow collect personal experiences on the study of *in vivo* neurochemistry and of its correlation with other neural events, contributed by representative scientists whose efforts have made possible the optimization of current techniques and the development of new ones. The chapters have been written and edited to facilitate the evaluation and comparison of the different techniques and experimental strategies used by the authors. Chapters in Part I concentrate on detailed descriptions of the probes and procedures used in this research and also provide a critical evaluation of the potentialities and limitations of the methodologies employed. Chapters in Part II exemplify the variety of experimental strategies in which these techniques have been used, gathering understanding on the chemical, bioelectrical, and behavioral aspects of brain function. They also illustrate interdisciplinary techniques for approaching problems of neuronal connectivity, neuroendocrinology, motor behavior, neuropathology, etc.

We think this is a timely review, not just for the specialist, who surely will find this a useful, updated reference text, but for neuroscientists and students who have not had contact with this field and who may now find that these developments could open new possibilities for their own research interests. The editors are grateful to the Dirección General de Asuntos del Personal Académico (DGAPA) and to the Coordinación de la Investigación Científica (CIC) of the Universidad Nacional Autónoma de México, without whose support this book could not have been written. We also thank Mrs. Martha Sarmiento for her patient clerical work.

Alejandro Bayón
René Drucker-Colín

In Vivo Perfusion and Release of Neuroactive Substances

Methods and Strategies

1

Introduction

ALEJANDRO BAYÓN

Departamento de Biología Molecular
Instituto de Investigaciones Biomédicas
Universidad Nacional Autónoma de México
Mexico City, Mexico

RENÉ DRUCKER-COLÍN

Centro de Investigaciones en Fisiología Celular
Universidad Nacional Autónoma de México
Mexico City, Mexico

METHODOLOGICAL ALTERNATIVES AND EXPERIMENTAL STRATEGIES FOR STUDYING THE *IN VIVO* PERFUSION AND RELEASE OF NEUROACTIVE SUBSTANCES IN THE CENTRAL NERVOUS SYSTEM

Twenty-seven years ago Fox and Hilton (*1*) designed a system of parallel needles to perfuse subcutaneous tissue, which was modified by J. H. Gaddum (*2*) into two concentric tubes—push–pull cannula—making it possible to perform *in vivo* experiments "to localize the site of liberation of substances in such tissues as the central nervous system, more precisely than by other means." In order to better understand the importance and consequences of this development, which revolutionized *in vivo* neurochemistry, one must compare it with alternate superfusion techniques. Perfusion methods, push–pull cannulae systems included, are based on the same working principle: controlled infusion and simultaneous withdrawal of an artificial physiological fluid through the nervous tissue. This procedure creates a stream that interfaces with tissular elements, allowing bidirectional diffusion

ISBN 0-12-083350-6

between the tissue and the exogenous fluid. The possibility of adding neuroactive chemicals to the infusion fluid, and the fractionation, collection, and analysis of the outcoming liquid have made perfusion techniques a milestone in neurobiology. However, both goals can be achieved *in vivo* by technical means other than Gaddum's cannulae, namely, surface cups and ventricular needles. Surface cups (mainly cortical cups) are chambers chronically adhered to the surface of the brain which contain inlet and outlet ports to allow infusion and withdrawal of perfusing medium. Ventricular needles or cannulae are probes implanted in separate regions of the brain ventricular system which act as inlet and outlet ports to perfuse the cerebrospinal fluid (CSF)-filled cavity between them. Cups and ventricular needles have been, and still are, valuable tools for *in vivo* neurochemistry; both were in use at the time Gaddum's cannula was developed and their power and limitations have been critically compared to those of concentric cannulae (3). Unfortunately, their use is restricted to the brain surfaces and cavities and do not allow the study of most deep-brain nuclei. The Gaddum cannula has found a much wider use: since the inlet and outlet ports (push–pull) are concentric (see Fig. 1 in the chapters that follow), the cannula can be implanted just as an electrode is, using stereotaxic techniques in order to reach discrete neural regions. Thus, the neuroanatomical selectivity and the versatility of its use are responsible for its success. Because of these advantages, and since the basic working principles of surface cups and ventricular needles are close to those of concentric cannulae, the latter will serve as a model for discussion of *in vivo* perfusion methodology. Some designs such as dialytrodes are also suitable for site-specific perfusions. Dialytrodes are probes based on the same working principles as other perfusion devices, but the diffusional exchange between the tissue and the perfusing medium is mediated by a dialysis membrane. The discussion of the advantages and limitations in brain neurochemistry of dialytrodes—and of electrochemical probes—deserve and need a separate treatment, given in Chapters 7, 8, and 9.

For the neuroscientist using push–pull perfusion methods it is not uncommon to meet colleagues who some time in their careers started using this type of method, but were discouraged very early because of technical difficulties and poor, unreliable results. This is the case, particularly, when no experienced advice backs up the setting of the experimental tools and procedures. In practice, the central and usually unexpected problem with these techniques is the difficulty in maintaining a steady flow of the perfusion medium at the interface with the tissue. Since flow obstructions and tissue damage are closely linked, we will first discuss the factors involving both problems, then present those related to damage in the absence of flow impairments.

Partial or total interruption of flow through the perfusion system has disastrous consequences (see Chapter 2) and will surely be observed in the course of the first perfusion sessions. There are several immediate causes for this occurrence, the most common being blood or plasma clogs obliterating fluid circulation. When the perfusion probe is acutely inserted into the brain, or if mechanical tissue damage is produced by cannula movements or hydrostatic pressure changes, the rupture of blood vessels is a highly probable event. The second important cause producing flow obstructions is the entrance of tissue fragments into the pull cannula. Tissue disruption rarely occurs under the normally used pressure and flow conditions (see the Methods sections in the following chapters), but extreme mechanical damage to the tissue will surely produce it. Flow impairments related to the malfunction of the perfusion system (failure of pumps, bent or twisted tubings, etc.) are less troublesome, and will be taken care of by constant maintenance and checking of the equipment prior to and during the experimental sessions.

Prolonged or abundant bleeding, and obstruction of flow by clogs that produce fluid accumulation in the brain, whatever their cause, will always lead to experimental failure. In these cases, terminating the perfusion will be a wiser decision than repeated cleaning of the system, since the latter leads to serious tissue damage. The use of alternative procedures may prevent or minimize this kind of problem. Chronic implantation of the probe avoids the bleeding sometimes observed after acute insertions; however, chronic implants may or may not be feasible depending on the experimental design and objectives (see, for instance, Chapters 6 and 15). Changing the stereotaxic routes in acute insertions can often make the cannula skip a large blood vessel frequently encountered when using a different trajectory (small vessels are always ruptured, but they usually present no problem and heal in a few minutes). One must remember that slight local edema may be produced during perfusion, even when CSF is used as the perfusion medium, and extravasation of plasma may produce clogs in the absence of visible red blood cells. When this problem (colorless clogs inside the cannula) is identified, the use of faster perfusion flowrates and/or lowering of the Ca^{2+} concentration in the medium may be indicated (see Chapter 15). The effect of using anticoagulants in the perfusing media will have to be tested and evaluated for particular experimental protocols.

Obstruction of flow by tissue fragments may be the immediate consequence of mechanical damage occurring during acute insertion of the probe. Introduction of a false cannula prior to the insertion of the actual probe is advisable when attempting to solve this problem. As indicated above, mechanical damage and consequent flow obstructions during the perfusion session should and can be minimized. Movement of the probe inside the animal's brain will lead to lesions and frequently to occlusions. Immobilization of the probe is a requisite met by chronic cannula implants cemented with acrylic; acute insertions into immobilized anesthetized animals also fulfill this requirement. However, the effects of these conditions on the experimental results and the needs and objectives of the experiment have to be carefully considered. When the experiment requires freely moving animals, a guide tubing is chronically implanted into the brain to allow the acute stereotaxic insertion of the perfusing cannula; a probe-fixating device (clamp or screw) is necessary in this case. Since the brain floats in the CSF and moves within the cranium of the behaving animal, care should be taken to prevent violent movements of the animal or collisions with the walls of the cage. Carrying out the perfusion in an environment that is isolated, nondisturbing, and familiar to the animal will help in this regard.

Extreme hydrostatic pressure within the perfused area is a factor that produces tissue damage and in some instances occlusions (see Chapters 2, 3, and 7). High positive pressure leads to accumulation of liquid, enlargement and disruption of the perfused area; negative pressure increases the erosion, lesions the tissue, and eventually may block the flow in the system. Thus, a good part of the success of *in vivo* perfusion systems lies in keeping a normal intracranial pressure. This requirement has been fulfilled using two different designs known as "closed" and "open" perfusion systems. The former uses precision delivery and withdrawal mechanisms (usually employing reciprocating syringe pumps) matched to keep a constant flow through the tissue and so requires isolation of the system from atmospheric pressure. The second system does not require high precision of the delivery and withdrawal mechanisms (peristaltic pumping, which is pulsatile and varies with tissue resistance, is frequently used); balance of inflow and outflow of fluid is achieved by opening the system to the atmospheric pressure (a small hole in the pull tubing; see Chapter 10). So, when the outflow is set faster than the inflow, it takes only the available liquid from the perfusion site and air enters the withdrawal system, avoiding excess negative pressure. Open systems and their equivalents (see Chapters 4 and 13) are more easily mastered and more reliable than closed systems because volumetric precision is not required and because, if accidental blockage occurs, it usually subsides by itself. However, closed systems incorporating pressure-buffering devices have advantages comparable to those of open systems (see Chapters 2 and 3). It is worth mentioning that in spite of these advances a theoretical hydrodynamic study of these perfusion systems is not yet available to neurobiologists.

Even in the absence of flow obstructions, some tissue erosion due to the passing stream of perfusion fluid seems to be unavoidable during push–pull perfusion. The extent of this erosion depends on the geometry of the tip of the push–pull cannula. When probes are used in which the push cannula protrudes out of the pull tubing (classical Gaddum cannula), the outflow stream of fluid collides against the tissue, increasing the erosion. With probes in which the push cannula is shielded within the pull tubing (see Chapters 4, 6, and 13) the stream does not circulate through the tissue. The eroded tissue is a minimal part of perfused tissue, but this phenomenon needs to be considered when studying the resting release of neurochemicals.

Given all these technical problems, what should be the starting strategies for those setting up their own perfusion system? The best practical advice is to begin by testing it *in vitro* in a fluid-filled beaker, then, inserting the probe in an isolated brain or using it in an anesthetized, immobilized animal, and, finally, using it in an implanted freely moving animal. Following this sequence the beginner will gain gradual experience in solving the problems inherent, first, in the hydraulic systems, second, in those due to the resistance of the tissue, and, finally, in those arising from the movement and physiology of the animal. Skipping one of these steps will lead to frustration and eventually will force the investigator to follow them in the inverse order. If this advice is followed, this overview and the chapters in this book will serve as useful guidelines for developing the various methods and strategies used in the multidisciplinary study of *in vivo* neurobiology.

Neuroscience is linked to the quests by scientists within traditional disciplines to raise questions about the nervous system as a whole. Morphological, chemical, and biophysical methods easily lend themselves to a convergence in the study of the substrates of neural activity; their finer techniques had been developed for postmortem or *in vitro* studies and allowed the creation of truly interdisciplinary subjects such as histochemistry and membrane biophysics. The higher level of complexity present *in vivo* and the methodological requirements of neurophysiological and behavioral studies made the integration of neurochemistry to their task more difficult; only some pharmacological and microsurgical techniques contributed to fill the gap. Further advances in the integration of the neurosciences require a more extensive development and use of methods which allow the simultaneous study of neurochemical and bioelectrical phenomena in the behaving animal, preserving neural connectivity and architecture, and providing anatomical precision. Techniques for the *in vivo* perfusion of the brain established the basis for this development.

Studying the modulation of the *in vivo* release of brain substances (both spontaneous and evoked by means of electrical, neurochemical, or pharmacological stimuli) is worthwhile in and of itself; the functional neurochemistry of defined brain regions and its association with neuronal activity and neural circuits and pathways first became accessible to us through the use of *in vivo* perfusion techniques (see, for instance, Chapters 10, 11, and 12). However, an outstanding and unique application of the *in vivo* brain perfusion has been in experiments directed to correlate neurochemistry to more elaborated physiological and behavioral events, approaching problems that go from neurovegetative and neuroendocrine functions (see Chapters 13, 14, and 15) to motor control, learning, sleep, and pathology (see Chapters 2, 16, and 17). Last, but not least, *in vivo* perfusion methods have been a unique potential path for the discovery of novel neurochemicals recovered from perfusates and tested through them for biological activity.

Given these potentialities and preceding discussion of the limitations of the uses of these techniques stands the question of when to use them. Briefly, they should be used whenever an *in vitro* study is not able to give the desired information because the anatomical, physiological, or behavioral integrity of the biological system are a part of the problem or a condition for its answer. The difficulties of these techniques make it inadvisable to use them when suitable alternatives can give us what we need. However, for technical reasons, push–pull perfusion can sometimes be the alternative of choice. For instance, the technique to be used for the administration of drugs into specific brain areas may present a dilemma: injection or perfusion? Since perfusion *in vivo* allows the administration of changing doses of pharmacological agents to the same animal during the same session, it may be better than injection (see Chapter 3).

The main limitation of current *in vivo* perfusion methods is resolution, both in space and in time. Even using a fixed geometry and size of the cannula tip, the volume of tissue perfused is not well delimited, since the diffusional gradient of perfused substances rapidly decreases around the cannula tip (see Chapter 16). This problem has to be studied and considered when assessing the anatomical specificity of the neural substrates affected by perfused substances and the neural origin of neurochemicals collected in superfusates. The resolution in time of neurochemical events by push–pull perfusion methods is also affected by the geometry and size of the cannula and connecting tubing, that is, the presence of dead-volume spaces where the perfusing stream can mix, diffuse, and dilute. Furthermore, however small the dead volumes in the flow system, neurophysiological events occur in a time scale far shorter than practical and possible flow rates and collected volumes.

Beyond these limitations, the contributions in this book show that *in vivo* perfusion techniques are being improved so that their development in the near future is a very promising one. On-line detection of neurochemicals can be achieved by high-pressure liquid chromatography coupled to the outflow system. The use of highly sensitive and specific immunoassays and receptor assays, frequently coupled to high-performance separation systems, now permits the measurement of neuropeptides and other complex neurochemicals. The development of better dialytrode systems allows the quantitative assessment of the release of neurochemicals in the extracellular medium. The study of the cellular uptake and binding of neurochemicals to receptors *in vivo* is also feasible with these techniques. The development of "chemitrodes" allows simultaneous perfusion and recording of single unit activity in freely moving animals. One can be sure that the *in vivo* neurochemical methods and strategies in the years to come will surpass our expectations.

REFERENCES

1. Fox, R., and Hilton, S. *J. Physiol. (London)* **142** (1958) 219.
2. Gaddum, J. H. Push–pull cannulae. *J. Physiol. (London)* **155** (1961) 1–2P.
3. Myers, R. D. Methods for perfusing different structures of the brain. *Meth. Psychobiol.* **2** (1972) 169–211.

I

Methods

2

Technical Issues Associated with Push–Pull Perfusion in Unanesthetized and Unrestrained Animals

PETER REDGRAVE

Department of Psychology
University of Sheffield
Sheffield, England

I. INTRODUCTION

The push–pull perfusion technique is often presented, by those who use it, as a technique of great versatility and promise. For example, it can be operated in two different modes: (1) as a device for chemically stimulating the brain and (2) as a method for measuring the local release of substances within the brain.

When used as a chemical stimulator it has several advantages over simple microinjections. First, it enables far greater control over the temporal aspects of stimulation. Second, it is possible to provide a systematic variation of stimulation intensity (in terms of different concentrations of substances within the push line) during a single experimental session. Third, it enables

IN VIVO PERFUSION AND RELEASE
OF NEUROACTIVE SUBSTANCES

ISBN 0-12-083350-6

stimulation with endogenous substances, e.g., acetylcholine and GABA, whose short half-line in brain often precludes their use in microinjection experiments.

As a technique for measuring the local release of substances from the brain, the main advantage of the push–pull perfusion is that it is an *in vivo* procedure which provides for repeated measures. There are two important consequences of this: (1) a preparation can be used as its own control and (2) release from exactly the same region of brain during experimental and control conditions is assured. When used in this mode there is, in principle, no limit to the variety of independent manipulations whose effects on local release can be measured with the push–pull perfusion.

In addition to providing greater temporal and spatial resolution than many comparable *in vivo* neurochemical techniques, the push–pull perfusion can be performed with unanesthetized and unrestrained animals. Thus, when used in either mode the push–pull perfusion enables direct correlations to be made between regional neurochemical events and behavior.

Given this considerable potential it is puzzling that in more than 20 years since Gaddum's original introduction of the technique (*3*), so few laboratories have attempted its use and even fewer retain it on a regular basis. For the purposes of this communication I commissioned a computer search of literature (IRS Dialtech) in which "push–pull" was the specified search term. In the neuroscience journals, over the past 10 years, 49 articles were identified which included "push–pull" either in the title or in the key words. These articles originated from 28 laboratories, only 11 of which have published articles since 1980. While these figures must be viewed with caution (there are several studies known to the author that use the push–pull technique yet fail to specify the term in the title or key words), they give some impression of the popularity of the technique. Interestingly, when the search term was relaxed to "perfusion" in association with "release" 265 neuroscience articles were identified. Clearly, even allowing for some underestimation in these figures, the push–pull perfusion can only have been used in a relatively small proportion of these studies.

One factor which may, in part, account for the disparity between the potential of the push–pull technique and its actual use, is that many potential users may have been put off by stories of tissue damage caused by push–pull perfusion. Certainly, while much time and effort has been spent on increasing the sensitivity and specificity of biochemical assay procedures used to analyze push–pull perfusate (e.g., *1, 7, 8, 9, 12, 13, 17, 18*), comparatively few studies have considered the problem of maintaining a constant flow of perfusate through the preparation (*4, 12, 14, 19*). In practice, the outflow or pull cannula sometimes becomes occluded at the tip, although this is not always easy to detect. If the pull cannula is blocked and the perfusion pump left running, fluid is inevitably lost into the brain. This can result in damage to tissue, which in turn places serious constraints on the subsequent interpretation of data (*2, 5*).

While the inadvertent destruction of brain tissue is an important concern of all investigators who use the push–pull technique, for those who attempt to perfuse unanesthetized animals, accidental neural damage often means the end of a preparation in which there has been considerable investment of time, effort, and expense.

The problem of fluid loss after an occlusion of the pull cannula will be considered in the following:

1. A Methods section in which a description of a system suitable for use with small unanesthetized animals is provided. The practical consequences of a blockage to the pull line of a closed system is considered, together with details of an improvement in technique that enables the immediate detection of such blockages.
2. Relevant empirical findings.
3. Implications of the technical changes on the future use of the technique.

II. METHODS

A. Cannula Construction

A convenient design of push–pull cannula suitable for use with smaller animals has been described by Myers (*11*) (see Fig. 1). Five simple steps are required to construct it.

1. An outer or pull tube is cut from 23-ga thin-walled stainless-steel tubing and soldered into the end of a 5–7 mm length of 18-ga tubing.
2. The end of the pull cannula can be beveled to reduce the occurrence of tissue occluding the tip of the cannula when it is first introduced into the brain.
3. The inner or push cannula is made from a length of 30-ga stainless-steel tubing and is also beveled at one end. The inner cannula is passed into the outer cannula until the lower lips of the beveled ends are at the same level (see Fig. 1). This arrangement minimizes blockages to the pull cannula (see below) but provides for a less than optimum exchange of constituents between the brain and the perfusing medium (*19*).
4. The outflow line is completed by passing a length of 25-ga needle tubing into the top of the "chamber" formed by the 18-ga collar.

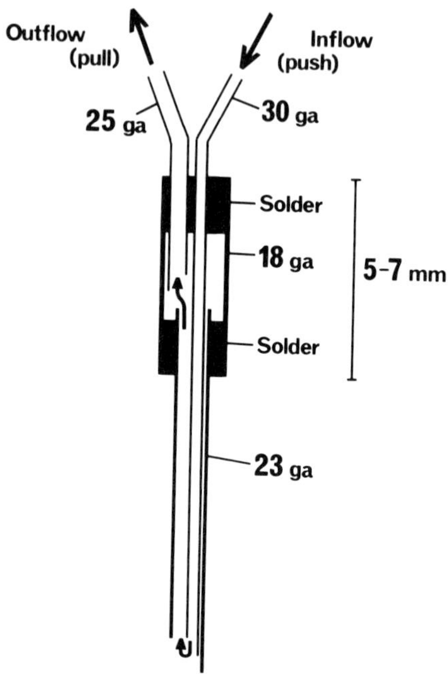

Fig. 1. Components of a push–pull cannula suitable for use with small unanesthetized animals. Only essential measurements are given; e.g., the overall length of the cannula will be determined by the depth of the intended structure and can be varied without affecting the performance of the system. The stainless-steel tubing can be obtained from Cooper's Needle Works (Redditch), Birmingham, England.

5. The top end of the 18-ga tube is closed with solder thereby permanently fixing the push cannula and the 25-ga outflow tube in place. A minimum amount of heat and solder are required to prevent the internal space of the 18-ga tube being completely filled.

B. Surgical and Perfusion Procedures

Standard stereotaxic procedures are used to implant a 10-mm, 20-ga thin-walled guide tube above the intended site of perfusion. The implant is chronically maintained by packing cranioplastic cement around the guide cannula and anchor screws embedded into the cranium. Except during perfusions, a stylet is always placed in the guide tube to prevent it from becoming blocked.

In the past (*11*), the push–pull perfusion has been achieved by connecting the inflow and outflow cannulae directly to reciprocally acting calibrated syringes with suitable lengths of polyethylene tubing (PP10-50). The cannulae, syringes, and tubing are normally filled with an artificial CSF (*12*). This produces a "closed" system into which no air is admitted. Typically, this system has been operated with a perfusion flow rate of 20–100 μl/min. At the beginning of a perfusion the animal is hand-restrained while the stylet is removed and replaced by the push–pull cannula which extends below the end of the guide tube into brain tissue. The perfusion is then continued for a time that is determined either by the requirements of the given experiment or by an interruption to the outflow.

III. FINDINGS

A. Modification of Experimental Procedures

1. THE CONSEQUENCES OF OUTFLOW BLOCKAGE

The negative pressure applied to the pull line of a closed system sometimes causes brain tissue to get sucked into the tip of the pull cannula, thereby preventing the removal of fluid from the brain. The first question is how much fluid is lost into the brain when the pull line gets blocked. A simple experiment was performed (*14*) in which (1) the time taken to detect a blockage in the pull line of a closed push–pull system was determined, and (2) the rate of flow, together with the detection time, was used to calculate the volume of fluid that would inevitably be lost into the brain after an occlusion. When all air is excluded from a closed push–pull system the first warning of a blockage is either the appearance of vacuum bubbles in the pull line or the drawing of air into the back of the pull syringe. The latter can be eliminated by applying a small amount of silicone grease to the plunger of the pull syringe (*19*). The experiment simply involved measuring the time taken for vacuum bubbles to appear following an artificial blockage of the pull line in a closed push–pull system. The pull line was occluded by clamping the polyethylene tubing close to the pull cannula with a pair of forceps. Table I presents the mean times taken to detect the first signs of the blockage under conditions of varying perfusion flow rates. Also included in this table are the mean volumes of fluid which would be unavoidably pumped into the brain by the push syringe during the time taken to detect the obstruction to the pull line.

From these data it is clear, even for the slower flow rates, that significant volumes of fluid are lost into the brain after a blockage in the pull line. Figure 2 gives an indication of the amount of tissue that would be displaced in a rat brain following the loss of comparable volumes of perfusate. (In order to give an impression of the extent of displacement, unrecovered fluid is shown to be contained in the immediate vicinity of the cannula tip. In

TABLE I

Time Taken for Vacuum Bubbles to Appear in a Closed Pull Line Following an Artificial Blockage and the Volume of Fluid Which Is Unavoidably Pumped into the Brain during Detection Time[a]

Perfusion flow rate	Mean detection time (min + SE)	Mean volume pumped into brain during detection time (μl + SE)
7.9	3.43 + 0.42	27.1 + 3.3
19.7	1.83 + 0.19	36.1 + 3.8
39.3	1.32 + 0.19	51.7 + 7.7
79.0	0.80 + 0.04	63.2 + 2.8
197.0	0.38 + 0.02	75.7 + 3.7

[a] $N = 5$ observations at each flow rate.

fact, the indicated volume would be assimilated into the tissue in an unpredictable manner.) Obviously, the consequences of losing these volumes into brain tissue are unacceptable.

In the absence of procedures for eliminating occasional blockages of the pull cannula, a significant improvement in technique would be the introduction of a system that gave immediate notice of an occlusion in the outflow line. In this event at least the infusion pump can be switched off. A very simple modification to the closed system in common use (*1, 4, 7, 9, 10, 11, 17, 19*), provides a successful means whereby the outflow of the push–pull system can be monitored (*14*).

2. MODIFIED PROCEDURES

Figure 3 illustrates the incorporation of a 3-way tap (Hamilton Valve 86503) and a calibrated monitor tube (PP10) into the normally closed push–pull system. The monitor tube is conveniently taped to the leg of the table on which the perfusion is performed. The 3–way tap permits the pull syringe (which is equal in volume to the push syringe) to pull either from the animal or from the monitor tube. Under normal circumstances, the total volume pushed through the system is pulled from the animal by setting the level of fluid in the monitor tube (ink marker) below the level of the animal. In fact, it is this hydrostatic pressure that creates the force required to extract perfusate from the brain. Now if the pull cannula becomes blocked, the pull syringe is no longer able to pull from the animal; instead, fluid is immediately pulled from the monitor tube. When this occurs the cannula assembly has to be removed from the animal and the material causing the blockage cleared by flushing before the perfusion is continued.

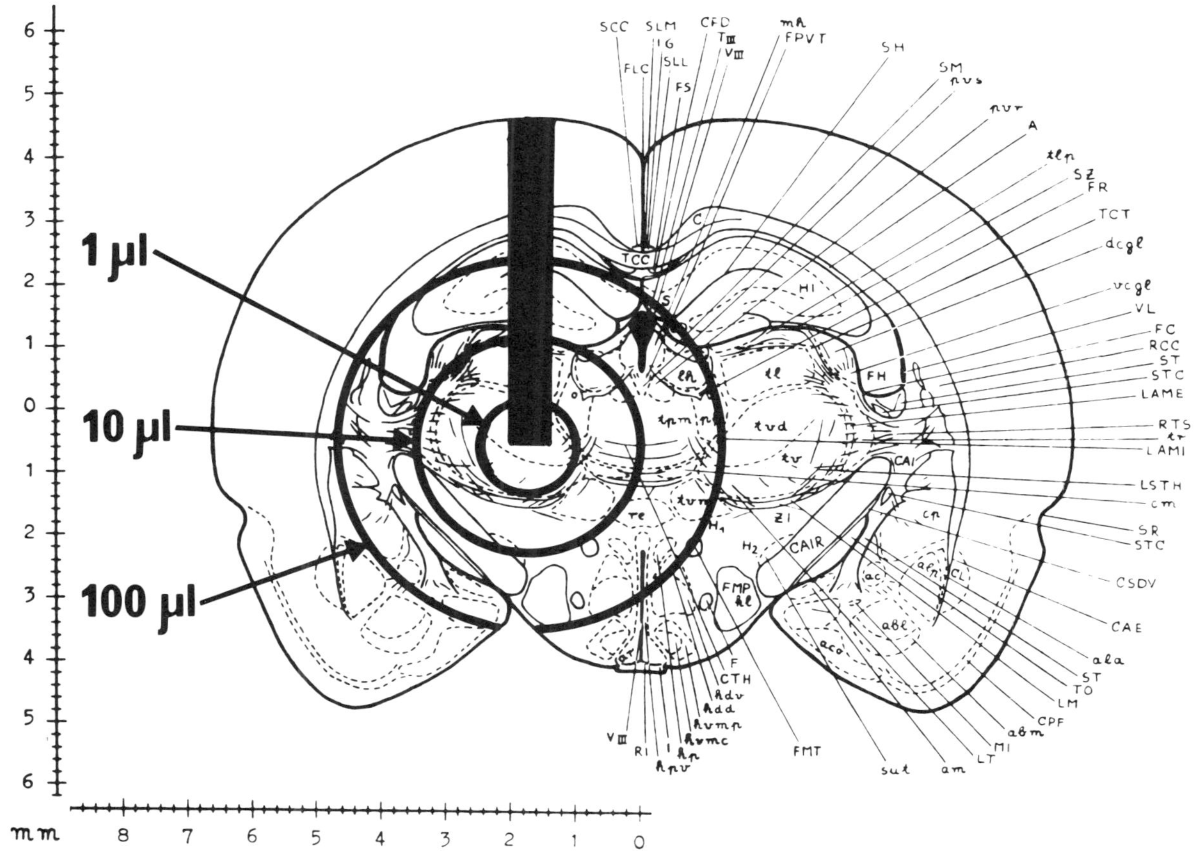

Fig. 2. An indication of the degree to which rat brain tissue would be displaced by different volumes of fluid. [The section of rat brain is from the atlas of Konig and Klippel © 1963, the Williams & Wilkins Co., Baltimore. (6).]

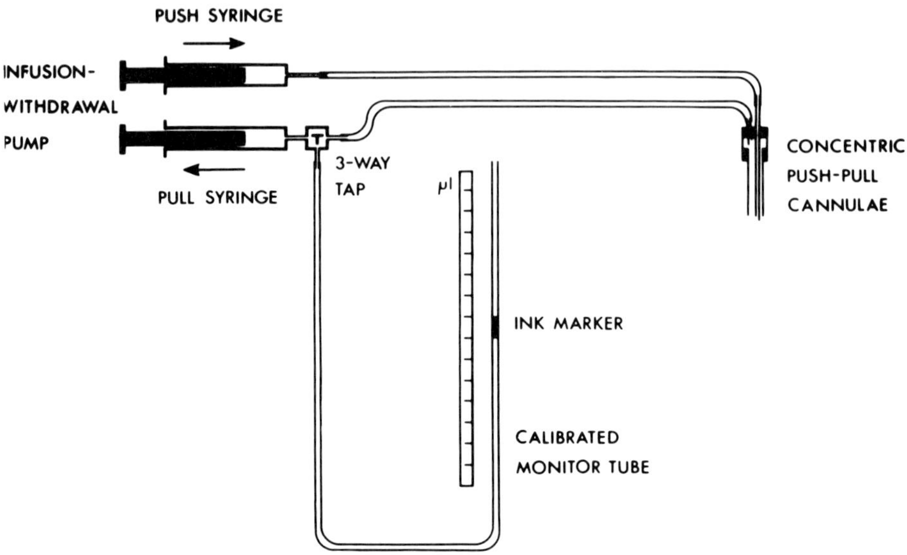

Fig. 3. A schematic representation of the modified push–pull system. A 3-way tap and a monitor tube have been incorporated into a normally closed push–pull system in order to facilitate the discovery of blockages in the pull side of the system.

This simple modification to the push–pull system has several advantages which can be listed as follows.

1. The inadvertent induction of expansion lesions and experimental hydrocephalus is now completely avoidable since immediate indication of a blockage is provided.
2. The amount of fluid unrecovered from the preparation after a blockage to the pull cannula can be quantified by calibrating the monitor tube (0.5-μl divisions is convenient). The unrecovered volume is indicated by the difference between the original and the final heights of the ink marker following a blockage. I consider a fall corresponding to 0.5–1.0 μl sufficient grounds to switch off the pump and determine the cause of the blockage.
3. The difference in height between the animal and the level of fluid in the monitor tube provides a measure (in millimeters of water) of the pressure applied to the pull side of the system; this is normally in the range 10–300 mm.
4. Commonly used flow rates of 20–200 μl/min can be reduced to 0.6–1.7 μl/min without affecting the probability of detecting occlusions. (As flow rate is increased in the present system, additional suction in terms of the difference in height between the animal and level of fluid in the monitor tube must also increase to remove the additional volume of fluid.)

5. Flow rates of 0.6–1.7 μl/min are less likely to cause mechanical disturbance to tissue compared with rates of 20–200 μl/min.

6. The actual incidence of occlusions seems to be reduced. A possible explanation for this may be in terms of the system's response to partial occlusions. When the outflow system is monitored partial blockages are sometimes detected, i.e., when less than the total volume pushed through the system is recovered from the brain. In such cases the fluid level in the monitor tube falls more slowly than when there is a complete occlusion. In the monitored system partial occlusions often tend to clear themselves without intervention (see below). However, in a closed system a partial occlusion would almost inevitably lead to a total blockage as rapidly increasing suction (up to atmospheric pressure) is applied by the pull syringe.

Two types of empirical evidence are considered which testify to the value of monitoring the outflow of the push–pull perfusion. Additional data are also provided concerning the frequency of occlusions in the monitored system.

The first and perhaps most important finding is that when the pull side of the push–pull system is carefully monitored, the useful life of the preparation is considerably extended without increasing the probability of physical trauma to the brain. For example, sections A and B in Fig. 4 are representative of the histology obtained from 6 out of 8 unanesthetized rats with chronic implants which were subjected to between 1 and 5 15-min perfusion attempts with a closed push–pull system with a flow rate of 20 μl/min. In contrast, sections C and D are representative of the histology obtained from rats which had received between 10 and 25 push–pull perfusions of 20- to 30-min duration spaced over a period of several weeks (*15, 16*). The flow rate was 1.0 μl/min and the pull system was monitored at all times. Clearly, the monitored system restricts damage to the track along which the cannulae pass. In no case has damage to the extent of that shown in sections A and B of Fig. 4 ever been observed in animals where the perfusion outflow has been monitored.

B. Neurobiological Applications

The monitored push–pull system has been used successfully to determine dose–response relationships between centrally administered neurotransmitters and intracranial self-stimulation behavior in rats (*15, 16*). In both studies advantage was taken of the temporal control afforded by the push–pull perfusion for chemically stimulating the brain. The first experiment (*16*) demonstrated that local administration of either acetylcholine or serotonin to the substantia nigra/ventral tegmental area produced a dose-dependent

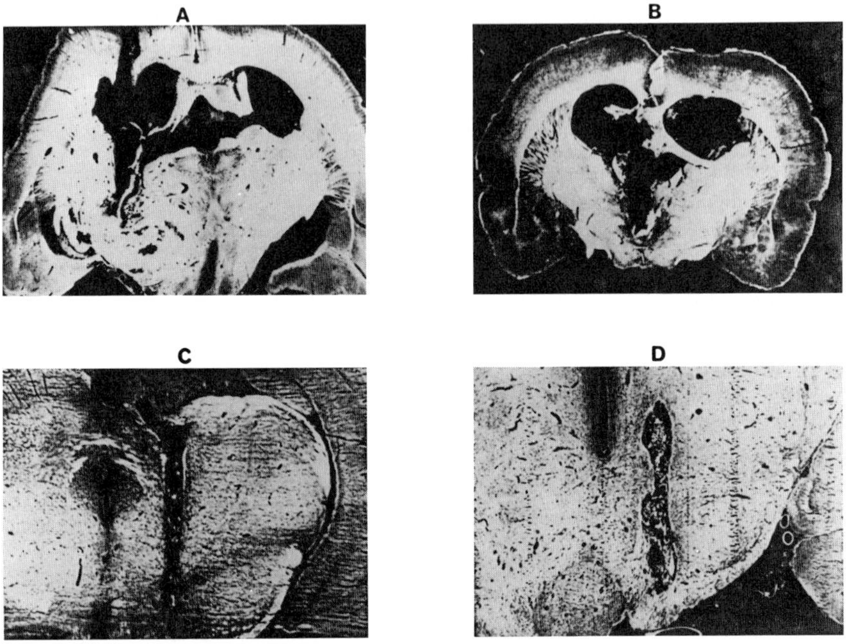

Fig. 4. Histological sections of rat brain. Sections A and B were obtained from brains subjected to push–pull perfusions in which a closed system was used. Sections C and D were obtained from brains subjected to similar perfusions except that the perfusion outflow was continuously monitored using the present modified system.

potentiation of self-stimulation on medial forebrain bundle electrodes. The second series of experiments (*15*) showed that similar increases in self-stimulation could be achieved by perfusing either dopamine or noradrenaline into dopamine terminal areas (corpus striatum and nucleus accumbens). Interestingly, serotonin at these sites produced a dose-dependent suppression of self-stimulation behavior. In these experiments some animals received as many as 30–40 individual 15-min perfusion sessions at each of several locations with the brain; while experiments with a single subject were spread over several months. Clearly, this kind of experimental regimen required procedures which minimized intracerebral trauma.

More recently, the monitored system has been used to measure the release of unlabeled GABA from the superior colliculus of rats (Redgrave, Dean, and Nahorski, unpublished observations). In these experiments animals were anesthetized and the superior colliculus perfused bilaterally for 90–120 min with a monitored push–pull system described above. There were a total of 92 perfusions; in 67.5% there were no blockages; in 13.0% there were partial blockages which cleared themselves before 1.0 μl was lost into the brain; and in 19.5% there were complete blockages which required attention. These results provide some indication of the frequency of blockages in the push–pull system as detected by the present monitoring facility.

IV. PERSPECTIVES AND DISCUSSION

The basic concern of this chapter is the problem of inadvertent damage caused to brain tissue during push–pull perfusion. It is suggested that this factor may, in part, explain why comparatively few investigators use the technique on a permanent basis. Insofar as undetected blockages at the tip of the pull cannula prevent the removal of perfusate from the brain, this is seen as the single most important event contributing to accidental damage to tissue.

The loss of unacceptably large quantities of fluid into the brain can compromise experiments in many ways. At one extreme, two of the animals whose histology is represented by sections A and B in Fig. 4 subsequently died as a result of perfusion. Less final effects of fluid loss can, however, seriously affect the reliability of results and interpretation of data.

1. Nonlethal mechanical damage to tissue at the tip of the push–pull cannula would clearly make data obtained from either stimulation or release experiments uninterpretable.
2. Several investigators (*4, 19*) have demonstrated that discontinuities in the flow of perfusate can seriously influence the uptake of substances from the extracellular space.
3. In chemical stimulation experiments a blockage in the pull line can result in the stimulating substances reaching unintended parts of the brain. In this context it is worth considering what happens to fluid that is "lost" after a blockage. In animals with chronic implants there is no place for the excess fluid to go other than into surrounding tissue or back up the cannula track into the cerebral ventricles (see sections A and B in Fig. 4). In acute experiments much less damage is typically caused since fluid can easily pass back along the cannula track onto the surface of the brain to mingle with fluid used to irrigate the wound. However, in both cases data would be difficult to interpret since unintended areas of the brain would have been exposed to the stimulating compound.

These considerations suggest that a technical modification which satisfactorily monitors flow in the pull line will reduce (1) accidental damage to the brain during push–pull perfusions, and (2) the wider than intended distribution of stimulating substances. Insofar as the present monitoring facility achieves these ends, the most compelling reasons for cautious attitudes toward use of the push–pull technique will be less sustainable.

ACKNOWLEDGMENTS

Grateful thanks are due to Paul Dean for his helpful comments on this manuscript, to Iona Hodges for her expert technical assistance, and to Dr. R. D. Myers who first introduced me to the problem.

REFERENCES

1. Bartholini, G., Stadler, H., Ciria, M. G., and Lloyd, K. G. The use of the push–pull cannula to estimate the dynamics of acetylcholine and catecholamines within various brain areas. *Neuropharmacology* **15** (1976) 515–519.
2. Chase, T. N., and Kopin, I. J. Stimulus-induced release of substances from olfactory bulb using the push–pull cannula. *Nature* (*London*) **217** (1968) 466–467.
3. Gaddum, J. H. Push–pull cannulae. *J. Physiol.* (*London*) **155** (1961) 1–2P.
4. Honchar, M. P., Hartman, B. K., and Sharpe, L. G. Evaluation of *in vivo* brain site perfusion with the push–pull cannula. *Am. J. Physiol.* **236** (1979) R48–R56.
5. Izquierdo, I., and Izquierdo, J. A. Effects of drugs on deep brain centers. *Am. Rev. Pharmacol.* **11** (1971) 189–208.
6. Konig, J. F. R. and Klippel, R. A. "The Rat Brain: A Stereotaxic Atlas of the Forebrain and Lower Parts of the Brain Stem," 1963. Williams & Wilkins, Baltimore, Maryland.
7. Korf, J., Boer, P. H., and Fekkes, D. Release of cerebral cyclic AMP into push–pull perfusates in freely moving rats. *Brain Res.*
8. Levine, J. E., and Ramirez, V. D. *In vivo* release of lutenizing hormone releasing hormone estimated with push–pull cannulae from the mediobasal hypothalami of ovariectomized steroid primed rats. *Endocrinology* **107** (1980) 1782–1790. **113** (1976) 551–561.
9. Loullis, C. C., Hingtgen, J. N., Shea, P. A., and Aprison, M. H. *In vivo* determination of biogenic amines in rat brain using HPLC and push–pull cannula. *Pharmacol. Biochem. Behav.* **12** (1980) 959–963.
10. Martin, G. E., and Haubrich, D. R. Striatal dopamine relase and contraversive rotation elicited by intranigrally applied muscimol. *Nature* (*London*) **275** (1978) 230–231.
11. Myers, R. D. Methods for perfusing different structures of the brain. *Meth. Psychobiol.* **2** (1972) 169–211.
12. Nieoullon, A., Cheramy, A., and Glowinski, J. An adaptation of the push–pull cannula method to study the *in vivo* release of tritiated dopamine synthesized from tritiated tyrosine in the cat caudate nucleus. Effects of various physical and pharmacological treatments. *J. Neurochem.* **28** (1977) 819–828.
13. Philips, S. R., Robson, A. M., and Boulton, A. A. Unstimulated and amphetamine stimulated release of endogenous noradrenaline and dopamine from rat brain *in vivo*. *J. Neurochem.* **38** (1982) 1106–1110.
14. Redgrave, P. A modified push–pull system for the localized perfusion of brain tissue. *Pharmacol. Biochem. Behav.* **6** (1977) 471–474.
15. Redgrave, P. Modulation of intracranial self-stimulation by local perfusions of dopamine,

noradrenaline and serotonin within the caudate nucleus and nucleus accumbens. *Brain Res.* **155** (1978) 277–295.
16. Redgrave, P., and Horrell R. I. Potentiation of central reward by localised perfusion of acetylcholine and 5-hydroxytryptamine. *Nature (London)* **262** (1976) 305–307.
17. Van der Heyden, J. A. M., Venema, K., and Korf, J. *In vivo* release of endogenous GABA from rat substantia nigra measured by a novel method. *J. Neurochem.* **32** (1979) 469–476.
18. Wolfensberger, M., and Amsler, U. Mass fragmentographic method for the determination of trace amounts of putative amino acid neurotransmitters and related compounds from brain perfusates collected *in vivo*. *J. Neurochem.* **38** (1982) 451–456.
19. Yaksh, T. L., and Yamamura, H. I. Factors affecting performance of the push–pull cannula in brain. *J. Appl. Physiol.* **37** (1974) 428–434.

3

Neuronal Responses to Neuroactive Substances Administered by Push–Pull Perfusion

EUGENE P. SCHOENER

Department of Pharmacology
Wayne State University
School of Medicine
Detroit, Michigan

I. INTRODUCTION

The technique of push–pull perfusion (PPP) using dual, coaxial cannulae for *in situ* investigation of cerebral tissue originated with Gaddum (*4*). It may be thought of best as a reciprocal of the *in vitro* paradigm, for instead of removing a tissue sample and placing it in a bath, here we insert a microbath into the tissue. It is a powerful method which has been exploited for several purposes, including discrete drug application to specific brain structures,

IN VIVO PERFUSION AND RELEASE
OF NEUROACTIVE SUBSTANCES

ISBN 0-12-083350-6

collection of endogenous substances released from brain tissue, and observation of systemic physiological and behavioral functions concomitant with application or collection of neuroactive substances.

We have employed this multifaceted technique in our laboratory for both biochemical and physiological analysis of neurotransmitter function *in vivo*. One of the systems we have chosen to study and the subject of this chapter is dopaminergic transmission in the striatum. Much has been accomplished on this model substrate with other *in vitro* and *in situ* methods of study, but we proposed at the outset that push–pull perfusion would enable us to conduct very different types of experiments on a single system. Integration of resulting data would therefore require little extrapolation and ultimately provide a more systematic description of neurotransmitter function at molecular, cellular, and behavioral levels. Our initial end points have been adenylate and guanylate cyclase activities, and single-neuron discharge patterns in response to specific dopaminergic challenge.

II. METHODS

A. Cannulae

Although the concept of PPP is universal, there is no international convention for its mode of application. Each laboratory has adopted its own unique approach based upon Gaddum's idea of coaxial, bidirectional perfusion. For the acute neurochemical and neurophysiological experiments in our laboratory, we designed an easily constructed cannula and incorporated this in a closed PPP circuit driven with a peristaltic pump. The cannula was manufactured using stainless-steel tubing (24 ga thin walled, and 30 ga), a male luer plug, two O rings, and a B-D polyethylene tubing adapter. A facsimile of the final product is illustrated in Fig. 1. Tip-to-port dead space of the device is approximately 5 μl for the inner tube and 8μl for the outer. The cannula is leak-proof, indefinitely reusable, and easily disassembled for regular cleaning. The longer tubing length that we employ serves to regulate perfusion fluid temperatures. Countercurrent flow through the cannula provides for heat exchange from outer barrel fluid leaving the brain to inner barrel fluid which is entering.

B. Surgical Procedures

Studies like those reported here are conducted in our laboratory on male Sprague-Dawley rats (weighing about 350 g) anesthetized with urethane (1 g/kg). The animals are tracheostomized and catheterized with arterial

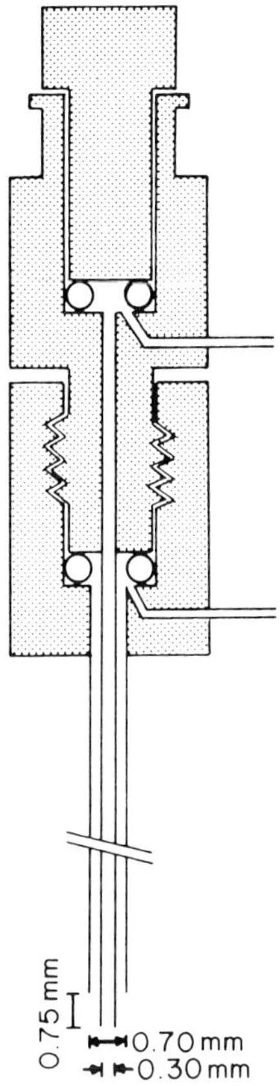

Fig. 1. Diagram of the push–pull perfusion cannula designed and constructed for stereotaxic use in acute experiments (not to scale).

and venous cannulae. Blood pressure, heart rate, and body (rectal) temperature are monitored continuously to assure that the preparation remains in viable condition. Ventilatory assist, fluids (dextran with dextrose), and body warming are provided, as needed, for homeostasis. Thus prepared, each animal is mounted in a cranial stereotaxic device to perform a limited, unilateral, frontoparietal craniotomy and permit accurate stereotaxic insertion of the push–pull cannula and extracellular recording electrode.

C. Perfusion and Recording Procedures

Use of a peristaltic pump to provide the head pressure for infusion and withdrawal in closed-circuit PPP may incur some difficulty, not the least of which is a constant pulsatile modulation of circuit pressure. Excessive pressure change, be it periodic or irregular, is intolerable in PPP, especially with neuron recording. Therefore, we have introduced two pressure damping modifications, as indicated in Fig. 2. The first of these is bifurcation of both inflow and outflow lines as they pass through the pump. Because the two sides of our pump (Harvard model 1203) are 180° out of phase with each other, the pressure waves algebraically summate and nullify each other upon recombination. The small pulsatile ripple that remains is completely eliminated by fluid transit through a "buffer chamber" which, in effect, becomes a pressure reservoir. In order to facilitate addition of test agents to the inflow and collection of neuroactive substances in the effluent, diversion circuits managed by Hamilton 3-way microvalves are included in both lines close to the cannula ports.

Collection of push–pull perfusate is accomplished by placing a small, stoppered tube in the line between microvalves. This sample vessel is kept on ice to lower the effluent temperature and delay spontaneous degradation of neuroactive substances. A standard perfusion medium used in all of these studies is comprised of Na (143.0 m*M*), K (5.87 m*M*), Ca (2.6 m*M*), Mg(1.2 m*M*), Cl (128.2 m*M*), SO_4 (1.2 m*M*), H_2PO_4 (1.2 m*M*), HCO_3 (25.0 m*M*), and glucose (5.6 m*M*). It is bubbled with gas containing 95% O_2 and 5% CO_2 to adjust and maintain pH. The rate of perfusion in most experiments is 25 μl/min. This, we have found, yields a preparation which is stable in less than 1 hr and remains so for at least 8–10 hr thereafter.

To accomplish the simultaneous recording of single-unit neuron activity and PPP, two micromanipulators are employed. One of them carries the PPP cannula to a preselected site in the striatum at a 15° angle. The other holds a glass-coated, platinum–iridium microelectrode in a vertical position. The electrode is mounted in a semifloating holder and advanced through the brain with a remote hydraulic drive. Figure 3 illustrates the experimental arrangement.

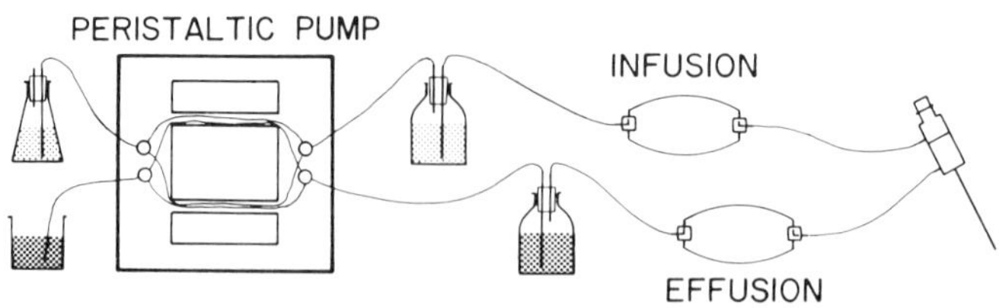

Fig. 2. Components of the push–pull perfusion circuit employed in this laboratory. (See text for further discussion.)

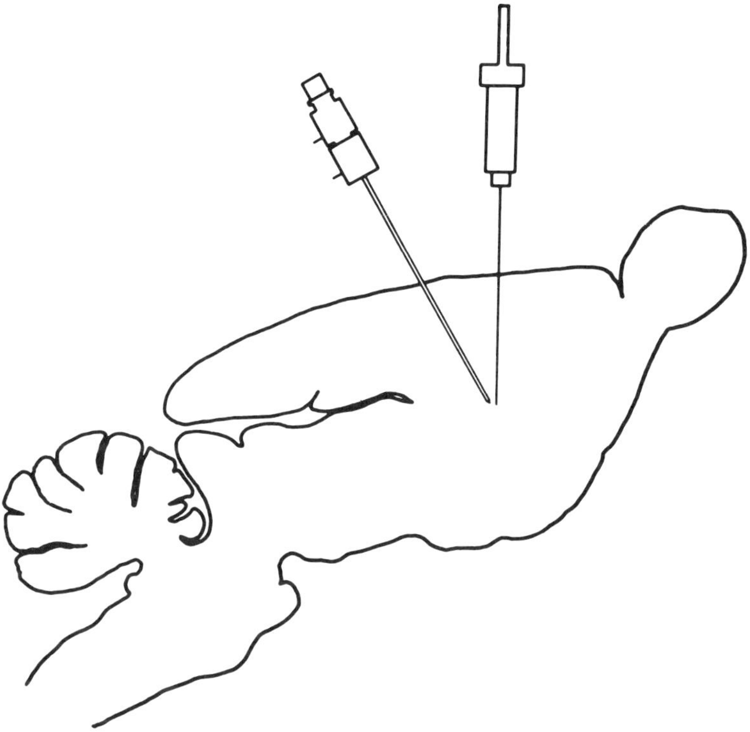

Fig. 3. Diagrammatic representation of the stereotaxic placement of both push–pull cannula and recording electrode in the rat neostriatum.

III. FINDINGS

A. Optimization of Experimental Procedures

In our experience, we have found that the most critical element in a closed perfusion circuit is stability of driving pressure. Initial experiments were performed with 10- or 20-ml syringes on an infusion withdrawal pump, but when a transducer was inserted in the line, we clearly observed that pressure, and thus flow was exceedingly irregular. Lubrication of the syringes reduced, but did not eliminate the unstable pattern of flow. Seeking a more reliable source of pressure, we tested the Harvard peristaltic pump. Like all pumps of this type, it produced a pulsatile wave of pressure; however, this regular sinusoidal pattern could be reduced to a negligible level (less than 1 mm Hg peak to peak) with the modifications previously discussed. We found this to be more acceptable than random pressure changes that occurred with the infusion–withdrawal instrument. In fact, our rate of successful perfusion has been greater than 90% with this approach.

B. Neurobiological Applications

In the past few years, we have directed some of our efforts toward the investigation of striatal function. Endogenous neuroactive substances have been collected (*5, 19*) and, more recently, cellular activity has been recorded (*17, 18*) in the perfused neostriatum. The primary concern of these studies has been the role of dopamine in cyclic nucleotide production/release and neuronal discharge.

C. Cyclic Nucleotides in the Striatum

Prior to our PPP experiments, dopamine (DA) had been shown to modulate the production of adenosine 3′,5′-monophosphate (cAMP) in tissue slices and homogenates of the striatum (*3, 11, 14, 15, 22*). One study had demonstrated increased tissue content of guanosine 3′,5′-monophosphate (cGMP) in response to DA (*16*). With the perfusion technique, we sought to demonstrate a dose-related, dynamic release of cyclic nucleotides *in situ* in response to a DA challenge. Rats anesthetized with urethane (1 g/kg ip) were used in the study. PPP was carried out at 25 μl/min and the accumulated effluent was collected every 10 min. Samples were stored at −80°C until they could be analyzed by radioimmunoassay using the methods of Steiner *et al.* (*20*) and Harper and Brooker (6). In the first experiments, theophylline was perfused to establish that cyclic nucleotides would accumulate in the perfusate when their metabolism was inhibited. This proved to be true, with cAMP showing a dose-related increase of approximately 10-fold over the pretest concentration range (1.0–5.0 m*M*). cGMP levels increased as well, but did so less reliably. Theophylline (5 m*M*) was included in the perfusion medium for all subsequent experiments, as it had been in experiments conducted by others on tissue slices and homogenates. Early studies indicated that initial tissue trauma from cannula implantation would provoke enhanced release of cyclic nucleotides which decreased and stabilized within 30 min. In all subsequent studies, therefore, control collections were made only after a 30-min stabilization period. When DA was added to the infusion fluid for 30-min periods at concentrations of from 5×10^{-6} to 5×10^{-3} *M*, both cAMP and cGMP levels in the effluent were altered. Levels of both were increased in a dose-dependent manner (see Figs. 4 and 5): cAMP rose from 0.9 n*M* under basal conditions to 3.8 n*M* at 5×10^{-3} *M* DA, while cGMP increased from a control of 0.4 n*M* to about 1.2n*M*. Careful inspec-

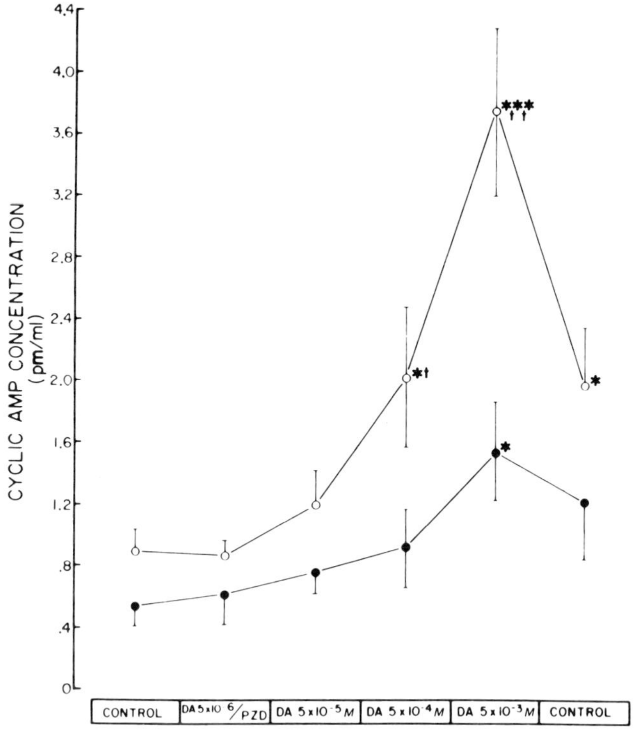

Fig. 4. Cyclic AMP concentration in push–pull perfusate with dopamine (5×10^{-6} to 5×10^{-3} *M*) added to perfusion medium. Each point represents an average of six experiments conducted either in the presence (solid circles) or absence (open circles) of dopamine antagonist pimozide. Symbols indicate values significantly different from control ($^{*}p < .05$, $^{***}p < .001$) or from the pimozide pretreated condition ($^{\dagger}p < .05$, $^{\ddagger}p < .01$). [Reprinted from ref. (*19*).]

tion of the individual cAMP response to DA application as a function of time revealed a bimodal effect, i.e., an initial decrease occurred during the first collection period, but this was followed by a more dramatic rise. Such behavior may suggest a complex mechanism of DA action involving presynaptic as well as postsynaptic phenomena.

The DA antagonist pimozide was used in a second set of studies to determine whether the DA/cyclic nucleotide effects were pharmacologically specific. The drug was administered intravenously at 0.5 mg/kg and control studies demonstrated that its presence had no appreciable effect on the amount of cyclic nucleotides appearing in the perfusate. However, it did cause a statistically significant reduction in both cAMP and cGMP evoked with DA perfusion. The patterns of response for cAMP and cGMP accumulation in the presence and absence of pimozide were sufficiently different to

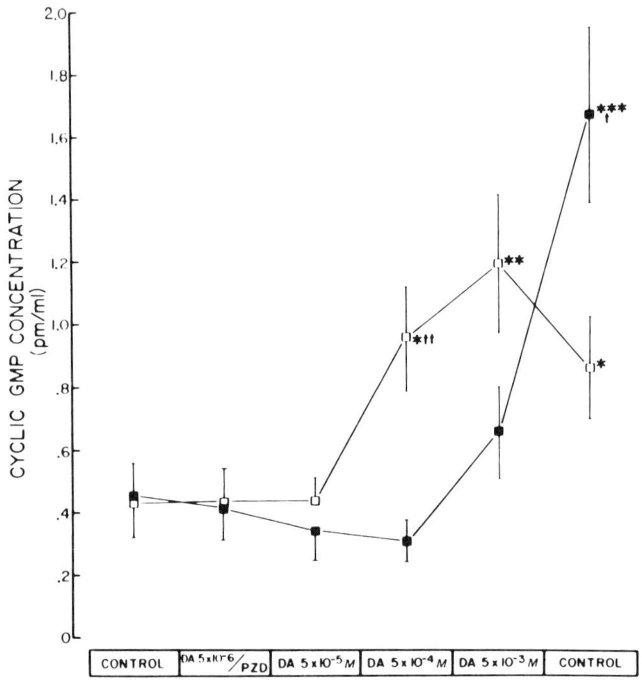

Fig. 5. Cyclic GMP concentration in push–pull perfusate with dopamine addition as described for Fig. 4. [Reprinted from ref. (*19*).]

suggest independent mechanisms of DA activation, although interactive effects were not experimentally discounted.

IV. EFFECTS OF DOPAMINE ON STRIATAL NEURON DISCHARGE

Physiological studies were conducted in our laboratory to assess the functional, cellular response to push–pull perfused DA. This, we felt, would permit some degree of interpolation between PPP-derived neurochemical data and electrophysiological observations made with iontophoretic techniques (*1, 6, 8, 9, 19*). Furthermore, it was hoped that such a study would, by virtue of its ability to investigate the dose-related nature of DA effects, disclose a mechanistic rationale for purportedly variable DA effects on neuronal discharge pattern.

Attempts were made in this series of experiments to maintain the experimental conditions much as they had been in the previous ones. Slight modifications were required by the need to insert two probes rather than the cannula alone, but the very same striatal region of urethane-anesthetized rats was examined. Pilot studies disclosed that the physiological endpoint of neuronal discharge was far more sensitive to DA than the neurochemical ones and required only brief exposure. DA was therefore infused for 3-min test periods in all of these studies. A total of 124 trials were made with DA over a test range of 10^{-10}–10^{-7} *M*. Sixty-two percent of the test neurons exhibited significant change in their discharge after DA, 88% were depressed, while 12% were excited. Ten percent of these units actually showed a bimodal response pattern. Figures 6 and 7 exemplify the type of data obtained in two individual cases.

The minority of neurons that were stimulated by DA exhibited no strict dose–response relationship. However, it was noted that this response favored lower challenge doses and, indeed, never occurred at the highest concentration employed (10^{-7} *M*). As a group, these units showed an average increase of 72% over the control rate of firing (4.8 spikes/sec), with an onset latency of 4.2 min. Neurons that responded to DA bimodally

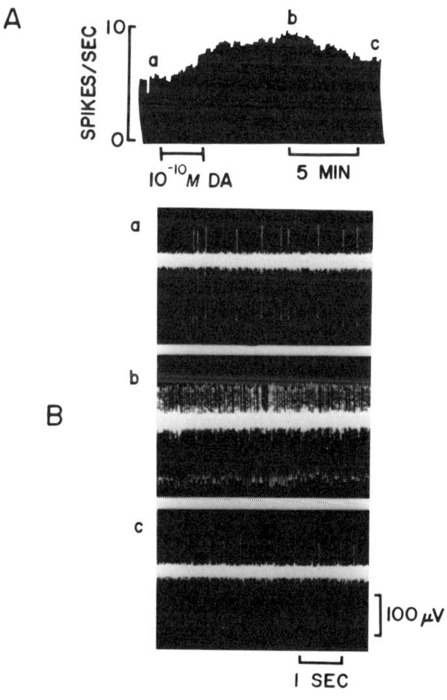

Fig. 6. Example of single-unit data obtained when recording in the rat neostriatum with perfusion of dopamine (10^{-10} *M*). The average frequency record (A) and oscillographic tracings (B) are shown.

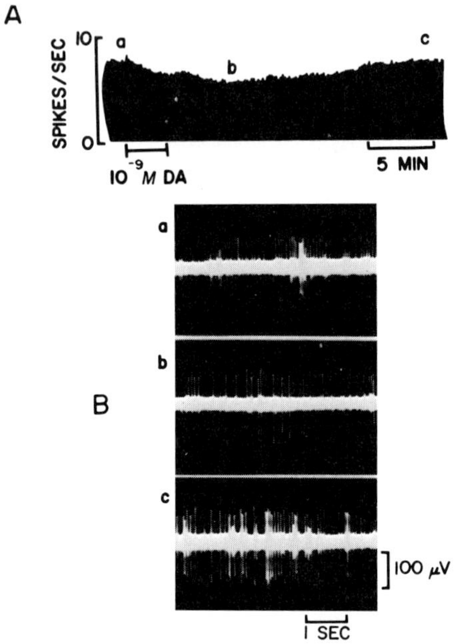

Fig. 7. Neuronal function data obtained when recording the activity of a single striatal unit with perfusion of dopamine ($10^{-9}M$). The average frequency record (A) and oscillographic tracings (B) are shown.

always did so with an initial excitation followed by depression. The elevated discharge was rapid in onset (1.4-min latency) and brief in duration (4.6 min), leaving the impression that it was a reflection of low dose action in the progressive accumulation of DA at its receptors.

The most prominent DA effect on neuronal discharge was inhibition. With a sufficiently large number of units in this population (50), a direct dose–effect relationship was clearly evident (see Table I). Interestingly, when the response was considered as a function of the basal discharge rate, we found that the low-frequency units were affected to a much greater extent than those with high frequency of discharge. In fact, when the DA response was plotted as a function of the initial discharge rate for each concentration tested, the disparity seemed to grow with increasing concentration (see Fig. 8). We theorized that this greater DA responsiveness of slower units reflected a greater proportion of DA receptors, viz., their total receptor complement. In fact, this reasoning may provide the very rationale for their inherently slow rate of discharge.

TABLE I

Dopamine Depression of Striatal Neurons

DA Conc. (*M*)	(N)	Initial firing rate	Decrease after DA (%Δ)	Latency to peak effect (min)	Duration (min)
10^{-10}	(9)	6.9 ± 1.2	35.4 ± 6.0	5.6 ± 0.7	8.2 ± 0.9
10^{-9}	(14)	5.7 ± 0.9	45.5 ± 7.3	6.4 ± 0.7	9.1 ± 1.2
10^{-8}	(16)	6.3 ± 0.8	44.6 ± 6.6	6.5 ± 0.7	10.0 ± 1.3
10^{-7}	(11)	5.6 ± 1.1	70.4 ± 9.1	7.1 ± 1.5	10.0 ± 1.5

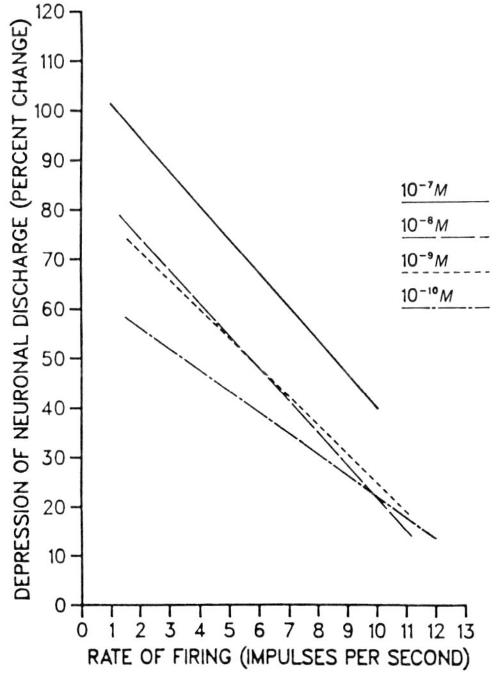

Fig. 8. Graphic representation of the effectiveness of dopamine depression as a function of the initial (control) discharge rate of neurons tested.

V. ETHANOL ACTION ON STRIATAL NEURONS

Cellular effects of ethanol have been noted before in various brain regions with systemic as well as local (iontophoretic, osmotic) administration. However, there has never been a systematic examination of the dose–effect relationship between ethanol concentration and single-unit neuronal response. Because of the theoretically important relationship between ethanol action and dopaminergic transmission (*8*), we proceeded to investigate striatal neuron response to ethanol administration over a wide concentration range. Precisely the same approach was employed as for the earlier experiments on DA. Test doses of ethanol at 10^{-9}–10^{-4} *M* were added to the infusion fluid for 3-min application periods. Neuronal discharge (single-unit activity) was recorded for at least 10 min before drug administration and for as long as possible thereafter, or until control activity was recovered.

The data obtained from 54 different striatal units were most conclusive in demonstrating a dose–effect relationship (see Table II). At the lowest concentration (10^{-9}*M*), all of the units tested were facilitated. As the concentration increased, there was a progressive decrease in the number of neurons excited, but a concomitant rise in those that were depressed. Interestingly, whereas the very lowest dose elicited an unequivocal positive response, at two and three orders of magnitude greater, about one third of the units showed no response at all. This apparent quiescence may have simply reflected the net result of opposing positive and negative forces, for at still higher test concentrations (10^{-5} and 10^{-4}*M*), depression clearly manifested itself. The crossover between stimulation and inhibition occurred at 10^{-7}–10^{-6}*M*. This was the range in which the number of units with no obvious change was greatest and, purportedly, is the level of endogenous ethanol due to microorganism metabolism in the gut (*13*). The only neurons which were bimodally responsive (excitation then depression) were observed at 10^{-6}*M* ethanol.

TABLE II

Ethanol Effects on Striatal Neuron Activity

Conc. ethanol (*M*)	Percent increased	Percent decreased	Percent no change	Neurons tested
10^{-9}	100.0	0	0	9
10^{-8}	85.7	14.3	0	14
10^{-7}	40.0	26.7	33.3	15
10^{-6}	7.7	61.5	30.8	13
10^{-5}	12.5	62.5	25.0	8
10^{-4}	0	83.3	16.7	6

TABLE III

Excitatory Effects of Ethanol on Striatal Neurons

Conc. ethanol (*M*)	(N)	Initial firing rate (ips)	Firing rate after ethanol (ips)	Increase in firing rate (ips)(%)	Latency to peak effect (min)
10^{-9}	(9)	10.6 ± 3.8	13.9 ± 4.3	3.3 ± 0.9 (31.1)	14.4 ± 3.2
10^{-8}	(12)	12.7 ± 3.6	20.2 ± 4.7	8.1 ± 1.6 (63.8)	27.9 ± 3.2
10^{-7}	(6)	12.5 ± 5.9	15.9 ± 6.6	3.4 ± 1.0 (27.2)	19.0 ± 3.9
10^{-6}	(1)	5	9	4 (80)	7
10^{-5}	(1)	6	8	2 (33.3)	16

Analysis of the distinct excitatory effects revealed that maximal ethanol facilitation occurred at 10^{-8} *M*, with approximately 64% increase in the average discharge rate (Table III). The change was highly significant ($p < .001$). At one log unit above and below this optimum test concentration, the facilitation fell off to about 30%. Interestingly, the time to attain peak effect was also reduced. One unit at each of the two higher ethanol concentrations employed was apparently stimulated, rather than depressed, as the majority of the others were. This may well have represented an *actual* low-dose effect due to greater distance of these units from the cannula tip (perfusion site).

Above $10^{-7}M$ ethanol the neuronal response was predominantly one of depression (Table IV), with a peak inhibition of 58% at $10^{-6}M$ ($p < .01$). Depression seen at $10^{-7}M$ ethanol was not as severe (48%) and, surprisingly, it was much less at the higher concentration of $10^{-5}M$. However, at the very highest dose of ethanol tested, depression once again intensified. This polymodal dose–effect relationship suggests the possibility that different mechanisms are implicated in the decrease of activity at moderate and

TABLE IV

Inhibitory Effects of Ethanol on Striatal Neurons

Conc. ethanol (*M*)	(N)	Initial firing rate (ips)	Firing rate after ethanol (ips)	Decrease in firing rate (ips)(%)	Latency to peak effect (min)
10^{-8}	(2)	21.0	15.5	5.5 (26.2)	18.0
10^{-7}	(4)	7.1 ± 2.2	3.8 ± 0.8	3.4 ± 1.6 (47.9)	12.8 ± 2.2
10^{-6}	(8)	17.1 ± 5.0	7.2 ± 2.8	9.9 ± 3.0 (57.9)	30.9 ± 8.9
10^{-5}	(5)	14.8 ± 3.0	12.7 ± 2.9	2.1 ± 0.3 (14.2)	18.6 ± 8.3
10^{-4}	(5)	12.3 ± 2.7	6.1 ± 1.4	6.2 ± 1.6 (50.4)	37.6 ± 15.0

higher dosage. As was true for the case of facilitation, the time to achieve maximal effect varied directly with its extent.

VI. PERSPECTIVES AND DISCUSSION

Push–pull perfusion, an imaginative contribution to neuroscience research, has enormous inherent value, not simply because it is a means of locally and discretely applying a test substance to a small brain region or collecting and analyzing tissue metabolites from such an area, nor because it can be employed *in vivo* in awake animals as well as acutely anesthetized ones to study behavior or systemic physiological activity, nor because it can be coupled with other sophisticated techniques like single-unit, extracellular recording to examine cellular responses to change in the immediate environment. No, this technique possesses such great potential precisely because it can do all of these things, and more. One of the greatest challenges of modern neuroscience is the integration of findings that have been generated in so many different ways on radically diverse model systems. With the aid of push–pull perfusion, we can now conduct experiments using multiple chemical, physiological, and behavior end points which directly and unequivocally establish mechanistic interrelationships between all of them.

Enthusiasm for PPP is realistically tempered by recognition of the uncertainties associated with it. The task that lies before us includes more adequate definition of diffusional kinetics, exact tissue concentration of test substances or tissue metabolites, and distribution volume surrounding the cannula tip. As we have done in some of our push–pull perfusion work, others in the field must confirm and corroborate PPP findings with those generated by more widely accepted techniques.

ACKNOWLEDGMENTS

Research reported here was supported in part by awards from the NIAAA and the Pharmaceutical Manufacturers Association.

REFERENCES

1. Bernardi, G., Marciani, M. G., Morocutti, C., Pavone, F., and Stantione, P. The action of dopamine on rat caudate nucleus neurons intracellularly recorded. *Neurosci. Lett.* **8** (1978) 235–240.

2. Buchwald, N. A., Price, D. D., Vernon, L., and Hull, C. D. Caudate intracellular responses to thalamic and cortical inputs. *Exp. Neurol.* **38** (1973) 311–323.
3. Clement-Cormier, Y. C., Parrish, R. C., Petzold, G. L., Kebabian, J. W., and Greengard, P. Characterization of a dopamine-sensitive adenylate cyclase in the rat caudate nucleus. *J. Neurochem.* **25** (1975) 143–149.
4. Gaddum, J. H. Push–pull cannulae, *J. Physiol.* (*London*) **155** (1961) 1–2P.
5. Gorell, J. M., Callahan, M. J., and Schoener, E. P. Regulation of acetylcholine release in the rat caudate nucleus. *Soc. Neurosci. Abstr.* **7** (1981) 575.
6. Harper, J. F., and Brooker, G. Femtomole sensitivity radioimmunoassay for cyclic AMP and cyclic GMP after 2′-*O*-acetylation by acetic anhydride in aqueous solution. *J. Cyclic Nucleotide Res.* **1** (1975) 207–218.
7. Herrling, P. L., and Hull, C. D. Iontophoretically applied dopamine depolarizes and hyperpolarizes the membrane of cat caudate neurons. *Brain Res.* **192** (1980) 441–461.
8. Hull, C. D., Bernardi, G., and Buchwald, N. A. Intracellular responses of caudate neurons to brain stem stimulation. *Brain Res.* **22** (1970) 169–179.
9. Hull, C. D., Bernardi, G., Price, D. D., and Buchwald, N. A. Intracellular responses of caudate neurons to temporally and spatially combined stimuli. *Exp. Neurol.* **38** (1973) 324–336.
10. Hunt, W. A. Neurotransmitter function in the basal ganglia after acute and chronic alcohol treatment. *Fed. Proc.* **40** (1981) 2077–2081.
11. Kebabian, J. W., Petzold, G. L., and Greengard, P. Dopamine-sensitive adenylate cyclase in caudate nucleus of rat brain and its similarity to the "dopamine receptor." *Proc. Natl. Acad. Sci. U.S.A.* **69** (1972) 2145–2149.
12. Kitai, S. T., Sugimori M., and Koscis, J. D. Excitatory nature of dopamine in the nigrocaudate pathway. *Exp. Brain. Res.* **24** (1976) 351–363.
13. Lester, D. Endogenous ethanol: a review, *Quart. J. Stud. Alc.* **22** (1961) 554–574.
14. Miller, R. J., Horu, A. S., and Iversen, L. L. The action of neuroleptic drugs on dopamine-stimulated adenosine cyclic 3′,5′-monophosphate production in rat neostriatum and limbic forebrain. *Molec. Pharmacol.* (1974) 759–766.
15. Mishra, R. K., Gardner, E. L., Katzman, R., and Makman, M. H. Enhancement of dopamine-stimulated adenylate cyclase in rat caudate after lesions in substantia nigra: evidence for denervation supersensitivity. *Proc. Natl. Acad. Sci. U.S.A.* **71** (1974) 3883–3887.
16. Puri, S. K., Coma, P., and Volicer, L. Cyclic nucleotide levels in the rat striatum and cerebellum: *in vivo* effects of dopamine and acetylcholine receptor agonists and antagonists. *Biochem. Pharmacol.* **27** (1978) 2333–2336.
17. Schoener, E. P. Ethanol effects on striatal neuron activity. *Alcoholism: Clin. Exp. Res.* **8** (1984) 266–268.
18. Schoener, E. P., and Elkins, D. P. Neuronal response to dopamine in rat neostriatum: a push–pull perfusion study. *Neuropharmacology* **23** (1984) 611–616.
19. Schoener, E. P., Hager, P. J., Felt, B. T., and Schneider, D. R. Cyclic nucleotides in the rat neostriatum: push–pull perfusion studies. *Brain Res.* **179** (1979) 111–119.
20. Steiner, A. L., Ferrendelli, J. A., and Kipnis, D. M. Radioimunoassay for cyclic nucleotides. *J. Biol. Chem.* **247** (1972) 1121–1124.
21. Vandermaelen, C. P., and Kitai, S. T. Intracellular analysis of synaptic potentials in rat neostriatum following stimulation of the cerebral cortex, thalamus and substantia nigra. *Brain Res. Bull.* **5** (1980) 725–733.
22. Walker, J. B., and Walker, J. P. Neurohumoral regulation of adenylate cyclase activity in rat striatum. *Brain Res.* **54** (1973) 386–390.

4

Superfusion and Electrical Stimulation of the Canine Brain with a Push–Pull Cannula

TOSHIHIKO IIJIMA AND KAZUO NUNOKI

Department of Pharmacology
Tohoku University School of Medicine
Sendai, Japan

I. INTRODUCTION

Since Gaddum (*2*) first reported the use of a push–pull cannula for collection of neurohumoral factors of an isolated region of the *in situ* brain, it has been used widely for neurological studies of the brain. Advantages of usage of the push–pull cannula are as follows:

1. Substances liberated from discrete areas of the brain can be detected under fairly normal conditions.
2. It is possible to localize the site of perfusion and/or stimulation more precisely.
3. The blood–brain barrier is circumvented.
4. Repeated perfusion of a given site of the brain structures is carried out under control and experimental conditions.

IN VIVO PERFUSION AND RELEASE
OF NEUROACTIVE SUBSTANCES

ISBN 0-12-083350-6

Most reports indicate that use of push–pull cannulae has been limited to small animals such as rats, cats, and rabbits. It is possible to minimize the relative dimensions of the damaged tissue, and to perfuse a much more discrete area if large-sized animals are used.

In this chapter, we describe the method for perfusing canine hypothalamus *in vivo*. This method enables us to obtain many site-specific responses.

II. METHODS

Several different kinds of cannulae have been used to perform the push–pull perfusion. Among them a concentric push–pull assembly is preferable because the lesion caused by the cannula is smaller than that produced by the side-by-side assembly. Myers (*4*) devised a push–pull cannula for the purpose of perfusing a single site several times. However, the requirement of a special infusion–withdrawal pump is a disadvantage. The pump should collect just the volume of fluid which is infused into it. A push–pull cannula developed by Philippu (*8*) consists of a concentric assembly and has a dipping side branch on the pull cannula. Artificial cerebrospinal fluid pumped into the push cannula which is opened at 0.5 mm above the orifice of the pull cannula superfuses the brain tissue and runs over from the side-branch cannula. The advantage of this assembly is that a withdrawal pump is not needed. The brain tissue can be superfused at constant hydrostatic perfusion pressure produced by the length of the pull cannula because the top and the side branch are opened to the air. We constructed the push–pull cannula to perfuse the canine hypothalamus in the same manner as Philippu's cannula. In order to apply the push–pull cannula to superfuse the canine hypothalamus, the length and diameter of the cannula had to be adjusted for the varying sizes of the canine hypothalamus. The push–pull cannula modified for the canine hypothalamus is shown in Fig. 1. The push (inner) cannula of 0.5 mm o.d. is 0.5 mm shorter than the pull cannula at the tip. The push cannula soldered with a collar is inserted into the pull (outer) cannula of 1.8 mm o.d. and fixed at the top of the pull cannula with the collar (Fig. 1). A stylet is used when the push–pull cannula is inserted into the brain to avoid sticking of brain tissue into the cannula and to minimize tearing of the tissue during insertion. The brass stylet of 1.5 mm o.d. just fitted into the pull cannula has a groove for the push cannula, and the tip of the stylet is sharpened conically. The outer surface of the pull cannula is insulated with an epoxy resin. After several coatings for full insulation of the cannula surface, the insulation is oven cured at 60°C for 6–

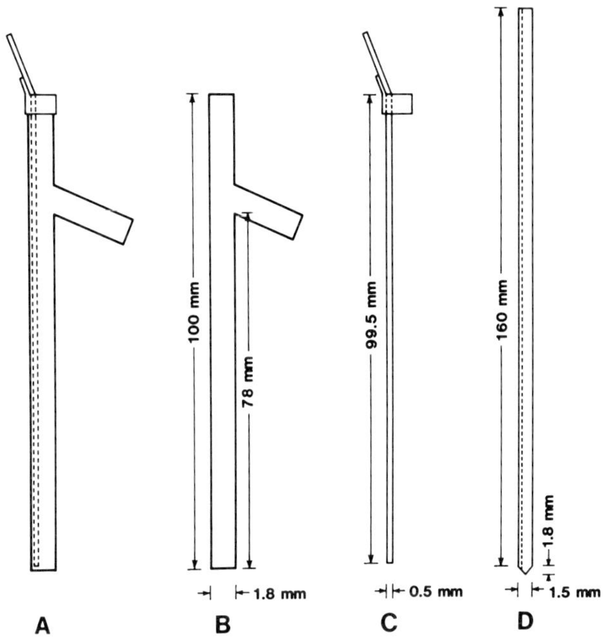

Fig. 1. Push–pull cannula assembly (A). When the push–pull cannula is inserted into the brain, the push cannula with collar (C) and the brass stylet (D) are inserted into the pull cannula (B).

8 hr. The tip of the cannula is exposed by polishing with an oilstone for electrical stimulation of the superfused area.

III. FINDINGS AND OPTIMIZATION OF EXPERIMENTAL PROCEDURES

A. Stereotaxic Technique

Stereotaxic instruments vary considerably in versatility. However, the stereotaxic instrument that has a rigid frame with two parallel bars extending back from a crosspiece is preferable for the dog because animals of small to moderate size can be fixed by simply changing positions of the ear bars and the mouth (snout) adaptor. It might be true that endless variations in the size and shape of dogs' heads make them unsuitable for research involving accurate cranioencephalic topography. However, "there is no valid reason why experiments should not be carried out in the dog's brain, and there are many good reasons why they should. By selecting short-haired hound-like dogs of limited weight (10 ± 2 kg) and without unduly short or long noses" (3), it is possible to use the dog in the Narishige stereotaxic headholder (SN-2) with a minor modification. A mongrel dog's head correctly mounted in a stereotaxic instrument with eye bars resting on the infraorbital ridge is shown in Fig. 2. The modified snout adaptor and the infraorbital bars are shown in Fig. 3. After the snout adaptor is applied over the upper jaw behind the canines, the head is rotated on the earpins until the infraorbital bars can be placed on the infraorbital margins and secured in this position by tightening the snout adaptor. A close-up view of the snout adaptor and the infraorbital bars applied on a dog is shown in Fig. 4. Then the push–pull cannula is fixed on the cannula holder, which is mounted on an electrode carrier (Narishige, SM-11). The push–pull cannula with the brass stylet of which the conically sharpened tip is projected from the pull cannula is inserted into the brain. The brass stylet is pulled out when the tip of the cannula reaches 1.5 mm above the desired position. The tip of the stylet just touches the desired position. Then the cannula is advanced vertically 1.5 mm more and reaches the position. By this procedure damaged tissues can be minimized.

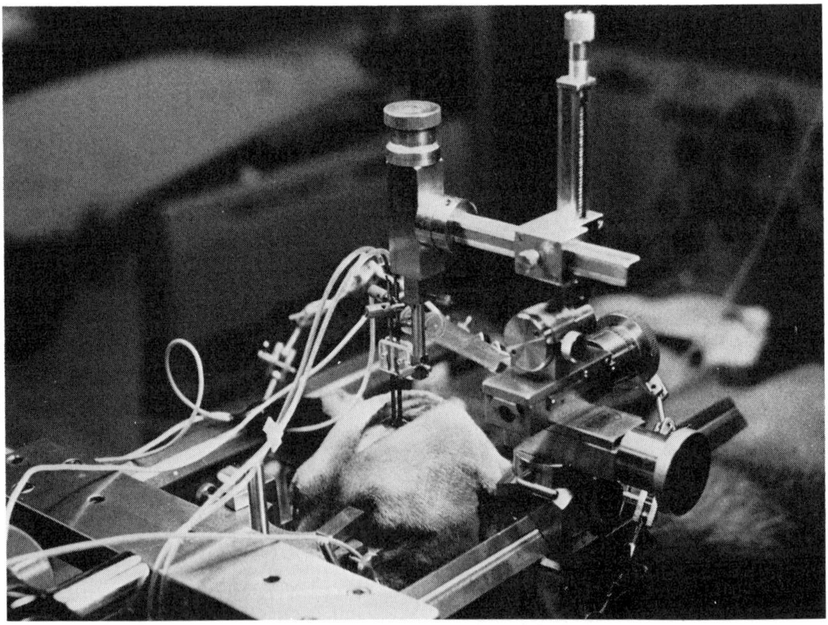

Fig. 2. A dog correctly mounted in a stereotaxic instrument with eye bars. The push–pull cannulae are inserted bilaterally into the hypothalamus.

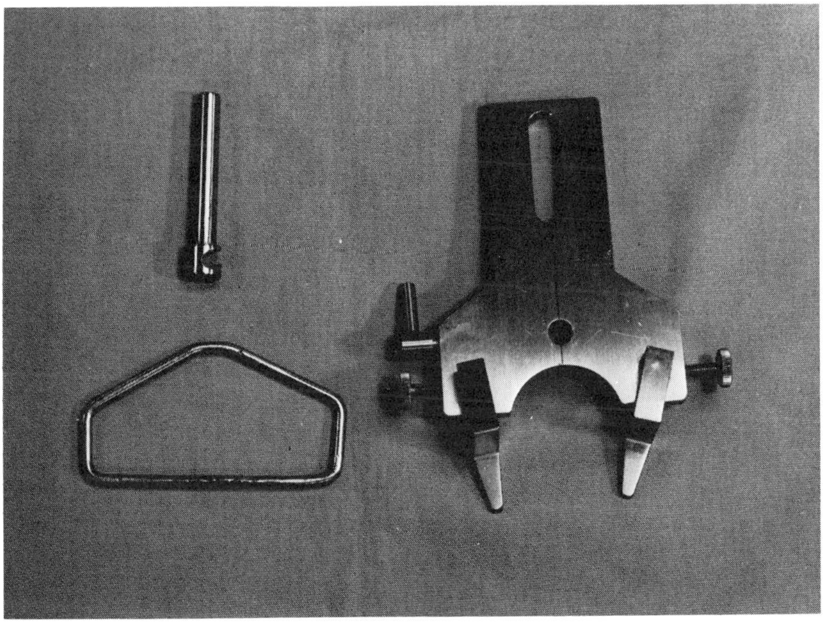

Fig. 3. The modified snout adaptor (left) and eye bars (right).

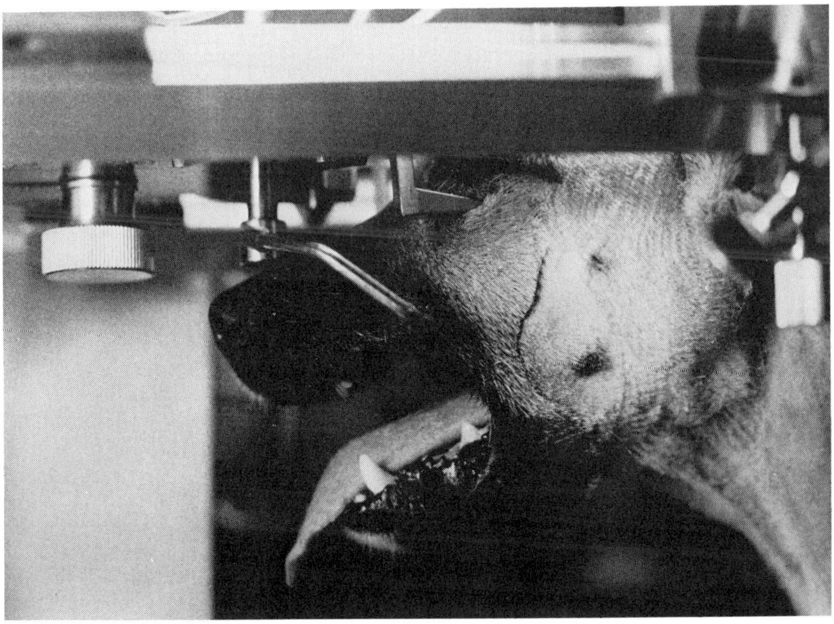

Fig. 4. Close-up view of the snout adaptor and the infraorbital bars applied on a dog.

B. Push–Pull Perfusion of the Hypothalamus

In regard to the pull side of the push–pull system, it has been reported that the use of gravity or anything other than a syringe for producing negative pressure does not provide constant pressure in the vacuum in the pull line over an extended interval (5). The push–pull cannula we have used has two openings on the pull cannula (Fig. 1). Effluent comes out from the side-branch cannula, which is 15 mm long, and trickles down into a collection tube. This means that perfusion pressure of the tissue attached to the orifice of the pull cannula is kept fairly constant at about 80 mm H_2O when the cannula is vertically inserted into the brain. Assuming a tissue (mean capillary) pressure of 150–200 mm H_2O, perfusion pressure for our system never exceeds tissue pressure. Even when bubbling arises in the side-branch cannula and effluent comes up to the top of the pull cannula, which is 20 mm apart from a branching point, the resulting perfusion pressure is about 100 mm H_2O.

During the superfusion special notice should be taken of the following. If the effluent becomes bloody, or if any signs of cerebral edema are observed, the experiment must be terminated. The rate at which the perfusate flows may also be an important factor. In our experiments a perfusion rate of 75 μl/min using a peristaltic pump (Ismatec, IP-4) is used and can be increased to 500 μl/min without any functional effects or damage to the tissue. When a rapid perfusion rate is used, perfusion fluid should be kept at 37°C in order to avoid the effects of temperature. Use of the perfusion rate of 50 μl/min or less always creates the risk of a block in flow.

C. Electrical Stimulation through the Cannula

Electrical stimulation of the hypothalamus has been performed through the uninsulated tip of the pull cannula. An electrode (cannula) and the surrounding tissue have a complex physicochemical relationship. Problems created by this interaction are electrolytic actions and the polarization process of the electrode tip. Electrolytic actions of the electrode tip may create undesirable difficulties but can be avoided by using stainless-steel tubings. The polarization process may seriously distort the stimulating processes. The constant current stimulator bucks polarization by achieving high voltage outputs. Since the degree of polarization can change rapidly, a continuous monitoring of the stimulation current is essential to avoid an unstable response. The current can be measured from a voltage drop across a known resistor on the indifferent side of the circuit. Figure 5 shows current traces obtained by cathodal stimulation of the hypothalamus with rectangular pulses of various duration at 40 Hz through the uninsulated tip of the cannula. The indifferent electrode was attached to the ipsilateral side of the

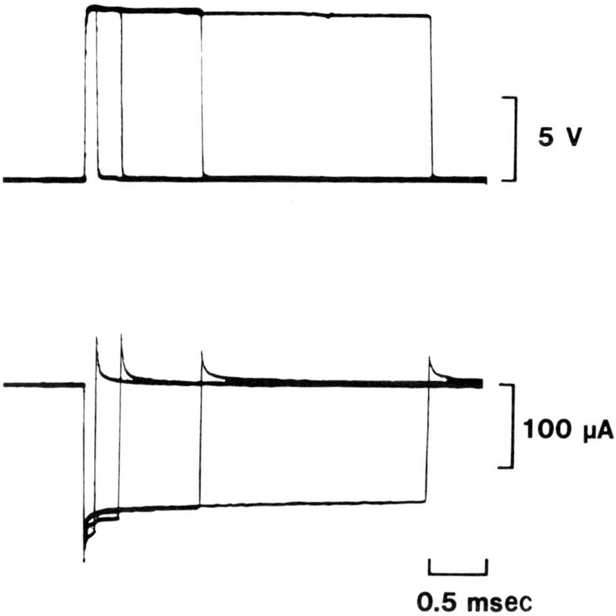

Fig. 5. Current flow during electrical stimulation of the hypothalamus with the push–pull cannula. Superimposed traces are stimulus voltage of 10 V with varied (0.1, 0.3, 1, and 3 msec) intervals (upper traces) and current measured from voltage drop across a 200 Ω resistor on the indifferent side of the circuit (lower traces). Stimulus pulses were applied at a rate of 40 Hz.

temporal skin. The amplitude of the current decreases with time by the capacitance and reaches a steady state. This means that polarization does not affect the stimulus current. The peak amplitude of the current decreases with increases of the stimulus pulse duration at a fixed rate (Fig. 5). Peak amplitude of the stimulus current is very important because an area stimulated by the current is mainly dependent on the amplitude of the current. In our experiments the peak amplitude has been less than 200 μA. Therefore estimated area stimulated is spherically less than 1 mm from the tip of the cannula (*10*). The points at which electrical stimulation elicited the depressor response associated with a decrease in heart rate (6), and the pressor response with an increase in heart rate (7) are plotted in Fig. 6.

It is also important to stimulate the hypothalamus with optimal parameters of electrical stimulation for eliciting reproducible responses. The optimal frequency to elicit the depressor response accompanying the decrease in heart rate for stimulation of the anterior hypothalamus of the dog was about 60 Hz (6). This result is consistent with that obtained in the cat (9). In general, pulse duration of 0.1–1.0 msec and frequencies of 60–100 Hz are most likely to be effective (*1*).

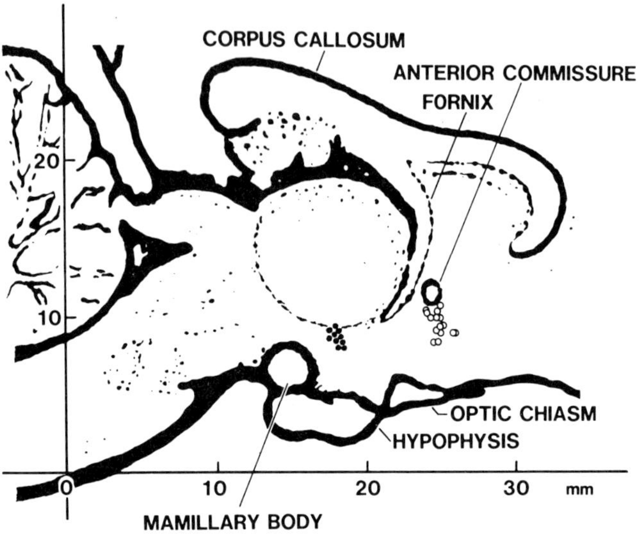

Fig. 6. The depressor (open circles) and the pressor (filled circles) areas of the canine hypothalamus obtained by monopolar electrical stimulation through the push–pull cannula.

IV. CONCLUSION

In this chapter we described the methods for superfusion and electrical stimulation of the canine hypothalamus with the push–pull cannula originally developed by Philippu. By the use of this cannula a small and restricted area of the internal portion of the brain can be superfused selectively. Moreover, it can be easy to obtain more site-specific responses with this cannula by using the dog.

ACKNOWLEDGMENTS

We wish to express our sincere thanks to Dr. A. Philippu for his generous supply of a prototype of the push–pull cannula, and for his advice. We also wish to thank Dr. N. Taira for his reading of this manuscript.

REFERENCES

1. Ervin, F. R., and Kenney, G. J. Electrical stimulation of the brain. *Meth. Psychobiol.* **1** (1971) 207–246.
2. Gaddum, J. H. Push–pull cannulae. *J. Physiol. (London)* **155** (1961) 1–2P.

3. Lim, R. K. S., Liu, C.-N., and Moffitt, R. L. "A Stereotaxic Atlas of the Dog's Brain," Thomas, Springfield, Illinois, 1960.
4. Myers, R. D. An improved push–pull cannula system for perfusing an isolated region of the brain. *Physiol. Behav.* **5** (1970) 243–246.
5. Myers, R. D. Methods for perfusing different structures of the brain. *Meth. Psychobiol.* **2** (1972) 169–211.
6. Nunoki, K., and Iijima, T. Decreases in arterial pressure and heart rate elicited by electrical stimulation of the anterior hypothalamus of pentobarbital anesthetized dogs. *Jpn. J. Pharmacol.* **32** (1982) 195–197.
7. Nunoki, K., and Iijima, T. Modification of the baroreceptor reflex by superfusion of the canine posterior hypothalamus with tetrodotoxin. *Naunyn-Schmiedeberg's Arch. Pharmacol.* **321** (1982) 185–189.
8. Philippu, A., Przuntek, H., and Roensberg, W. Superfusion of the hypothalamus with gamma-aminobutyric acid: effect on release of noradrenaline and blood pressure. *Naunyn-Schmiedeberg's Arch. Pharmacol.* **276** (1973) 103–118.
9. Philippu, A., and Schartner, P. Inhibition by locally applied alpha-adrenoceptor blocking drugs of the depressor response to stimulation of the anterior hypothalamus. *Naunyn-Schmiedeberg's Arch. Pharmacol.* 295 (1976) 1–7.
10. Ranck, J. B., Jr. Which elements are excited in electrical stimulation of mammalian central nervous system. *Brain Res.* **98** (1975) 417–440.

5

Push–Pull Perfusion Studies on the *in Vivo* Release of Endogenous Transmitter and Nontransmitter Amino Acids in the Rat Brain

JAN A. M. VAN DER HEYDEN,*
KOR VENEMA, AND JAKOB KORF

**Department of Pharmacology*
Duphar B.V.
Weesp, The Netherlands

Department of Biological Psychiatry
University Psychiatric Clinic
Groningen, The Netherlands

I. INTRODUCTION

The biochemical possibilities to measure the neurotransmitter activity of amino acids in the central nervous system *in vivo* are rather limited (*8*). Endogenous levels of amino acids tell us little or nothing about the release

IN VIVO PERFUSION AND RELEASE
OF NEUROACTIVE SUBSTANCES

ISBN 0-12-083350-6

because they are mainly determined by the sizes of various pools to which the amino acids are confined. In addition to neurotransmission these pools are also involved in general metabolism or precursor function (2). In the case of GABA it is possible to measure the rate of synthesis as reflected by accumulation after inhibition of its degradation (*4, 13, 26*) or by the labeling pattern following precursor loading (*5*). The first approach will reflect release only if the cellular site of synthesis and degradation have a different localization. Indeed, a different subcellular distribution of glutamic acid decarboxylase (GAD) and GABA-transaminase (GABA-T) has been reported but localization of at least some GABA-T in the same neuronal compartment as where synthesis occurs cannot yet be entirely excluded (*27, 36, 39*). Studies on the labeling pattern of the amino acids are limited because the methods of detection are complicated and the precise relationship between the various pools involved are complex.

A more direct approach to assess the neuronal activity of transmitter amino acids *in vivo* is the measurement of their efflux from the perfused brain region *in vivo* (*7, 9, 14, 15, 20, 24, 31*). In this way the possible neurotransmitter function of various amino acids can be studied following local depolarization, electrical stimulation of afferent fibers, or addition of drugs to the perfusion medium. A major disadvantage of *in vitro* release studies on amino acids is the necessity to preload the tissue with the labeled compound. This may result in loading and subsequent release of these compounds from different pools, compared to the *in vivo* situation. Some major drawbacks of measurement of the *in vitro* release of endogenous amino acids include postmortem artifacts (e.g., increased GABA concentration, uncontrolled diffusion, and disturbed compartmental distribution), interrupted neuronal circuitry, and finally, the impossibility to correlate neurochemical alterations with behavioral and physiological parameters. We present data here demonstrating that the release of endogenous neurotransmitter amino acids is of neuronal origin and mutually independent and that it can be differentiated from the efflux of nontransmitter amino acids.

II. METHODS

A. Cannulae

Two types of cannulae were used. The first type consisted of two concentric stainless-steel tubes with external diameters of 1.0 and 0.4 mm, respectively. The extent of protrusion of the inner cannula was adjustable. In all experiments a protrusion of 1.3 mm was chosen for optimal efficiency of

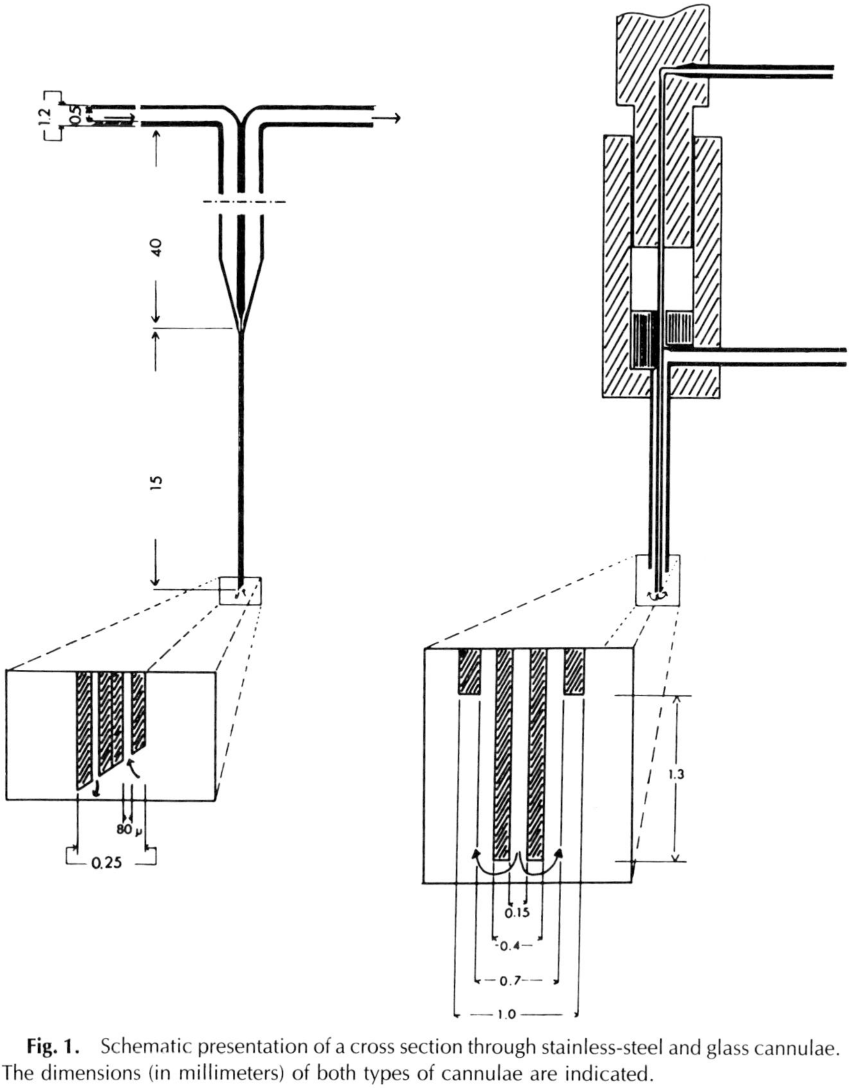

Fig. 1. Schematic presentation of a cross section through stainless-steel and glass cannulae. The dimensions (in millimeters) of both types of cannulae are indicated.

collection. The other type was made of two adjacent glass micropipettes with an internal diameter of the tip of 50–80 μm. Both cannulae were made in our laboratory. A cross section of both types of cannulae is shown in Fig. 1. Essentially, we started using the glass cannula to perfuse a smaller brain area. Histological control revealed that this goal was achieved. We observed no difference in the content of amino acids in the perfusate.

B. Surgical Procedures

The rats were anesthetized with chloral hydrate (400 mg/kg i.p.) and placed in a stereotaxic instrument (Kopf). A burr hole was made in the skull. The push–pull cannula was slowly inserted until the tip reached the targeted brain area. When the stainless-steel cannula was in use, the outer cannula was then slowly raised until the inner cannula protruded 1.3 mm. The perfusion was then started.

C. Perfusion Procedure

The cannula was continuously supplied with freshly prepared artificial cerebrospinal fluid (CSF). The composition of the artificial CSF was 120 m*M* NaCl, 15 m*M* $NaHCO_3$, 5 m*M* KCl, 1.5 m*M* $CaCl_2$, 1 m*M* $MgSO_4$, and 6 m*M* glucose, adjusted to pH 7.2 with an O_2–CO_2 (95–5 v/v) mixture. Two peristaltic infusion pumps (Varioperpex, LKB) were used with silicone tubing (internal diameter 0.5 mm). We used a closed perfusion system. The pooled perfusate samples were weighed and stored at −20°C until analysis (within 1 week). The amount of flow collected was always equal to the amount perfused. At the end of the experiments the brain was removed and the position of the cannula was examined histologically. The damage to the tissue when using the stainless-steel cannula was equal to the diameter of the pull cannula and was not beyond the depth of the inner cannula. When the glass cannula was used, the tissue damage was also equal to the outer diameter of the cannula. Only the results of successful experiments are presented, i.e., correct location of the cannula and a constant flow during the experiments.

The amino acid content of the perfusate was measured using either cation-exchange high-performance liquid chromatography (HPLC) followed by postcolumn derivatization with *o*-phthalaldehyde (OPA), or by reversed-phase HPLC preceded by an automated precolumn derivatization of the samples with OPA (Fig. 2; for detailed descriptions see *31, 38*). The former technique enabled us to measure the fluorophores formed by GABA, lysine, and ethanolamine, whereas a considerably larger number of amino acids could be fluorimetrically determined using the precolumn derivatization technique.

III. FINDINGS

A. Experimental Procedure

Except for the size of the brain area perfused, the performance of the glass cannula did not differ from the stainless-steel cannula. The success rate, i.e.,

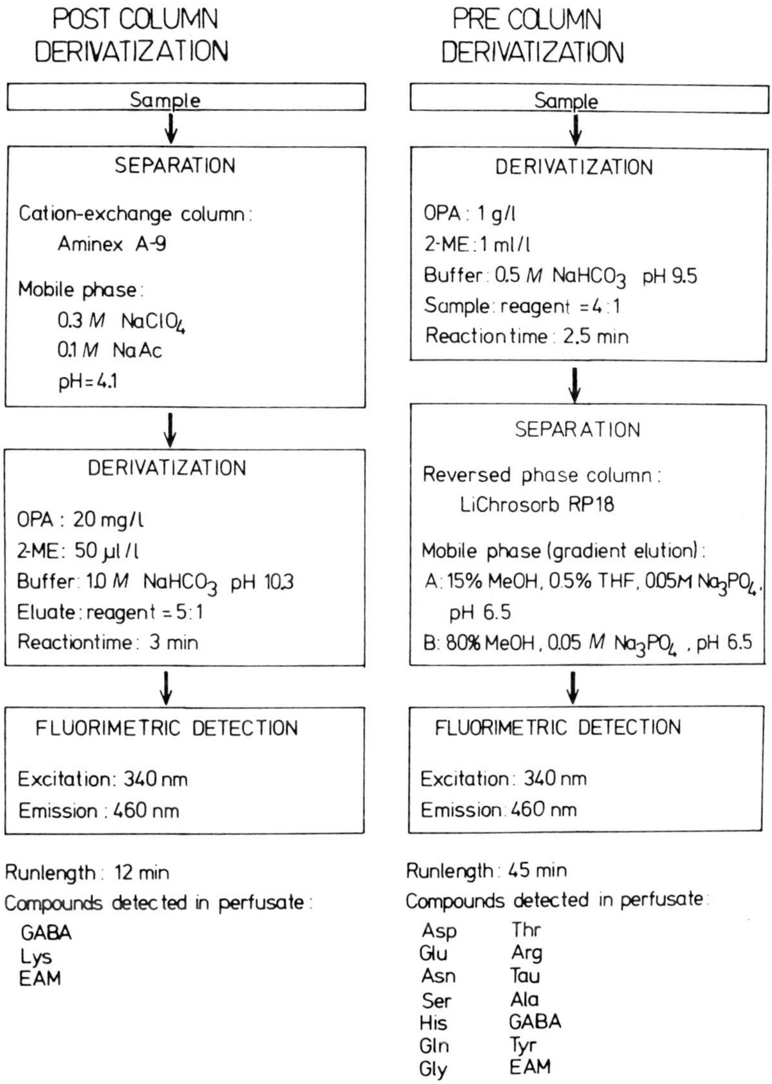

Fig. 2. Schematic presentation of the HPLC procedures used for the determination of the indicated amino acids. OPA, *o*-phthalaldehyde; 2-ME, 2-mercaptoethanol; THF, tetrahydrofuran. (For more detailed descriptions, see *30, 37*.)

the percentage of perfusions with a constant flow during the experiment, was 60–70% with both cannulae. A possible disadvantage of the glass cannula was its fragility.

The efflux of GABA and other amino acids rapidly declined after onset of the perfusion and reached a steady state after approximately 30 min. The release of GABA was studied in several brain areas, including the substantia nigra, the corpus striatum, and the ventral thalamus. The amount of GABA released in these areas was found to be approximately 7.5, 1.6, and 1.0 pmol/min, respectively (under steady-state conditions) and corresponded to the GABA concentrations in these brain regions: 207, 33, and 23 pmol/mg protein, respectively (*17, 30, 31, 34*).

Increasing the perfusion rate from 6.6 to 66 μl/min in the substantia nigra revealed that the amount of GABA released per minute showed an almost linear increase which is likely due to a decreased uptake of the amino acid (data not shown). Increasing the flow rate from 6.6 to 20 μl/min also resulted in an increased lysine and ethanolamine release which was less pronounced when the flow rate was further increased to 66 μl/min.

B. Neurobiological Findings

1. *IN VIVO* RELEASE OF GABA, A TRANSMITTER AMINO ACID

As has been described elsewhere (*31, 34*), the GABA released into the perfusion medium originates from a newly synthesized neuronal pool. Thus, inhibition of the synthesis of GABA by 3-mercaptopropionic acid resulted in an immediately decreased GABA output whereas inhibition of the GABA degradation by aminooxyacetic acid increased the GABA output only after a latency time of approximately 15 min. The latter observation can be explained by assuming that GABA is accumulated and subsequently released from structures such as glial cells after a delay.

The rate of GABA release from the substantia nigra is dependent upon the neuronal activity of the GABA neurons (Fig. 3), since electrical stimulation of afferent fibers increases the output whereas inhibition of the neuronal activity by local application of tetrodotoxine results in a decreased GABA output. The GABA release was greatly enhanced by addition of depolarizing concentrations of potassium in the perfusion medium in all brain areas studied. A calcium dependency of this effect cannot be shown *in vivo* by omitting calcium from the perfusion medium. Apparently the perfused brain area is supplied with calcium from the surrounding tissue and blood. This is shown by the findings that omission of calcium and magnesium from the perfusion medium did not alter the spontaneous or potassium-stimulated release, and that increasing the magnesium concentration in the absence of

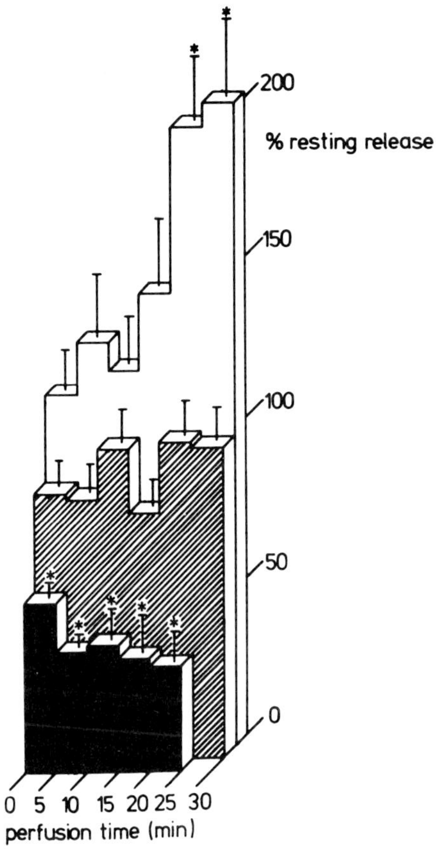

Fig. 3. Effect of 0.5 m*M* 3-mercaptopropionic acid (MPA) (■) and 1 m*M* aminooxyacetic acid (AOAA) (□) on the release of GABA from the substantia nigra. GABA release (ordinate) is expressed as the percentage of the average spontaneous release before drug application. Data are the mean ± SEM during consecutive 5-min periods. Number of control (▨), MPA, and AOAA experiments: 7, 3, and 5 respectively. *, $p < .05$.

calcium (thus allowing a competition for the calcium binding sites) significantly reduced the potassium-stimulated GABA release (Table I).

2. *IN VIVO* RELEASE OF TRANSMITTER AND NONTRANSMITTER AMINO ACIDS

In the ventral thalamus we found of all amino acids measured in our procedure that only the *in vivo* release of GABA, glutamate, and aspartate was enhanced by potassium, whereas the release of glutamine was significantly decreased. Similar results have been obtained measuring the release of endogenous amino acids from the rat hippocampus *in vitro* (*11*). These

TABLE I

Calcium Dependency of Potassium-Induced GABA Release from the Substantia Nigra

Medium containing (m*M*)			Number of experiments	Percentages GABA release[a]
K^+	Ca^{2+}	Mg^{2+}		
5	1.5	1	10	99 ± 9
40	1.5	1	5	517 ± 42
40	0	0	2	483 ± 8
40	0	8	2	136 ± 4
5	0	0	3	103 ± 15[b]

[a] The GABA release during a period of 5 min is expressed as a percentage (mean ± SEM) of the resting release (mean value of the three 5-min fractions preceding the altered composition of the perfusion medium). The perfusion medium was kept isotonic by variation of the Na^+ ions.

[b] Percentage vs following period containing 1.5 m*M* Ca^{2+} and 1 m*M* Mg^{2+}.

results enable us to distinguish the release of transmitter from that of non-transmitter amino acids from the brain.

It was considered possible that the release of several amino acids was interrelated because of a metabolic relationship. Such a possibility was investigated by studying the effect of local drug application and/or estimation of pool sizes of these amino acids. The potassium-induced decrease in glutamine release is unlikely to be due to a rapid conversion into glutamate since we observed that the glutamate release was increased by local application of desmethylimipramine (DMI) without a concomitant reduction of the glutamine release (Table II).

The observed decline in glutamine efflux following exposure to a high potassium concentration, similar to that from the cerebral cortex (*1, 21*), may be explained by an increased uptake of this amino acid. Evidence for such an increased glutamine uptake has been found with *in vitro* preparations where the release of this amino acid was also found to be independent from glutamate synthesis (*10*).

We also showed that increased aspartate release was not due to some metabolic relationship to the other transmitter amino acids since addition of adenosine to the perfusion medium increased the aspartate efflux without affecting the release rate of glutamate and GABA (preliminary observations).

We estimated pool size of glutamate and other amino acids in GABA containing neurons as follows: after lesioning the well-defined striatonigral pathway by injecting kainic acid into the striatum, we subsequently measured the amino acid content of the substantia nigra and striatum (*18*).

TABLE II

Efflux of Several Endogenous Amino acids from the Rat Thalamus in the Presence of DMI or High Potassium Concentration[a]

Treatment	Fraction no.	Percentage amino acid release										
		Asp	Glu	Asn	Ser	Gln	His	Arg	Ala	Tyr	GABA	EAM
Control	I	114 ± 12	103 ± 3	109 ± 7	114 ± 7	106 ± 2	107 ± 3	104 ± 3	112 ± 6	112 ± 5	100 ± 6	107 ± 3
	II	86 ± 12	97 ± 3	91 ± 7	87 ± 7	94 ± 2	94 ± 3	96 ± 3	88 ± 6	94 ± 6	100 ± 6	93 ± 3
No drug	III	199 ± 99	128 ± 35	137 ± 55	262 ± 170	147 ± 58	79 ± 8[b]	122 ± 33	211 ± 119	93 ± 11	100 ± 9	128 ± 39
	IV	106 ± 24	117 ± 25	118 ± 26	139 ± 45	163 ± 76	112 ± 38	104 ± 22	129 ± 31	164 ± 43	96 ± 17	123 ± 32
	V	136 ± 46	109 ± 25	116 ± 29	148 ± 48	136 ± 55	84 ± 22	110 ± 26	136 ± 33	178 ± 69	87 ± 19	91 ± 9
Control	I	99 ± 2	100 ± 2	103 ± 3	103 ± 2	100 ± 1	95 ± 6	98 ± 2	105 ± 2	106 ± 2	102 ± 2	97 ± 2
	II	100 ± 2	100 ± 2	97 ± 3	97 ± 2	100 ± 1	105 ± 6	102 ± 2	95 ± 2	94 ± 2	98 ± 2	103 ± 2
500 μ*M* DMI	III	564 ± 102[d]	269 ± 42[d]	112 ± 7	155 ± 40[b]	103 ± 3	139 ± 48	105 ± 7	119 ± 31	134 ± 29	319 ± 50[d]	105 ± 4
	IV	637 ± 76[d]	388 ± 5[d]	114 ± 18	137 ± 29	98 ± 4	113 ± 12	89 ± 15	122 ± 28	102 ± 14	488 ± 82[d]	95 ± 5
	V	602 ± 112[d]	313 ± 61[d]	116 ± 17	118 ± 17	98 ± 4	122 ± 24	99 ± 14	126 ± 25	108 ± 20	517 ± 90[d]	96 ± 9
Control	I	113 ± 10	111 ± 6	110 ± 5	109 ± 8	105 ± 2	112 ± 5	112 ± 3	118 ± 5	107 ± 7	106 ± 4	104 ± 2
	II	87 ± 10	89 ± 6	90 ± 5	91 ± 8	95 ± 3	88 ± 5	88 ± 3	82 ± 5	93 ± 7	93 ± 7	96 ± 2
60 m*M*K+	III	273 ± 40[d]	252 ± 22[d]	118 ± 25	130 ± 25	83 ± 11	96 ± 8	94 ± 8	118 ± 16	114 ± 18	596 ± 126[d]	95 ± 11
	IV	196 ± 32[c]	313 ± 88[d]	98 ± 12	87 ± 15	53 ± 10[d]	77 ± 16	80 ± 10	106 ± 18	78 ± 16	746 ± 107[d]	96 ± 8
	V	160 ± 11[d]	219 ± 55[d]	95 ± 10	74 ± 15	46 ± 9[d]	75 ± 9[b]	63 ± 6[d]	106 ± 22	74 ± 10[b]	466 ± 71[d]	86 ± 9

[a] The efflux of amino acids during three 5-min periods (III to V) is expressed as a percentage (mean ± SEM of 5 experiments) of the resting release (two 5-min periods I and II). The concentration of DMI in the perfusion medium was 500 μ*M*, and that of potassium 60 m*M* (replacing sodium).

[b] $p < .05$ vs preceding control period.

[c] $p < .02$ vs preceding control period.

[d] $p < .002$ vs preceding control period.

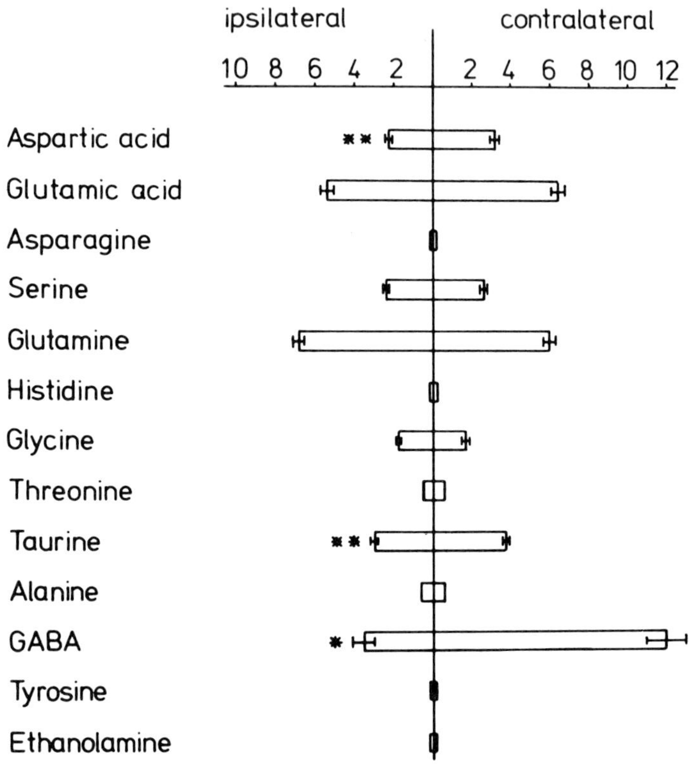

Fig. 4. Effect of striatal kainic acid lesion on the amino acid contents of the substantia nigra. Kainic acid (2 μg) was injected into the striatum 2 weeks before sacrifice. Postmortem increases in the levels of GABA were prevented by administering 1.5 mmol/kg MPA 2 min before decapitation (*29*). The amino acid levels are expressed in μmol/g wet weight (mean of 12 experiments ± SEM). *, ** indicate a significant difference between the ipsi- and contralateral side of $p < .002$, and $p < .02$, respectively.

With the exception of threonine, ethanolamine, and tyrosine, the striatal content of the amino acids was significantly lower in the lesioned striatum, whereas in the substantia nigra only the levels of GABA, aspartate, and taurine were significantly decreased (Fig. 4). Moreover, the ratio of the content of glutamate and glutamine was significantly ($p < .002$) lowered from 1.10 ± 0.05 (mean of 16 observations ± SEM, control side) to 0.88 ± 0.04 (lesioned side). In these experiments glutamine levels tended to increase, whereas the content of glutamate was slightly lower at the affected side.

These and other findings (*25*) suggest a rather small size (i.e., <10%) of the glutamate pool in GABAergic nerve endings. This rules out a major contribution of the glutamate present in this pool to the potassium-induced increased release of GABA, unless under such conditions the formation of glutamate is very rapid and the subsequent conversion to GABA is relatively slow, which seems unlikely. The decreased nigral levels of aspartate and taurine after a kainic acid lesion of the striatum cannot be explained by a direct metabolic relationship with GABA and therefore point to a neurotransmitter or cotransmitter function of these amino acids in a striatonigral pathway.

3. *IN VIVO* INTERACTIONS OF GABAergic SYSTEM WITH OTHER TRANSMITTERS: DRUG EFFECTS

We have previously shown that the release of GABA is influenced by several other transmitter systems (*31–35*). We found that the GABA release from the substantia nigra was slightly enhanced after addition of low concentration (10 μM) of dopamine to the perfusion medium, but that the predominant action of dopamine (at higher concentrations) was inhibitory (Table III).

The latter effect was also observed from addition of ADTN or low concentrations of apomorphine. Dopamine and apomorphine also inhibited the GABA release in the striatum. We found that addition of a high concentration of apomorphine (100 μM) to the perfusion medium did not affect the striatal GABA release, whereas a fourfold increase was obtained in the substantia nigra. It is not clear whether the latter effect is mediated by

TABLE III

Effect of Local Application of Various Drugs on GABA Release from Substantia Nigra and Striatum[a]

	Substantia nigra		Corpus striatum	
Drug applied	Con	+ Haloperidol	Con	+ Haloperidol
None	0	(−)	0	0
Dopamine	+/−−	nd[b]/0	−−	++
Apomorphine	−/++++	nd/++	−−	nd
Noradrenaline	nd	nd	−−	−−
Serotonin	nd	nd	0	nd
Oxotremorine	nd	nd	+	0
Morphine	nd	nd	−−	−−
Muscimol	nd	nd	−−	nd

[a] The changes in the GABA release are indicated as an increase (+), a decrease (−), or no effect (0). The magnitude of the change is indicated by the number of symbols.

[b] nd, Not determined. A more detailed description of the effects of these drugs appears elsewhere (*32–34*).

stimulation of dopamine receptors, though haloperidol both antagonized the dopamine-induced inhibitory effects and the apomorphine-induced stimulation of the GABA release. In most of these experiments no statistically significant change was observed in the release of lysine and ethanolamine. The changes in the release of these two compounds that was observed in some experiments did not show any correlation with the direction or magnitude of the altered GABA release rate.

The influence of the cholinergic, noradrenergic, and opioid system upon GABAergic transmission was studied in the striatum. Thus, addition of oxotremorine produced a small increase in GABA output which could be antagonized both by atropine and haloperidol. Noradrenaline resulted in a diminished GABA release that could be mimicked both by the α- and β-receptor agonists clonidine and isoprenaline, respectively, and by electrical stimulation of the locus coeruleus. The action of noradrenaline could not be antagonized by haloperidol. We observed a decreased GABA release after infusion of morphine that was antagonized by nalorphine but not by haloperidol (Table III). These data provide us with information about the regulation of GABA release and also show that the effect of acetylcholine is most likely mediated by dopamine. The finding that muscimol and pictrotoxine decrease and increase striatal GABA release, respectively, suggests the existence of either GABA autoreceptors or the presence of GABAergic afferents regulating the release of GABA.

Local infusion of noradrenaline uptake inhibitor DMI enhanced the release of GABA in the striatum and thalamus. In the striatum we observed that the stimulated GABA release due to DMI or potassium was diminished if it had been preceded by potassium or DMI, respectively (*19*). We also found that DMI- and potassium-induced increased GABA efflux in the thalamus was dependent upon the presence of calcium (Fig. 5), though calcium dependency of potassium-induced GABA release was more pronounced than that of DMI.

These results suggest that the same presumably neuronal pool of GABA was involved for both potassium and DMI. Other structurally related antidepressant drugs such as imipramine and trimipramine (a drug that does not inhibit uptake of noradrenaline or serotonin) also greatly enhanced thalamic GABA release (Table IV). Similar results were obtained with two other lipophilic drugs (i.e., log $p > 3$): propranolol and haloperidol.

Our results were obtained after local application of rather high concentrations (μ*M* range) of the drugs. However, it should be taken into account that in animal studies it has been shown that systemic administration of 5–25 mg/kg of antidepressant drugs results in brain levels as high as 10–70 μ*M* (*23, 32*). The brain levels of antidepressant drugs in patients have been

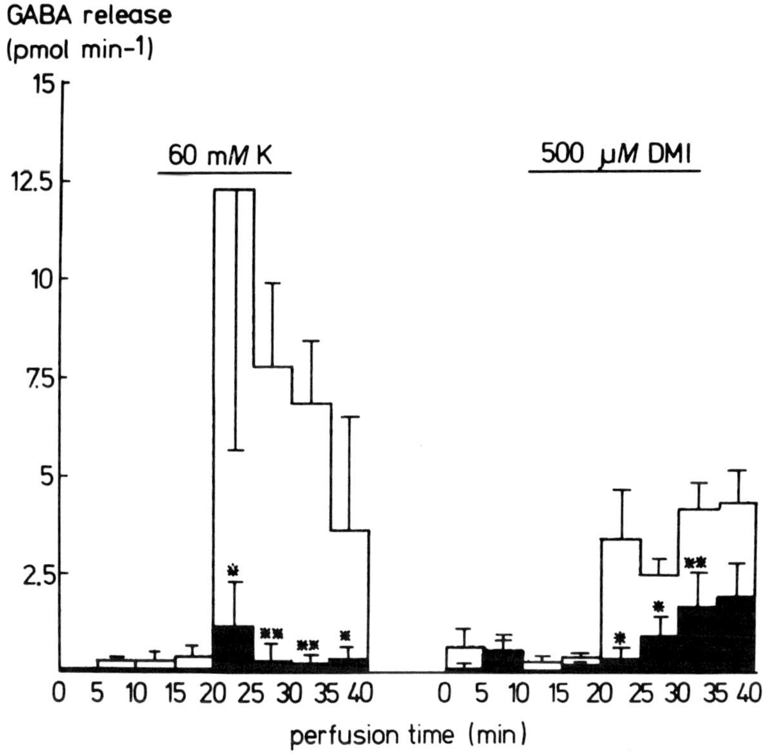

Fig. 5. Calcium dependence of potassium- and DMI-induced GABA release from the rat thalamus. GABA release is expressed as pmol/min (mean ± SEM) during consecutive 5-min periods following a wash period of 35 min. The calcium dependency was established by omitting this ion from the perfusion medium and increasing the magnesium concentration to 8 m*M* (replacing sodium ions). *, ** indicate a statistically significant difference from normal perfusion medium containing either 60 m*M* potassum (4 experiments) or 500 μ*M* DMI (10 experiments) of $p < .05$ and $p < .01$, respectively. (■), no Ca^{2+}; (□), control.

estimated to be 7–100 μ*M* (*6, 16,* the latter levels from fatal intoxications). The results of these studies suggest that the central levels of antidepressants, both in men and animals, are sufficiently high to affect the release of amino acid neurotransmitters, and that some side effects of these drugs (e.g., seizures) may be attributed to the findings reported here.

DMI promotes the net efflux of the amino acid neurotrasmitters glutamate and aspartate similarly to that observed after high potassium concentrations (Table II). Unlike potassium, DMI did not decrease the output of glutamine

TABLE IV

Release of Endogenous GABA from the Rat Thalamus Exposed for 5 Min to Drug[a]

Drug added (10 μM)	Percentage GABA release		
	Predrug	Drug	Postdrug
None	89 ± 8	73 ± 9	74 ± 6
Desmethylimipramine	115 ± 17	857 ± 364[c]	121 ± 34
Imipramine	92 ± 13	305 ± 97[b]	152 ± 45
Trimepramine	174 ± 57	539 ± 270[c]	162 ± 48
Propranolol	104 ± 28	470 ± 189[c]	113 ± 32
Haloperidol	132 ± 60	978 ± 412[c]	196 ± 64

[a] GABA release is expressed as a percentage (mean ± SEM of 5–10 experiments) of the resting release. The release during 5 min, before, during, and after drug application (predrug, drug, and postdrug, respectively) is presented.

[b] $p < .01$ vs predrug period.

[c] $p < .0005$ vs predrug period.

from the thalamus, clearly indicating the independence of glutamine and glutamate with regard to the release under these conditions.

Considering the present results, the question arises as to whether the drug-increased efflux of the amino acids is due to inhibition of the uptake or to provoking release from nerve terminals. Most of the drugs used by us inhibit the uptake of GABA in brain slices or subcellular particles (*12, 40*). Thus, inhibition of high-affinity uptake of GABA in brain slices was virtually complete in the presence of 0.2–1 m*M* of DMI, haloperidol, imipramine, or propranolol and appeared to be noncompetitive for DMI (*12*). An increase in the release of GABA from subcellular particles (possible synaptosomes) has been observed at concentrations of 100 μ*M* imipramine and higher (*40*). *In vivo,* the release of GABA was higher in the presence of uptake inhibitors (*12, 15*) and recently a five fold increase of GABA output was found in the presence of 5 m*M* 2,4-diaminobutyric acid (*22*). Inhibition of the uptake of glutamate or aspartate by DMI has not been reported, but the structural requirements of drugs to affect neuronal uptake of these amino acids *in vitro* seem to be rather specific (*3*). Thus, inhibition of uptake or induction of release of neurotransmitter amino acids or both may produce the present results. It is of interest here to mention that several of the drugs used are local anesthetics and may alter the fluidity of cellular membranes, leading to an increased diffusion of the transmitter from and inhibition of uptake into the nerve terminal (*28*).

IV. PERSPECTIVES AND DISCUSSION

The push–pull cannula technique is very useful for obtaining information about the *in vivo* release of endogenous neurotransmitters. It is possible to study the regulation of the neuronal activity of a transmitter *in situ,* i.e., without major prior destruction of the neuronal connections. Thus, the effect of chemical or electrical stimulation of afferent fibers upon the release of a transmitter can directly be measured. Especially with regard to amino acids, this technique enables us to measure the activity as a neurotransmitter as opposed to the metabolic and precursor functions. One of the prominent differences between *in vitro* and *in vivo* release studies appeared to be the calcium dependency of an altered release rate. Under our *in vivo* conditions we observed that omission of calcium from the perfusion medium does not influence the spontaneous or potassium-stimulated release which is most probably due to a major calcium transport from the direct environment of the perfused area. A calcium dependency could only be shown by concomitantly increasing the magnesium concentration. We observed that tricyclic antidepressant drugs greatly enhanced the release of GABA after local application, a property that was shared by two unrelated lipophilic compounds. *In vitro* studies have revealed that various lipophilic drugs inhibit the uptake of exogenous GABA. Since the effect of DMI was shown to be calcium dependent, the GABA released is most probably of neuronal origin. It is uncertain, however, whether this effect is mediated by specific receptors located on the GABA terminals. When assessing the influence of locally applied drugs, a careful choice of the concentration to be added to the perfusion medium is necessary. The rather strong accumulation of antidepressant drugs in the brain after systemic administration illustrates the difficulties encountered in choosing the appropriate concentration.

It will be very interesting to study the effect of systemically applied drugs on the *in vivo* release of endogenous transmitters, though the constant perfusion of a brain area might prevent the required accumulation of a drug at its site of action. Our study also clearly shows that the release of several metabolically closely related neurotransmitter amino acids is independently regulated, again supporting the neuronal origin of these amino acids released into the perfusion medium.

REFERENCES

1. Abdul-Ghani, A.-S., Coutinho-Netto, J., and Bradford, H. F. *In vivo* superfusion methods and release of glutamate. *In* "Glutamate: Transmitter in the Central Nervous System," (P. J.

Roberts, J. Storm-Mathisen, and G. A. R. Johnston, eds.), 1981, pp. 155–208. Wiley, New York.

2. Bachelard, H. S. Biochemistry of centrally active amino acids. *In* "Amino Acid Neurotransmitters," Vol. 29 (F. V. DeFeudis and P. Mandel, eds.), 1981, pp. 475–498. Raven, New York.
3. Balcar, V. J., and Johnston, G. A. R. The structural specificity of the high affinity uptake of L-glutamate and L-aspartate by rat brain slices. *J. Neurochem.* **19** (1972) 2657–2666.
4. Bernasconi, R., Maitre, L., Martin, P., and Raschdorf, F. The use of inhibitors of GABA-transaminase for the determination of GABA turnover in mouse brain regions: an evaluation of amino oxyacetic acid and gabaculine. *J. Neurochem.* **38** (1982) 57–66.
5. Bertilsson, L., Mao, C. C., and Costa, E. Application of principles of steady-state kinetics to the estimation of γ-aminobutyric acid turnover rate in nuclei of the rat brain. *J. Pharmacol. Exp. Ther.* **200** (1977) 277–284.
6. Bickel, M. H. Poisoning by tricyclic antidepressant drugs; general and pharmacokinetic considerations. *Int. J. Clin. Pharmacol.* **11** (1975) 145–176.
7. Dietl, H., and Philippu, A. *In vivo* release of endogenous GABA in the cat hypothalamus. *N. S. Arch Pharmacol.* **308** (1979) 143–147.
8. Fonnum, F. The turnover of transmitter amino acids, with special reference to GABA. *In* "Central Neurotransmitter Turnover," (C. J. Pycock and P. V. Taberner, eds.), 1981, pp. 105–124. Croom Helm, London.
9. Gauchy, M., Kemel, M. L., Glowinski, J., and Besson, M. J. *In vivo* release of endogenously synthesized [^{3}H]GABA from the cat substantia nigra and the pallido-entopeduncular nuclei. *Brain Res.* **136** (1980) 129–141.
10. Hamberger, A. C., Han Chiang, G., Sandoval, E., and Cotman, C. W. Glutamate as a CNS transmitter. II. Regulation of synthesis in the releasable pool. *Brain Res.* **168** (1979) 531–541.
11. Hamberger, A., Jacobson, I., Lindroth, P., Mopper, K., Nystrom, B., Sandberg, M., Molin, S.-O., and Svanberg, U. Neuron–glia interactions in the biosynthesis and release of transmitter amino acids. *In* "Amino Acid Neurotransmitters," Vol. 29 (F. V. DeFeudis and P. Mandel, eds.), 1981, pp. 509–518. Raven, New York.
12. Harris, M., Hopkin, J. M., and Neal, M. J. Effect of centrally acting drugs in the uptake of γ-amino butyric acid (GABA) by slices of rat cerebral cortex. *Br. J. Pharmacol.* **47** (1973) 229–239.
13. Iadarola, M. J., and Gale, K. Dissociation between drug-induced increases in nerve terminal and non-nerve terminal pools of GABA *in vivo*. *Eur. J. Pharmacol.* **59** (1979) 125–129.
14. Iversen, L. L., Mitchel, J. F., and Srinivasan, V. The release of γ-aminobutyric acid during inhibition in the cat visual cortex. *J. Physiol. (London)* **212** (1971) 519–534.
15. Kondo, Y., and Iwatsubo, K. Increased release of preloaded [^{3}H]GABA from substantia nigra *in vivo* following stimulation of caudate nucleus and globus pallidus. *Brain Res.* **154** (1978) 395–400.
16. Korf, J. Central molecular aspects of tricyclic antidepressant drug action. *Rev. Pure Appl. Pharmacol. Sci.* **4** (1983) 139–212.
17. Korf, J., and Venema, K. Desmethylimipramine enhances the release of endogenous GABA and other neurotransmitter amino acids from the rat thalamus. *J. Neurochem.* **40** (1983) 946–950.
18. Korf, J., and Venema, K. Amino acids in the substantia nigra of rats with striatal lesions produced by kainic acid. *J. Neurochem.* **40** (1983) 1171–1173.
19. Korf, J., van der Heyden, J. A. M., Venema, K., and Postema, F. Distribution and release of GABA in the basal ganglia. *In* "GABA and Basal Ganglia," (G. DiChiara and G. L. Gessa, eds.), 1981, pp. 105–117. Raven, New York.

20. Moroni, F., Corradetti, R., Casamenti, F., Moneti, G., and Pepeu, G. The release of endogenous GABA and glutamate from the cerebral cortex in the rat. *N. S. Arch. Pharmacol.* **316** (1981) 235–239.
21. Moroni, F., Corradetti, R., Casamenti, F., Moneti, G., and Pepeu, G. The release of GABA and glutamate from the cerebral cortex is an index of the activity of underlying aminoacidergic neurons. *In* "Glutamate as a Neurotransmitter," (G. DiChiara and G. L. Gessa, eds.), 1981, pp. 157–167. Raven, New York.
22. Moroni, F., Mulas, A., Moneti, G., and Pepeu, G. *In vivo* changes in γ-aminobutyric acid output from the cerebral cortex induced by inhibitors of γ-aminobutyric uptake and metabolism. *J. Neurochem.* **39** (1982) 582–584.
23. Nagy, A. Blood and brain concentrations of imipramine, clomipramine and their monomethylated metabolites after oral and intramuscular administration to rats. *J. Pharm. Pharmacol.* **29** (1977) 104–107.
24. Obata, K., and Takeda, K. Release of γ-aminobutyric acid into the fourth ventricle induced by stimulation of the cat's cerebellum. *J. Neurochem.* **16** (1969) 1043–1047.
25. Patel, A. J., Johnson, A. L., and Balazs, R. Metabolic compartmentation of glutamate associated with the formation of γ-aminobutyrate. *J. Neurochem.* **23** (1974) 1271–1279.
26. Pericic, D., Walters, J. R., and Chase, T. N. Effects of diazepam and pentobarbital on amino-oxyacetic acid-induced accumulation of GABA. *J. Neurochem.* **29** (1977) 839–846.
27. Salganicoff, L., and De Robertis, E. Subcellular distribution of the enzymes of the glutamic acid, glutamine and γ-aminobutyric acid cycle in rat brain. *J. Neurochem.* **12** (1965) 287–309.
28. Seeman, P. The membrane actions of anaesthetics and tranquilizers. *Pharmacol. Rev.* **24** (1972) 583–655.
29. van der Heyden, J. A. M., Venema, K., and Korf, J. Regional levels of GABA in the brain: rapid semi-automated assay and prevention of postmortem increase by 3-mercaptopropionic acid. *J. Neurochem.* **31** (1978) 197–203.
30. van der Heyden, J. A. M., de Kloet, E. R., Korf, J., and Versteeg, D. H. G. GABA content of discrete brain nuclei and spinal cord of the rat. *J. Neurochem.* **33** (1979) 857–861.
31. van der Heyden, J. A. M., Venema, K., and Korf, J. *In vivo* release of endogenous GABA from rat substantia nigra measured by a novel method. *J. Neurochem.* **32** (1979) 469–476.
32. van der Heyden, J. A. M., Venema, K., and Korf, J. Biphasic and opposite effects of dopamine and apomorphine on endogenous GABA release in the rat substantia nigra. *J. Neurochem.* **34** (1980) 119–125.
33. van der Heyden, J. A. M., Venema, K., and Korf, J. *In vivo* release of endogenous GABA from rat striatum: inhibition by dopamine. *J. Neurochem.* **34** (1980) 1338–1341.
34. van der Heyden, J. A. M., Venema, K., and Korf, J. *In vivo* release of endogenous GABA from rat striatum: effects of muscimol, oxotremorine and morphine. *J. Neurochem.* **34** (1980) 1648–1653.
35. van der Heyden, J. A. M., Venema, K., Lebrun, P., Sebens, J. B., and Korf, J. Release of endogenous GABA from the rat brain: methodological aspects and the effects of catecholamines. *In* "Amino Acid Neurotransmitters," Vol. 29, (F. V. DeFeudis and P. Mandel, eds.), 1981, pp. 193–203. Raven, New York.
36. van Kempen, G. M. J., van den Berg, C. J., van der Helm, H. J., and Veldstra, H. Intracellular localization of glutamate decarboxylase, γ-aminobutyrate transaminase and some other enzymes in brain tissue. *J. Neurochem.* **12** (1965) 581–588.
37. van Wijk, M., and Korf, J. A quantitative study in the rat on the relationship between imipramine levels in brain and serum. *Psychopharmacology* **76** (1982) 48–51.
38. Venema, K., Leever, W., Bakker, J. O., Haayer, G., and Korf, J. An automated precolumn

derivatization device to determine neurotransmitter and other amino acids by reversed-phase high-performance liquid chromatography. *J. Chromat.* **260** (1983) 371–376.
39. Vincent, S. R., Lehman, J., and McGeer, E. G. The localization of GABA-transaminase in the striato-nigral system. *Life Sci.* **27** (1980) 595–601.
40. Weinstein, H., Varon, S., and Roberts, E. Effects of imipramine on the Na^+ dependent exchange and retention of γ-aminobutyric acid by mouse brain subcellular particles. *Biochem. Pharmacol.* **20** (1971) 103–117.

6

Push–Pull Perfusion Studies on the *in Vivo* Release of Proteins, Enzymes, and the Neuroactive Peptides–Enkephalins from the Rat Brain

ALEJANDRO BAYÓN, SARA SOLANO, BENITO ANTÓN, IRENE CASTAÑO, AND DAVID DÍAZ-PONTONES

Departamento de Biología Molecular
Instituto de Investigaciones Biomédicas
Universidad Nacional Autónoma de México
Mexico City, Mexico

I. INTRODUCTION

The fundamental role that *in vitro* neurochemical techniques have played in understanding the chemical coding of brain function has made us aware of some of their limitations. Thus, surgically isolated brain regions and mechanically fractionated cellular and subcellular structures facilitate the

IN VIVO PERFUSION AND RELEASE
OF NEUROACTIVE SUBSTANCES

ISBN 0-12-083350-6

control of the experimental conditions in which they are studied, but as a consequence of this isolation, their normal connections with the brain, the whole organism, and the environment are lost. Therefore, to study the physiological regulation of neurochemical events and their integration into neural function, an *in vivo* approach is needed. The most obvious one is to create a superfusion system analogous to those used *in vitro,* but instead of the tissue sample being placed inside a bath, the bath is implanted in the brain tissue of a live animal. Cups, needles, concentric cannulae, and dialysis bags and fibers all introduce a stream of artificial physiological fluid in the brain, allowing the administration and sampling of chemicals into and from defined neural structures.

Because of this common working principle some of the basic technical problems and limitations of the *in vivo* perfusion methods were previously revealed by methods *in vitro* . These difficulties, which must be controlled before any scientific questions can be asked, are lesion of the tissue produced by the perfusing device, by hydrodynamic accidents, or by the constant circulation of fluid through the tissue; the decrease of neural responsiveness of the tissue to stimulation and to pharmacological manipulations along perfusions; and the efficiency of the diffusional exchange between the tissue and the perfusion medium. The initial part of this chapter deals with the use of biochemical markers (proteins, peptides, and nonpeptide transmitters) to assess tissue damage and viability. In this context we describe an improved design of the tip of the concentric push–pull cannula, the probe most widely used for *in vivo* perfusion. Compared to the classical Gaddum cannula, this design (slot-tip cannula) produces less tissue damage during perfusion, keeps tissue responsiveness stable for several hours, and allows a tissue–medium exchange similar to that observed with the traditional model. In contrast with dialytrodes, which also reduce tissue damage during perfusion, slot cannulae allow the diffusion into the perfusates of both small chemicals and macromolecules (proteins and enzymes) released from brain tissue.

The body of this chapter deals with the *in vivo* release of proteins and peptides from the brain. In addition to classical transmission, other possible roles of these neurochemicals in brain function are a subject of increasing interest in neurobiology. Current evidence indicates that their availability at the release sites has a close dependence on the entire structure of the neuron, differing from nonpeptide messengers whose metabolism is mostly centered on the synaptic apparatus. Therefore, it seems to be particularly important to study peptide and protein release in integral pathways and circuits. Thus, we present data on the *in vivo* release of protein material and several enzyme activities from the brain; we also show evidence of the *in vivo* release of the neuropeptides enkephalins, presenting results on the physiological regulation of this release in freely moving animals.

II. METHODS

A. Cannula

The basic design of the push–pull cannula used in these experiments (Fig. 1) is that of Gaddum (*20*), as adapted by Myers (*41*). Early work with this cannula in our laboratory gave a relatively high incidence of flow obstructions during perfusion (see Section III), which were found to be due to the presence of tissue fragments or clogs obliterating the tip or the shaft of the

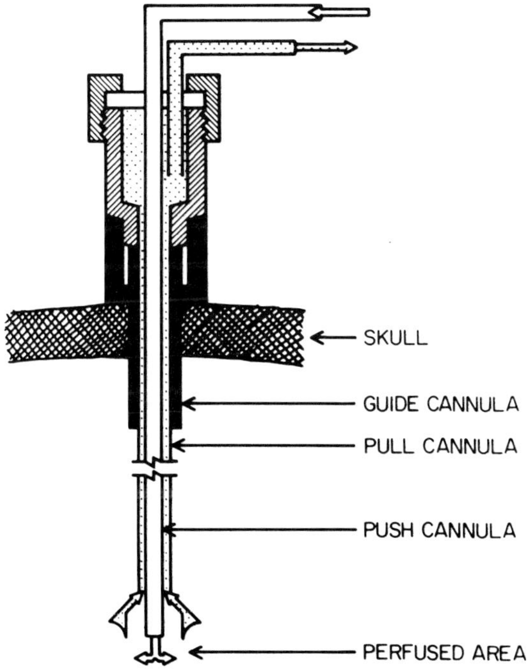

Fig. 1. Gaddum–Myers push–pull cannula. The inlet (white) and outlet (dotted) tubing systems are concentric along the shaft of the cannula but separate after entering the upper chamber, which is constructed of two stainless-steel screwed pieces (dashed) and a rubber septum (white). The guide cannula used in our laboratory incorporates a clamping device (black) to fix the push–pull cannula. Note that the push cannula protrudes from the tip of the pull cannula.

pull part of the cannula. These obstructing materials are produced mainly by negative pressures developed at the perfused region and by the tissue-eroding effect of the stream of superfusing medium. The former effect is mostly dependent on the pressure balance of the pumping systems and can be successfully dealt with using a pull line open to atmospheric pressure (*43*). The erosion depends mainly on the geometry of the cannula tip and has been minimized by keeping the end of the inner push cannula within the outer pull tubing (*30, 44, 45*). Although this type of design shields the tissue from the direct mechanical effects of the outflowing stream, it reduces the diffusion interface at the cannula tip to the size of the cross-sectional area of the outer cannula, making it necessary to use wider probes that are unsuitable for small laboratory animals.

We have designed a new cannula tip (Fig. 2) which, besides providing the shielding effect previously noted, allows for a larger interface between the tissue and the perfusing medium, even using small-gauge cannulae. The push–pull cannula is constructed from 21-ga (thin wall) and 29-ga stainless-steel tubing (Small Parts Inc., Miami, Florida). Before assembling the outer and inner tubing to form a concentric Gaddum–Myers system, the 21-ga pull tubing is obstructed at the tip with soldering material and two slots are drilled under microscopic control on the sides of the shaft, just above the tip. The number and length of the slots can be varied depending on the size of the region to be perfused. Unilateral perfusion of restricted areas of the wall of the third ventricle (i.e., the periventricular vascular organ of the chick) has been possible using a single-slotted cannula. This probe has also been successfully used to perfuse large (caudate putamen) and small (substantia nigra) regions of the rat brain. In the sections that follow we present results obtained perfusing the area of the globus pallidus, where most of our tests of the performance of this cannula have been carried out.

B. Surgical Procedures

Albino rats—local Wistar strain—weighing 150–200 g were anesthetized with sodium pentobarbital. Surgery, under aseptic conditions, is limited to the stereotaxic implantation of a stainless-steel 18-ga cannula which is chronically fixed with acrylic cement to the skull, serving as a guide for the acute insertion of the push–pull cannula (see Fig. 1). The lower end of the guide cannula is placed several millimeters above the brain region that will be reached by the tip of the push–pull cannula at the time of perfusion; this strategy avoids the gliosis which is found in the perfused area when the perfusing probe itself is chronically implanted into the brain (*24*). The upper end of the guide cannula (Fig. 1) was modified by adding a clamping device to impede rotational or axial movements of the push–pull cannula after it is

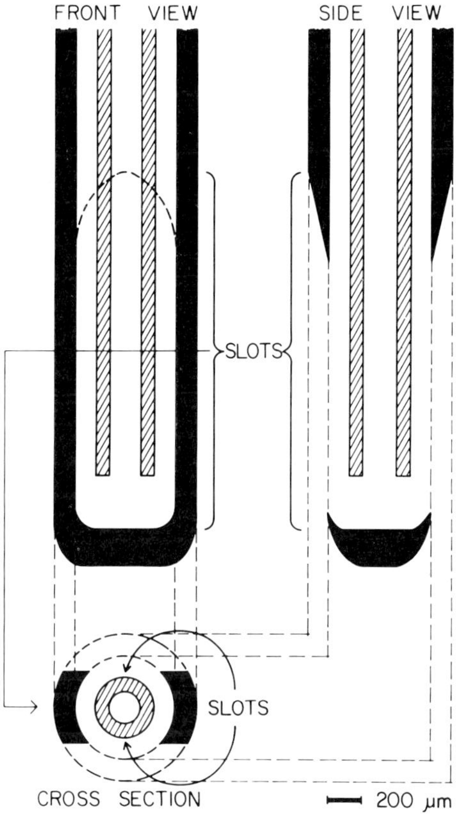

Fig. 2. Orthogonal projection of slot-tip modification of the push–pull cannula shown in Fig. 1. The design is drawn to scale, showing the double-slotted cannula used in this work. See text for construction details. (■), thin-walled 21-ga tubing; (▨), 29-ga tubing.

inserted; a tight fit between the outer pull cannula and the guide avoids other movements of the probe. After implantation, the lumen of the guide is temporarily blocked with a tight-fitting rod until the day of perfusion—1 week after surgery. During this time the implant is protected by a plastic cap covering the guide. The coordinates used for the globus pallidus and other brain regions were taken from the atlas of Konig and Klippel (*34*).

C. Perfusion Procedures

Implanted animals were placed in transparent plastic cages—their usual housing—in a quiet, isolated room 2 hr before the beginning of the session and remained in a freely moving situation throughout the perfusion. The animals were subjected to a single perfusion session. The protective mandrel was removed from the guide and the perfusing cannula slowly inserted and clamped in place. During early work in our laboratory the push and the pull ends of the cannulae were connected through polyethylene tubing to infusion and withdrawal syringes positioned in a Harvard reciprocating pump (*5, 7*). Currently, a continuous superfusion system has been adopted, using small-bore, thick-wall sylastic tubing and polystaltic cassette pumps (Manostat). This latter system is easier to handle than syringe pumping and also helps to prevent extreme pressure changes in the perfused area, such as those observed when changing syringes.

The standard perfusion medium is a Krebs–Ringer bicarbonate buffer: 127 m*M* NaCl, 3.73 m*M* KCl, 1.8 m*M* $CaCl_2$, 1.18 m*M* KH_2PO_4, 1.18 m*M* $MgSO_4$, 20 m*M* $NaHCO_3$, D-glucose 2 g/liter. Bovine serum albumin (BSA) (0.1%), and bacitracin (30 μg/ml) were included in the medium as protective agents for enkephalin release studies (*1*). Chemical stimulation of the perfused tissue was produced by substituting K^+ for Na^+ ions in the standard medium to reach a 50 m*M* K^+ concentration. From the onset of the sessions the flow rate was held constant (25 μl/min) and effluent fractions collected every 15 min. During the experiments, infused and collected fluid volumes were routinely measured, and there was constant monitoring for the presence of blood in the effluent. Abnormal animal behavior (motor disturbances, persistent drowsiness, hyperactivity, excessive grooming, salivation, etc.) was also recorded. At the end of the perfusion, the position of the tip of the cannula was verified by inspection of frontal sections of the brain under a dissection microscope.

During study of enkephalin release into the effluent medium, fractions were collected in plastic tubes containing 0.5 ml of 2.0 *N* ice-cold acetic acid in order to stop enzymatic degradation; these fractions were then boiled for 15 min, lyophilized, and resuspended in phosphate saline buffer for the enkephalin radioimmunoassay (RIA). When release of protein, enzyme activities, or radioactive tracers were studied, the perfusate fractions were aliquoted, frozen, and promptly assayed.

D. Assay of Biological Samples

Protein release was determined by the method of Lowry *et al.* (*38*), using BSA as the standard; the reaction volume was reduced and the sample volume increased in order to improve the sensitivity of the assay. Lactic acid dehydrogenase (LDH) activity was determined using pyruvate as substrate (*10*). Also, in order to increase the sensitivity of the assay, incubation volume was reduced, sample volume increased, and reaction time extended to 24 hr. When assaying perfusate samples with low LDH activities the initial velocities were linear for at least 12 hr and plots of enzyme concentration vs reaction velocity gave straight lines. Similar assay modifications also produced higher sensitivities when measuring acetylcholinesterase (AChe) [using acetylthiocholine iodide as substrate (*17*)] and protease activities [Hide powder azure as substrate (*49*)]. Units of enzyme activity are expressed in nanomoles of substrate/hr. Only protease activity is expressed in absorbance units/24 hr.

In order to study the release of exogenous GABA, tritiated γ-aminobutyric acid ([^{3}H]GABA, specific activity 34 Ci/mmol, Amersham) was added to the standard perfusion medium at the beginning of the perfusion ($4-20 \times 10^6$ cpm in 750 μl, perfused in 30 min). The [^{3}H]GABA and metabolites not retained or taken up by the tissue were washed out during the 1–2 hr that followed. During this process and throughout the rest of the perfusion, 10-μl aliquots from each collected fraction were counted in tritosol (*19*) to determine the resting and the evoked release of [^{3}H]GABA. The fraction of the tritiated material in the perfusates which was contributed by [^{3}H]GABA was determined by analysis of the samples in ion-exchange chromatography, followed by TLC (*51*). In spite of the fact that no inhibitor of GABA metabolism was added to the perfusing media 60% of the tracer released during the third hour of perfusion was GABA. This proportion was reduced to 30% after the sixth hour. When release was evoked by depolarization, the fraction of counts coeluting with GABA was more than 50% higher than that found in perfusates obtained during resting conditions. Since these ratios remained constant in the different experimental conditions presented in this work, release data were calculated from uncorrected total counts per minute in the perfusate fractions.

The release of endogenous immunoreactive enkephalin was determined by RIA. In addition to the Leu-enkephalin RIA that we have previously reported (*5, 7, 50*), two new assays have been developed. Glutaraldehyde conjugates of BSA-Met-enkephalin and BSA-Leu-enkephalin were purified by gel filtration and emulsified in complete Freund's adjuvant. Antisera were raised in rabbits during a 3-month immunization schedule. Either ^{125}I- or ^{3}H-labeled enkephalins were used as tracers and the free and bound enkephalins were separated with activated charcoal–dextran suspensions. When a final antiserum dilution of 1:1500 was used, the lowest detectable amounts of unlabeled enkephalins were 10–50 pg using ^{3}H-labeled tracers, and 2–5 pg using ^{125}I-labeled tracers. Leu-enkephalin cross-reacts 8% in the Met-enkephalin assay and Met-enkephalin cross-reacts 0.3% in the Leu-enkephalin assay; enkephalin fragments and endorphins cross-react less than 0.1% in the Met-enkephalin assay and less than 0.001% in the Leu-enkephalin assay. Both the Met- and the Leu-enkephalin assays have been validated with tissue samples. In order to facilitate the comparison of the results presented here with previous reports from our laboratory, we show only the data obtained with Leu-enkephalin RIAs; nevertheless, similar results were obtained using a Met-enkephalin assay. Since the Leu-enkephalin RIAs also read Met-enkephalin, an "enkephalin unit" has been defined: it is the enkephalin immunoreactive material that produces a displacement of tracer in the assay equal to that observed with 1 picogram of synthetic Leu-enkephalin (*50*). All perfusate samples were assayed at two dilutions and in duplicate.

III. FINDINGS

A. Optimization of Experimental Procedures

1. RELEASE OF PROTEIN, LACTATE DEHYDROGENASE, PROTEASES, ACETYLCHOLINESTERASE, [^{3}H]GABA, AND ENKEPHALINS AS BIOCHEMICAL MARKERS OF TISSUE VIABILITY DURING *IN VIVO* PUSH–PULL PERFUSION OF THE STRIATUM

In vivo push–pull perfusion techniques fall into the kinds of methods that conspicuously affect the subject under study. The need to assess the effect of perfusion on tissue viability has been fulfilled by using histological or electrophysiological controls of damage and functionality. However, it is often overlooked that biochemical markers released in the perfusate can give information on the tissue damage occurring during a perfusion session (*28*, *57*). Biochemical measurements also help to assess the functionality of the tissue during the course of a perfusion session, testing its capability for releasing exogenous and endogenous neurotransmitters. Thus, we have explored the suitability of several enzyme activities, total protein material, and representative peptide (enkephalin) and nonpeptide (GABA) transmitters as biochemical indicators of tissue damage and tissue responsiveness during *in vivo* perfusion of striatal regions. Gaddum and slot cannulae were indistinctly used in this part of the work.

We initially studied the release of two possible lesion markers during *in vivo* perfusion. Protein release into perfusates has been used earlier as a lesion marker (*57*). However, protein is always present and easily measured in perfusates because its normal level in the extracellular fluid of the nervous tissue is high (*26*). For this reason, only marked surges of protein content in perfusates have been used as indicators of tissue damage. LDH is a soluble cytoplasmic enzyme, also normally found in plasma, which is the most widely used marker of tissue damage both in biochemistry and in clinical medicine. Its level in perfusates is expected to increase as a consequence of cell lysis (by tissue erosion or by accidental mechanical damage) or after extravasation of serum (by edema or by rupture of capillaries). Figure 3 shows the release of LDH activity and total protein into perfusate fractions obtained during perfusion of the globus pallidus of the rat. Acute insertion of the cannula, disrupting the tissue, releases a high amount of LDH and protein into the perfusates. Mechanical damage by withdrawal and reinsertion of the cannula—intentionally produced just before terminating the perfusion session—induces an outflow of both putative lesion markers. Accidental lesions occurring during individual perfusions are also reflected in the release of these markers: bleeding episodes or flow obstructions leading to serious volume deficits (higher than 5% per collected fraction) invariably produce significant surges of LDH and protein in the perfusates. Four out of the ten animals perfused to compose Fig. 3 had severe flow obstructions during the second hour of perfusion (see fractions 5–8). These results indi-

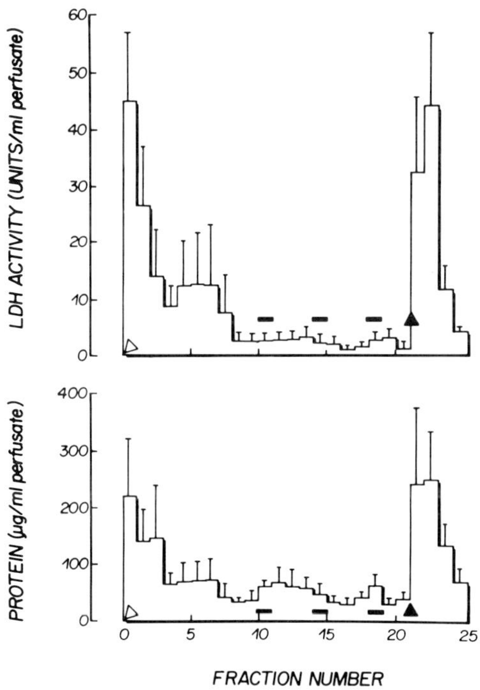

Fig. 3. Release of LDH activity and total protein during push–pull perfusion of the globus pallidus in freely moving rats. Insertion of the cannula is marked (▽) at the beginning of perfusion. In fractions 11, 15, and 18 (■), the perfusing medium contained 50 m*M* K^+. Close to the end of the perfusion session the cannula was removed and then reinserted in place in order to produce mechanical damage to the tissue (▲). The LDH assay (upper panel) and protein determination (lower panel) were as described in Section II. The bars represent the mean ± SEM of fractions collected in 10 perfusion sessions with different animals.

cate that tissue damage is marked by surges of protein and LDH. Moreover, about 10% of the surges of LDH and protein detected in individual perfusions occur in the absence of any obvious perfusion problems, suggesting that these biochemical markers are more sensitive in detecting tissue damage than physical observations—bleeding or volume deficits in perfusates.

However, increases in these markers produced by causes other than tissue lesions were not discarded a priori (*16*). Results in Fig. 3 already indicate that protein release, but not LDH release, is increased by chemical stimulation of the globus pallidus. Therefore, we compared the relase of proteins, LDH activity, and also of the putative lesion markers AChe and proteases, under conditions of chemical depolarization (50 m*M* K^+) and mechanical lesion. Proteolytic activity, mainly associated with lysosomes, and AChe activity, mostly membrane bound (but some soluble intracellularly and also present in blood), would also be expected to increase in perfusates after severe tissue disruption (*37*). Table I shows that high K^+ concentrations stimulate the release of protein both in the globus pallidus and in the caudate putamen of the rat and, only in the caudate, the release of AChe activity. Depolarization-induced release of LDH or protease activities was not observed. In contrast, mechanical damage elicited an increased release

TABLE I

Release of Enzyme Activities and Total Protein from Striatal Regions Evoked by Chemical Depolarization or by Mechanical Damage[a]

	Globus pallidus		Caudate putamen	
	Depolarization-induced release (% of control)	Mechanically induced release (% of control)	Depolarization-induced release (% of control)	Mechanically induced release (% of control)
LDH	105 ± 23	2010 ± 616	114 ± 16	1870 ± 720
Proteases	125 ± 25	216 ± 65	108 ± 19	156 ± 18
AChe	134 ± 14	284 ± 113	240 ± 60	660 ± 400
Protein	250 ± 62	1700 ± 580	275 ± 24	2500 ± 600

[a] Release was induced by depolarization with 50 m*M* K^+ in the perfusing medium or mechanically by withdrawal and reinsertion of the push–pull cannula. Data are expressed as % ± variation coefficient ($N = 4$) of the resting release values per milliliter of perfusate. In the globus pallidus these control values were: LDH, 6.5 ± 2.7 units; proteases, 12 ± 1 units; AChe, 2.6 ± 0.4 units, and protein, 30 ± 4 μg. In the caudate putamen resting values were: LDH, 16.0 ± 4.2 units; proteases, 12.5 ± 2.0 units; AChe, 5.0 ± 0.9 units, and protein, 60 ± 20 μg.

of all four markers in the caudate and in the pallidum. It is worth noting that the mechanically induced release was always higher than that evoked by depolarization.

The results presented here indicate that LDH activity and, less conspicuously, protease activity can be used as reliable markers of tissue damage during push–pull perfusion. This is not so for protein and AChe activity. Greenfield et al. (*22, 23*) had already shown that protein and AChe activity are released after chemical depolarization from the subtantia nigra and the caudate nucleus in the anesthetized cat. Our results confirm and extend these observations to the caudate-pallidal region in the freely moving rat. Although the origin of these proteins released from the brain by chemical stimulation is not yet clear, preliminary experiments (Oksenberg *et al.*, in preparation) indicate that at least some of them can be synthesized from labeled precursors injected in the striatum. Thus, these substances, first proposed as lesion markers, have become the subjects of neurobiological inquiries regarding their possible roles in neurochemical signaling.

The ability to detect tissue damage occurring during *in vivo* perfusions is not enough for validating the use of a particular perfusion system; tests of the functionality of the preparation during perfusion are required to assess the value of these techniques. The ability of the tissue to release chemical transmitters can be used for this purpose. Figure 4 shows the resting and the stimulated *in vivo* release of [^{3}H]GABA and endogenous enkephalins, the two transmitters known to be most abundant in the globus pallidus of the rat (*21, 58*). As described in Section II, after a washout period the release of tritiated GABA was evoked by high K^+ concentrations in the perfusing medium, repeated stimulations releasing lower amounts of tracer (Fig. 4, upper panel). This decrease can be related to the metabolism of [^{3}H]GABA and its exhaustion in the tissue pools (see Section II) and does not reflect progressive tissue damage. This conclusion is supported by the observation that a stable evoked release of endogenous enkephalin is observed after repeated stimulation (Fig. 4, lower panel) during perfusion sessions similar to those shown for GABA. This stability of the enkephalin-releasing systems during an *in vivo* perfusion session is particularly significant considering that earlier studies showed that enkephalin tissue stores in the pallidum are particularly labile to tissue damage. Thus, slicing of pallidal tissue decreases its enkephalin content by 30% (*5*). Also, enkephalin release *in vivo* is markedly reduced by the gliosis produced in animals that have been previously perfused in this region (*5, 7*). In our experiments the release of enkephalin and GABA in response to chemical stimulation was always blocked after severe mechanical damage to the tissue; partial recovery was seldom observed. Thus, changes in the release of endogenous enkephalin from the

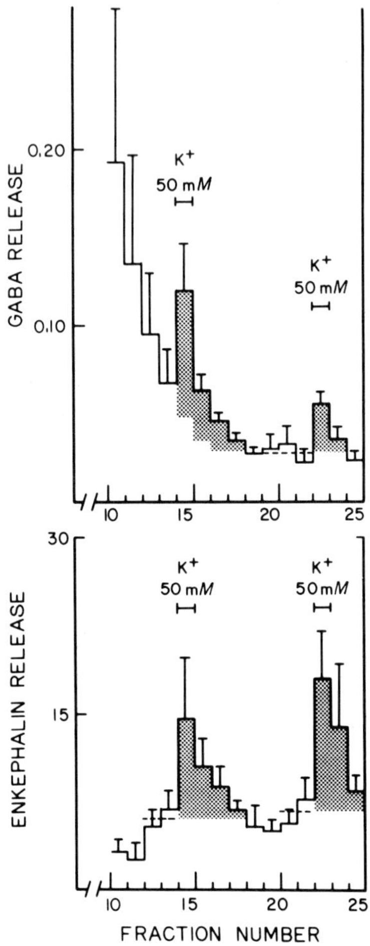

Fig. 4. Resting and stimulated release of [^{3}H]GABA and endogenous enkephalin during *in vivo* push–pull perfusion of the globus pallidus of the rat. Upper panel: After insertion of the cannula, perfusions were started using the standard perfusing medium. For studying the release of exogenous GABA, [^{3}H]GABA was added to the perfusing medium and circulated through the tissue within the first 30 min of the experiment. The profile of [^{3}H]GABA released in the perfusate fractions is expressed as the percentage of the [^{3}H]GABA uptake. The initial exponential washout phase is followed by a steady resting-release process [horizontal dashed line; see Kondo and Iwatsuro (*33*) for the calculation of this baseline]. [^{3}H]GABA release (shaded areas) was stimulated depolarizing the tissue with perfusing medium containing 50 m*M* K^+. Lower panel: For studying the release of endogenous enkephalin the fractions were processed, as described in Section II, for a Leu-enkephalin RIA, the results being expressed in enkephalin units (see Section II). Since the resting release of endogenous enkephalin varies during perfusion, in order to determine the enkephalin release stimulated by 50 m*M* K^+ (shaded areas), prestimulation values were defined as the average enkephalin content of the two collections preceding the stimulation (dashed lines). Values in this figure are the average ± SEM of fractions collected in 6 perfusion sessions performed from 4:30 P.M. to 10:30 P.M.

globus pallidus appear to be a suitable indicator of changes in the functionality and responsiveness of the region during perfusion. Exogenous GABA will be used as a secondary marker and as a control for the sampling efficiency of a probe.

2. COMPARISON OF THE PERFORMANCE OF THE GADDUM AND THE SLOT CANNULAE DURING *IN VIVO* PERFUSION

In order to evaluate the advantages or disadvantages of the modification of the tip of the push–pull cannula (described in Section II) compared to the traditional design, we have first analyzed the frequency of flow obstructions and vascular accidents observed during perfusions using these probes. Table II shows that with use of the modified slot model the bleeding episodes are reduced to those that occasionally, but almost unavoidably occur after the acute insertion of the cannulae; flow obstructions are also seen less frequently when using the slot cannula. Surges of LDH and protein were always associated with insertions and flow obstructions. However, the possibility was considered that this improvement in the hydrodynamics of *in vivo* perfusion could be due to a short circuit of the circulating fluid inside the tip of the slot cannula (see Fig. 2). Since this would produce an undesirable reduction of contact and diffusion between the tissue and the medium, we compared the efficiency of the slot and of the Gaddum cannula for sampling a tissue marker during perfusion. The protein present in perfusates obtained under resting conditions mostly represents a sampling of extracellular fluid. Perfusions were no indication that tissue damage was present—bleeding, volume deficits, or LDH surges—in these experiments. Figure 5 shows that no significant difference exists in the basal levels of protein in perfusates obtained using either one of these probes. This observation shows that the possible flow shunt previously mentioned, if present, does

TABLE II

Comparison of the Performance of the Gaddum and the Slot Cannulae:
Frequency of Accidents during Perfusion[a]

	Bleeding episodes	Flow obstructions requiring cannula withdrawal
Gaddum	4 in 6 perfusions (2 on cannula insertion, 2 during perfusion)	5 in 6 perfusions
Slot	1 in 6 perfusions (on cannula insertion)	1 in 6 perfusions

[a] Results from a series of 12 6-hr perfusion sessions carried out to compare the Gaddum and slot cannulae. All bleeding episodes and severe flow obstructions are accompanied by increases in protein and LDH content in the corresponding perfusate fractions (see text).

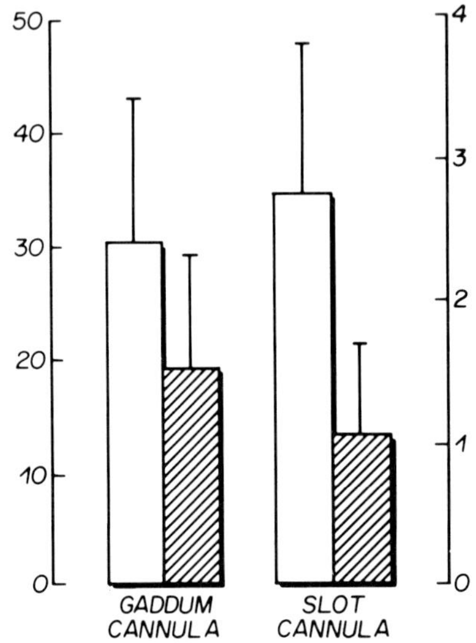

Fig. 5. Resting release of protein and LDH during perfusions using the Gaddum or the slot cannula designs. The values shown were obtained in 6 perfusion sessions (the vertical lines represent the SEM). (□), Resting content of protein in perfusates (μg/ml); (▨), resting activity of LDH in perfusates (units/ml).

not affect the efficiency of the slot cannula. In addition, the efficiency of both probes to deliver solutes into the perfused tissue was shown to be similar, since GABA uptake was about 30% using either cannula (data not shown).

Systems using the slot or the Gaddum cannulae were also compared in relation to the damage and to the viability of the tissue in the absence of perfusion accidents. LDH was used as the lesion marker. Figure 5 shows that the average basal LDH activities in perfusates obtained with the Gaddum cannula are not significantly different from those obtained using the slot design. The functionality of the tissues during perfusion with either one of these two probes was compared using the release of neurotransmitters as the index; also, only perfusion sessions where no major accidental damage occurred were used for this purpose. Figure 6 shows that the stimulated release and also the resting release of GABA and enkephalin were similar with the Gaddum and the slot cannulae after 5 hr of perfusion. Thus, in spite of the marked differences in the frequency of accidental lesions observed during perfusion with these two probes, the damage steadily produced during the perfusion, in the absence of accidents, was relatively small or limited to certain tissue elements so that quantitative differences in the functional parameters we measured cannot be detected. This is in contrast with the effects of more extensive lesions produced by perfusion accidents which, as indicated before, impaired release processes. In summary, the slot cannula reduces the incidence of vascular accidents and flow occlusions occurring during a perfusion session, keeping the same tissue sampling efficiency of the traditional design. Consequently, the number of successful perfusion sessions is considerably increased. These improvements allowed us to carry out long perfusion sessions needed for the studies of biological rhythms which we later present.

B. Neurobiological Applications

1. *IN VIVO* RELEASE OF ENKEPHALIN FROM THE GLOBUS PALLIDUS; RELATIONSHIP TO GABA-RELEASING SYSTEMS

The search for a model system to study the neurobiology of the enkephalins in the central nervous system (*29*) has led researchers to the striatum, which has one of the highest enkephalin concentrations in the brain (*27, 58*) and is also one of the few macroscopic regions of the brain where the chemically related endorphin systems are not present (*2, 3, 9*). Additionally, within the striatum, enkephalin perikarya and fibers are segregated: the globus pallidus is rich in fibers and terminals and all cell bodies are found in the caudo-putamen nucleus (*4, 15*). These advantages are exploited only in part when studying the release of enkephalin from the pallidum *in vitro* (*1*); the use of an *in vivo* preparation to study the charac-

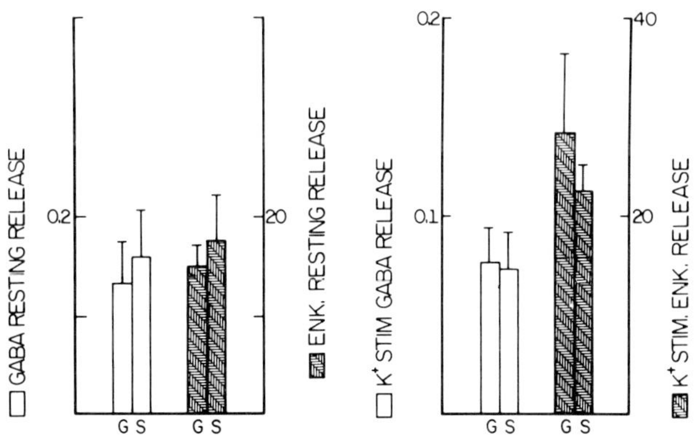

Fig. 6. Resting and stimulated release of exogenous GABA and endogenous enkephalin using the Gaddum (G) and slot (S) cannulae. In experiments to study $[^3H]$GABA release its uptake was also measured: with perfusion of 3.5×10^6 cpm of tritiated GABA the fraction remaining in the tissue after the washout period was 28 ± 5% with the Gaddum cannula and 29 ± 6% with the slot cannula. Results are the average of 6 experiments (± SEM).

teristics of enkephalin release takes advantage of the high density and anatomical segregation of enkephalin-containing terminals in the pallidum, while the integrity of pallidal connections with other brain regions is preserved. Previous studies have demonstrated that endogenous immunoreactive enkephalin is released *in vivo* from the globus pallidus; this release is calcium dependent and is enhanced during local or caudate nucleus stimulation (*5, 7, 13*) (see also Fig. 4, lower panel).

In order to understand the physiological mechanisms regulating the *in vivo* release of enkephalin in this model system, we have first studied the effects of putative transmitters present in the pallidum on the release of enkephalins. Since the globus pallidus is one of the brain region's richest in glutamate decarboxylase (*21*), we investigated the relationship between the GABA-containing system and the release of enkephalin in this area. Experiments were initially carried out in the globus pallidus of the cat because perfusion procedures are facilitated in larger species (*6*). Our present results have extended these studies to the rat, where neurochemical data are more abundant.

Figure 7 shows the effects of GABA and of the GABA-receptor antagonist picrotoxin on the pallidal release of enkephalin. The addition of GABA ($10^{-4}M$) to the perfusing medium did not produce a measurable change in the resting enkephalin release (Fig. 7a), although it significantly inhibited the release stimulated by veratrine (Fig. 7b). In contrast, picrotoxin ($5 \times 10^{-4}M$) had marked effects, increasing about threefold the resting release of enkephalin, both in the presence and in the absence of exogenous GABA (Fig. 7b and a, respectively). This effect of picrotoxin alone suggests that an endogenous GABAergic input tonically inhibits the *in vivo* release of enkephalin from the pallidum. Although in the experiment shown GABA ($10^{-4}M$) could not inhibit the effect of picrotoxin ($5 \times 10^{-4}\,M$), the increase in enkephalin release produced by lower concentrations of picrotoxin was blocked by millimolar concentrations of exogenous GABA, indicating that the picrotoxin effect is mediated by GABA receptors. In spite of the fact that these GABA receptor-mediated effects are initiated in the pallidum, the circuitry involved in regulating enkephalin release cannot be defined on this basis. However, since only enkephalin terminals, not cell bodies, are present in the pallidum, and this region is profusely innervated with glutamate decarboxylase-containing terminals (*48*), the simplest mechanism to explain this tonic inhibition is a presynaptic control of enkephalin release by GABA.

An inhibitory effect of GABA on enkephalin release had been previously shown using striatal slices (*25*). In this *in vitro* preparation, which includes the pallidal region, GABA inhibits the K^+-stimulated but not the resting release of enkephalin. Although this effect was blocked by picrotoxin, the

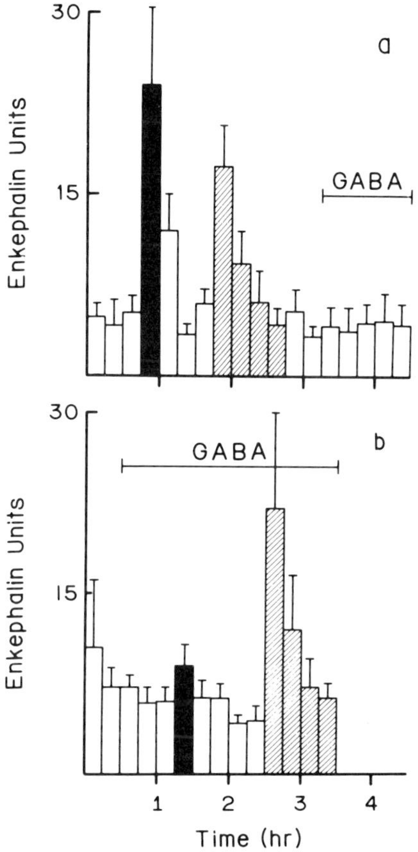

Fig. 7. Effect of GABA and picrotoxin on endogenous enkephalin release from the globus pallidus. Perfusions were conducted as described before but veratrine (60 μg/ml) was used as the depolarizing agent to stimulate the release of enkephalin (black bars). Exogenous GABA (10^{-4} *M*) added to the perfusing media is indicated by the horizontal lines. Picrotoxin (5×10^{-4} *M*) was present in the fractions represented by dashed bars. Results in each panel are the average ± SEM of 4 perfusions.

latter had no effect by itself. This finding would be in accordance with our proposition if the tonic GABA inhibition on enkephalin release would not be present *in vitro*. In this respect it is worth noting that the leakage of enkephalin observed in slices of globus pallidus is not observed *in vivo* (*1, 5, 7*). *In vivo* perfusion studies on the regulation of enkephalin release in the striatal regions of the anesthetized cat (*11*) have also shown an inhibition by GABA of pallidal release of enkephalin. However, in these experiments biphasic effects were observed with GABA, muscimol, diazepam, and the antagonist picrotoxin: their initial effect was inhibitory but a rebound release of enkephalin was observed after they were removed from the perfusion medium. We were not able to observe these biphasic drug effects in the freely moving rat; however, it is possible that the higher concentrations of GABA and picrotoxin we used—similar to those employed for the *in vitro* studies—revealed only in part the complexity of the effects of these drugs.

2. DIURNAL RHYTHM OF ENKEPHALIN *IN VIVO* RELEASE FROM THE GLOBUS PALLIDUS

Circadian rhythms and other periodic changes of the systems that produce or recognize endogenous opiates have already been documented (*12, 18, 35, 36, 42, 46, 54, 56*). Some of the early failures to observe circadian changes in opiate peptides were due to very restricted sampling schedules (*14, 55*). Since many of these opiate rhythms have already been linked to physiological, endocrinological, or behavioral changes, the search for oscillations of opiate-mediated communication in well-defined neural systems promises to shed some light on their functional roles.

In the course of our investigations on the regulation of the *in vivo* release of enkephalin from the globus pallidus of the rat it was observed that this release was consistently higher in the late afternoon and evening than in the morning hours. The analysis of resting enkephalin release levels at selected time intervals during morning and evening perfusion sessions showed a clear diurnal oscillation, the lowest levels being observed after noontime and increasing thereafter through the late evening hours (Fig. 8). Given the link previously established between the GABA and the enkephalin systems in the pallidum, we decided to study and compare possible diurnal variations in the *in vivo* release of these messengers in this region (*8*). The experimental protocols for *in vivo* perfusion were as those used in Fig. 4. Six perfusion sessions were carried out from 8:00 A.M. to 2:30 P.M. (daytime perfusions) and six from 4:00 P.M. TO 10:30 P.M. (evening perfusions). Resting enkephalin release increased 100% between 2:00 P.M. and 10:00 P.M., while [^{3}H]GABA resting release decreased by 60% (Fig. 9). This change in GABA resting release was not due to diurnal differences in uptake (Fig. 9). The release of [^{3}H]GABA and enkephalin was also studied under depolarizing conditions (Fig. 10). The diurnal differences, already observed during resting release, were more marked after stimulation: between daytime and evening perfusions the K^+-stimulated enkephalin release increased 6-fold while the K^+-stimulated [^{3}H]GABA release decreased more than 10-fold.

Other possible causes for these changes in transmitter release were considered early in this work and precautions were taken to follow the same

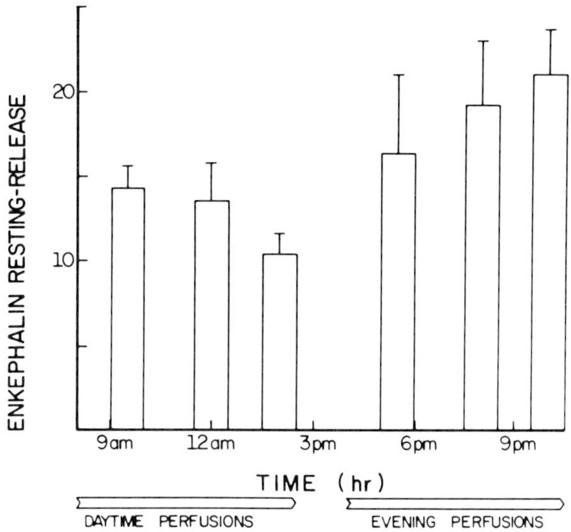

Fig. 8. *In vivo* resting enkephalin release from the rat globus pallidus during the course of daytime and evening perfusion sessions. Six perfusion sessions were carried out from 8:00 A.M. to 2:30 P.M. (daytime) and 6 from 4:00 P.M. to 10:30 P.M. (evening). In each perfusion the average resting release of enkephalin was determined at times close to the beginning, the middle, and the end of the session. Each value is the mean (± SEM) of the enkephalin contents in perfusate fractions collected during 1 hr. The resting enkephalin release values observed at the end of the daytime perfusions and at the end of the evening perfusions were significantly different ($p < .05$).

experimental procedures during morning and evening sessions. Since Cesselin *et al.* (*13*) reported that the enkephalin content and release in the globus pallidus of the cat was higher in the anterior portion than in the caudal part of this structure, the possibility that differences in the implantation sites of rats perfused in the morning or in the evening could simulate a rhythm was analyzed. Our results indicated that there was no correlation between enkephalin or [^{3}H]GABA release and the localization of the cannula tracks or the perfusion sites within the pallidum. The steady decrease in [^{3}H]GABA release observed during the course of a perfusion session (see Section III, A) was also considered when analyzing the perfusion data. Therefore, the comparison of resting and stimulated GABA release between morning and evening perfusions was made using perfusate fractions obtained with the same delay after the infusion of [^{3}H]GABA. Also, it was found that the uptake of [^{3}H]GABA (Fig. 9) and the fraction of radioactive tracer in the perfusates contributed by [^{3}H]GABA (see Section II) were not different in the morning and evening sessions, and therefore do not account

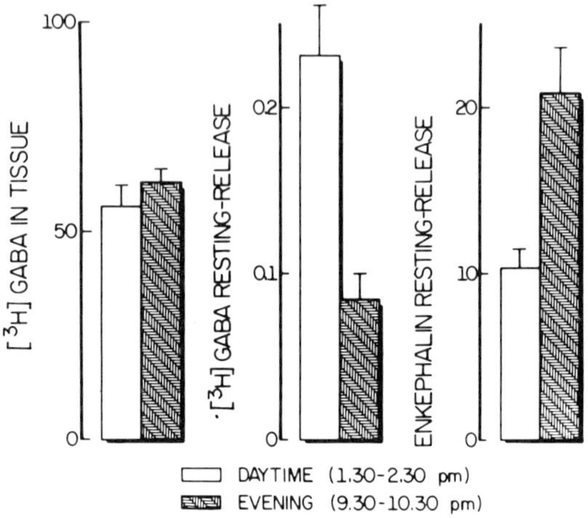

Fig. 9. Resting release of endogenous enkephalin and [3H]GABA between daytime and evening hours. The [3H] GABA uptake was similar between these hours (left panel). GABA release decreased significantly ($p < .05$) between 2:00 P.M. and 10:00 P.M. (center panel). The enkephalin release between these times showed an opposite, statistically significant difference (right panel, $p < .05$). Resting GABA and enkephalin release are defined as indicated in Fig. 4. Values are the average ± SEM of 6 experiments.

for the rhythm observed. Nevertheless, it must be noted that since the GABA we measured is exogenous, the anatomical structures and the mechanisms involved in its release may differ from those participating in the release of endogenous GABA (*32, 33, 53*).

The diurnal rhythm observed in the release of enkephalin from the nerve terminals in the pallidum is not due to changes in the pallidal or caudate enkephalin content. Wesche and Frederickson (*56*) reported that in heat-stressed mice, but not in normal controls, the enkephalin levels, specifically in the globus pallidus, increased from 7:30 A.M. to 3:30 P.M. In our experiments the levels of enkephalin in the globus pallidus and in the caudate ($5 \pm 1 \times 10^3$ units and $2 \pm 0.2 \times 10^3$ units, respectively) were not significantly different at 8 A.M., 2 P.M. or 10 P.M., the lowest and highest points observed in the rhythm.

The diurnal rhythms in the release of enkephalin and GABA follow opposite patterns, suggesting the possibility of reciprocal controlling mechanisms. We have already presented evidence for the existence of an inhibitory GABAergic mechanism upon the release of enkephalin from the pallidum. No evidence is available of an influence of opiates on the GABA systems in this region. However, the complexity of the multiple opiate–GABA interactions in the striatum is already being documented. Moroni *et al.* (*39, 40*) have shown that an increased turnover of GABA is observed in the pallidum after the administration of opiates in the caudate. This effect appears to be due to an opiate-mediated inhibition of striatal GABAergic neurons, which in turn activate GABA neurons in the caudo-pallidal pathway. Clearly, the efforts to understand the mechanisms of the oscillation of GABA and enkephalin release in the pallidum will have to go beyond the pallidal circuitry.

In relation to the functional role of these opposed diurnal rhythms of enkephalin and GABA release it is noteworthy that their actions in the globus pallidus also have opposite effects on the motor activity of the rat: bilateral injection of enkephalin analogs in the pallidum leads to hyperactivity, an action which is blocked by naloxone (*31*). In contrast, bilateral administration in the pallidum of drugs promoting GABAergic transmission produces akinesia and catalepsy, while the opposite is observed with drugs antagonizing this transmitter (*47, 52*). The increased enkephalin release and the decreased GABA release at night hours in the pallidum would lead to hyperactivity. Since the rat is a nightly active animal we suggest that the enkephalin-GABA transmission in the pallidum may be an important link in the neural control of the diurnal rhythms of motor activity in the rat.

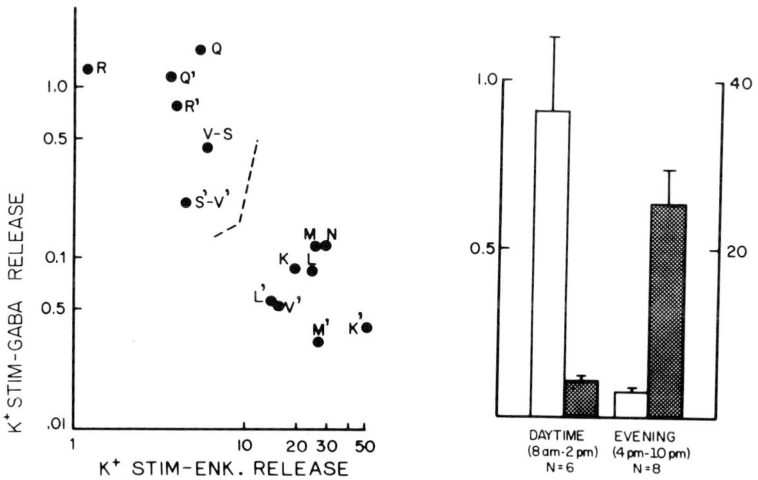

Fig. 10. K+-stimulated release of exogenous GABA and endogenous enkephalin from the globus pallidus in daytime and evening perfusion sessions. Left panel: Release values of these transmitters obtained in parallel are plotted in log-enkephalin vs log-GABA scales. Points above and to the left of the dashed lines correspond to individual data obtained from morning perfusions; points below and to the right of this line come from evening perfusions. Right panel: The same data are compared (in a linear scale) showing that the K+-stimulated GABA release (□) decreased 10-fold, while the enkephalin release ▩ increased 6-fold between the morning and the evening hours. Values are expressed as the mean ± SEM.

IV. PERSPECTIVES

Although recent developments allow the *in vivo* and *in situ* measurement of a gamut of substances in the brain, the stereochemical complexity of proteins and of most peptides demands highly specific and sensitive analysis, best performed in the assay tube. Furthermore, the enzymatic or biological activity of neural proteins can only be analyzed after these substances have been isolated from the brain. Although *in vivo* perfusion methods would have an important role in the future development of neurochemistry solely on this basis, the permanent need for these methods resides in their use within an old strategic approach: the identification of unknown substances released from the brain under physiological conditions. Some of the work presented here points in that direction.

ACKNOWLEDGMENTS

The authors are grateful to Dr. W. J. Shoemaker and Mrs. R. Azad-Fryer from the A. V. Davis Center of the Salk Institute for the preliminary tests of our anti-enkephalin sera. Synthetic enkephalins were a generous gift from Dr. N. Ling.

This work was supported in part by grants from CONACyT, México, Instituto Mexicano de Psiquiatría and Fondo de Estudios e Investigaciones, R. J. Zebada.

REFERENCES

1. Bayón, A., Rossier, J., Mauss, A., Bloom, F. E., Iversen, L. L., Ling, N., and Guillemin, R. *In vitro* release of methionine-enkephalin and leucine-enkephalin from the rat globus pallidus, *Proc. Natl. Acad. Sci. U.S.A.* **75** (1978) 3503–3506.
2. Bayón, A., Shoemaker, W. J., Bloom, F. E., Mauss, A., and Guillemin, R. Perinatal development of the endorphin and the enkephalin-containing systems in the rat brain. *Brain Res.* **179** (1979) 93–101.
3. Bayón, A., Koda, L., Battenberg, E., Azad, R., Guillemin, R., and Bloom, F. E. Regional distribution of endorphin, methionine-enkephalin and leucine-enkephalin in the pigeon brain. *Neurosci. Lett.* **16** (1980) 75–80.
4. Bayón, A., Koda, L., Battenberg, E., and Bloom, F. E. Redistribution of endorphin and enkephalin immunoreactivity in the rat brain and pituitary after *in vivo* treatment with colchicine or cytochalasin B. *Brain Res.* **183** (1980) 103–111.
5. Bayón, A., Drucker-Colín, R., Lugo, L., Shoemaker, W. J., Azad, R., and Bloom, F. E. Enkephalin release from the globus pallidus: *In vitro* and *in vivo* studies. *In* "Regulatory Mechanisms of Synaptic Transmission," (R. Tapia and W. Cotman, eds.), 1981, pp 29–41. Plenum, New York.
6. Bayón, A., Drucker-Colín, R., Lugo, L., Shoemaker, W. J., Azad, R., and Bloom, F. E. *In vivo* release of enkephalin from the globus pallidus is tonically inhibited by endogenous GABA. *Soc. Neurosci. Abstr.* **7** (1981) 800.

7. Bayón, A., Shoemaker, W. J., Lugo, L., Azad, R., Ling, N., Drucker-Colín, R., and Bloom, F. E. *In vivo* release of enkephalin from the globus pallidus. *Neurosci. Lett.* **24** (1981) 65–70.
8. Bayón, A., Anton, B., and Díaz-Pontones, D. *In vivo* enkephalin release from the globus pallidus of the rat; diurnal rhythm and relationship with GABA-releasing systems. *Soc. Neurosci. Abstr.* **9** (1983) 588.
9. Bloom, F., Battenberg, E., Rossier, J., Ling, N., and Guillemin, R. Neurons containing β-endorphin in rat brain exist separately from those containing enkephalin: immunocytochemical studies. *Proc. Natl. Acad. Sci. U.S.A.* **75** (1978) 1591–1595.
10. Bergmeyer, H. U. "Methods of Enzymatic Analysis" (2nd edition), Vol. 2, 1974, pp. 574–579. Academic Press, New York.
11. Bourgoin, S., Cesselin, F., Artaud, F., Glowinski, J., and Hamon, M. *In vivo* modulation by GABA-related drugs of Met-enkephalin release in basal ganglia of the cat brain. *Brain Res.* **248** (1982) 321–330.
12. Campos, A. E., Luján, M., López, E., Figueroa-Hernández, J. L., and Rodríguez, R., Circadian variation in the lethal effect of morphine in the mouse. *Proc. West. Pharmacol. Soc.* **26** (1983) 101–103.
13. Cesselin, F., Soubrie, P., Bourgoin, S., Artaud, F., Reisine, T. D., Michelot, R., Glowinski, J., and Hamon, M. *In vivo* release of Met-enkephalin in the cat brain. *Neuroscience* **6** (1981) 301–313.
14. Childers, S. R., and Snyder, S. H. Diurnal variation, post-mortem degradation and effect of cycloheximide. *In* "Endorphins in Mental Health Research," (E. Usdin, W. E. Bunney, and N. S. Kline, eds.), 1979, pp. 181–188. Macmillan, London.
15. Cuello, A. C., and Paxinos, S. G. Evidence for a long Leu^5-enkephalin strio-pallidal pathway in rat brain. *Nature (London)* **271** (1978) 178–180.
16. Drucker-Colín, R. Endogenous sleep peptides. *In* "Psychopharmacology of Sleep," (D. Wheatley, ed.), 1981, pp. 53–72. Raven, New York.
17. Ellman, G. L., Courtney, K. D., Andres, V., and Featherstone, R. M. A new and rapid colorimetric determination of acetylcholinesterase activity. *Biochem. Pharmacol.* **7** (1961) 88–95.
18. Frederickson, R. C. A., Burgis, V., and Edwards, J. Hyperalgesia induced by naloxone follows diurnal rhythm in responsivity to painful stimuli. *Science* **198** (1977) 756–758.
19. Fricke, U. Tritosol: a new scintillation cocktail based on Triton-X-100. *Anal. Biochem.* **63** (1975) 555–558.
20. Gaddum, J. H. Push–pull cannulae. *J. Physiol. (London)* **155** (1961) 1–2.
21. Gottesfeld, Z., and Jacobowitz, D. M. Neurochemical and anatomical studies of GABAergic neurons. *In* "Interactions between Putative Neurotransmitters in the Brain," (S. Garattini, J. Pujol, and R. Samanin, eds.), 1978, pp. 109–126. Raven, New York.
22. Greenfield, S., Cheramy, A., Leviel, V., and Glowinski, J. *In vivo* release of acetylcholinesterase in the cat substantiae nigrae and caudate nuclei. *Nature (London)* **284** (1980) 355–357.
23. Greenfield, S., Cheramy, A., and Glowinski, J. Evoked release of proteins from central neurons *in vivo*. *J. Neurochem.* **40** (1983) 1048–1057.
24. Hamberger, A., Berthold, C.-H., Jacobson, I., Karlsson, B., Lehmann, A., Nyström, B., and Sandberg, M. *In vivo* brain dialysis of extracellular nontransmitter and putative transmitter amino acids. This volume, Chapter 8.
25. Herz, A., Duka, T., Gramsch, C., Höllt, V., Osborne, H., Przewlocki, R., Schultz, R., and Wüster, M. Pharmacologic manipulation of brain and pituitary endorphin content and release. *In* "Neural Peptides and Neuronal Communication," (E. Costa and M. Trabucci, eds.), 1980, pp. 323–333. Raven, New York.

26. Hofstein, R., Hesse, G., and Shashoua, V. E. Proteins of the extracellular fluid of mouse brain: extraction and partial characterization. *J. Neurochem.* **40** (1983) 1448–1455.
27. Hökfelt, T., Elde, R., Johansson, O., Terenius, L. and Stein, L. The distribution of enkephalin immunoreactive cell bodies in the rat central nervous system. *Neurosci. Lett.* **5** (1977) 25–31.
28. Honchar, M. P., Hartman, B. K., and Sharpe, L. G. Evaluation of *in vivo* brain site perfusion with the push–pull cannula. *Am. J. Physiol.* **236** (1979) R45–56.
29. Hughes, J., Smith, T. W., Kosterlitz, H. W., Fothergill, L. H., Morgan, B. A., and Morris, H. Identification of two related pentapeptides from the brain with potent opiate agonist activity. *Nature (London)* **255** (1975) 577–579.
30. Iijima, T., and Nunoki, K. Superfusion and electrical stimulation of the canine brain with a push–pull cannula. This volume, Chapter 4.
31. Joyce, E. M., Koob, G. F., Strecker, R., Iversen, S. D., and Bloom, F. E. The behavioural effects of enkephalin analogs injected into the ventral tegmental area and globus pallidus. *Brain Res.* **221** (1981) 359–370.
32. Kemel, M. L., Gauchi, C., Glowinski, J., and Besson, M. J. Spontaneous and potassium evoked release of ^{3}H-GABA newly synthesized from ^{3}H-glutamine in slices of the rat substantia nigra. *Life Sci.* **24** (1979) 2139–2150.
33. Kondo, Y., and Iwatsuro, K. Increased release of preloaded (^{3}H)GABA from substantia nigra *in vivo* following stimulation of caudate nucleus and globus pallidus. *Brain Res.* **154** (1978) 395–400.
34. Konig, J. F. R., and Klippel, R. A. "The Rat Brain," 1967, 162 pp. Krieger, New York.
35. Kumar, M. S. A., Chen, C. L., and Muther, T. F. Changes in pituitary and hypothalamic content of Met-enkephalin during the estrous cycle of rats. *Life Sci.* **25** (1979) 1687–1696.
36. Kumar, M. S. A., Chen, C. L., Sharp, D. C., Liu, J. M., Kalra, P. S., and Kaira, S. R. Diurnal fluctuation in methionine-enkephalin levels in the hypothalamus and preptic area of the male rat: effects of pinealectomy. *Neuroendocrinology* **35** (1982) 28–31.
37. Lajtha, A. H. "Handbook of Neurochemistry" (2nd edition), Vol. 4, Enzymes in the Nervous System. 1983, 549 pp. Plenum, New York.
38. Lowry, O. H., Rosebrough, N. J., Farr, A. L., and Randall, R. J. Protein measurement with the folin-phenol reagent. *J. Biol. Chem.* **193** (1951) 265–275.
39. Moroni, F., Cheney, D. L., Peralta, E., and Costa, E. Opiate receptor agonists as modulators of γ-amino butyric acid turnover in the nucleus caudatus, globus pallidus and substantia nigra of the rat. *J. Pharmacol. Exp. Ther.* **207** (1978) 870–877.
40. Moroni, F., Peralta, E., Cheney, D. L., and Costa, E. On the regulation of γ-aminobutyric acid neurons in caudatus, pallidus and nigra: effects of opioids and dopamine agonists. *J. Pharmacol. Exp. Ther.* **208** (1979) 190–194.
41. Myers, R. D. An improved push–pull cannula system for perfusing an isolated region of the brain. *Physiol. Behav.* **5** (1970) 243–246.
42. Naber, D., Cohen, R. M., Picker, D. X., Kline, W. H., Davis, G., Pert, C. B., and Bunney, W. E., Jr. Episodic secretion of opioid activity in human plasma and monkey CSF: evidence for a diurnal rhythm. *Life Sci.* **28** (1981) 931–935.
43. Neouillon, A., Cheramy, A., and Glowinski, J. An adaptation of the push–pull cannula method to study the *in vivo* release of (^{3}H)dopamine synthesized from (^{3}H)tyrosine in cat caudate nucleus: effect of various physical and pharmacological treatments. *J. Neurochem.* **28** (1977) 819–828.
44. Philippu, A. The use of push–pull cannulae for superfusing various hypothalamic areas in anesthetized and conscious freely moving animals. This volume, Chapter 13.
45. Philippu, A., Przuntek, H., and Roensberg, W. Superfusion of the hypothalamus with

gamma-aminobutyric acid: effect on the release of noradrenaline and blood pressure. *Naunyn-Schmiedeberg's Arch. Pharmacol.* **276** (1973) 103–118.

46. Przewlocki, R., Lason, W., Konecka, A. M., Gramsch, C., Herz, A., and Reid, L. D. The opioid peptide dynorphin, circadian rhythms and starvation. *Science* **219** (1983) 71–73.
47. Pycock, C., Horton, R. W., and Marsden, C. D. The behavioural effects of manipulating GABA function in the globus pallidus. *Brain Res.* **116** (1976) 353–359.
48. Ribak, C. E. The GABAergic neurons of the extrapyramidal system as revealed by immunocytochemistry. *In* "GABA and the Basal Ganglia," (G. DiChiara and G. L. Gessa, eds.), 1981, pp. 23–36. Raven, New York.
49. Rinderknecht, H., Geokas, M. C., Silverman, P., and Haverback, B. J. A new ultrasensitive method for the determination of proteolytic activity. *Clin. Chim. Acta* **21** (1968) 197–203.
50. Rossier, J., Bayón, A., Vargo, T. M., Ling, N., Guillemin, R., and Bloom, F. E. Radioimmunoassay of brain peptides: evaluation of a methodology for the assay of β-endorphin and enkephalin. *Life Sci.* **21** (1977) 847–852.
51. Sandoval, M. E., Torner, C. A., and Medrano, L. High affinity uptake and Ca^{2+}-dependent release of glutamic acid in the developing cerebellum. *Neuroscience* **11** (1984) 867–875.
52. Scheel-Krüger, J., Magelund, G., and Olianas, M. C. Role of GABA in the striatal output system: globus pallidus, nucleus entopeduncularis, substantia nigra and nucleus subthalamicus. *In* "GABA and the Basal Ganglia," (G. DiChiara and G. L. Gessa, eds.), 1981, pp. 165–186. Raven, New York.
53. van der Heyden, J. A. M., Venema, K., and Korf, J. *In vivo* release of endogenous γ-aminobutyric acid from rat striatum: effects of muscimol, oxotremorine and morphine. *J. Neurochem.* **34** (1980) 1648–1653.
54. von Knorring, L., Almay, B. G. L., Johansson, F., Terenius, L., and Wahlstrom, A. Circannual variation in concentrations of endorphins in cerebrospinal fluid. *Pain* **12** (1982) 265–272.
55. Wesche, D. L., and Frederickson, R. C. A. Diurnal differences in opioid peptide levels correlated with nociceptive sensitivity. *Life Sci.* **24** (1979) 1861–1868.
56. Wesche, D. L., and Frederickson, R. C. A. Diurnal rhythm in response to noxious stimuli—increase of Met-enkephalin in globus pallidus. *In* "Advances in Endogenous and Exogenous Opioids" (Proc. Int. Narcotic Res. Conf.), 1981, pp. 232–234. Kodansha, Tokyo.
57. Yaksh, T. L., and Yamamura, H. I. Factors affecting performance of the push–pull cannula in brain. *J. Appl. Physiol.* **37** (1974) 428–434.
58. Yang, H.-Y., Hong, J. S., and Costa, E. Regional distribution of Leu- and Met-enkephalin in the rat brain. *Neuropharmacology* **16** (1977) 303–307.

7

Use of Dialytrodes in Brain Neurochemistry

JOSÉ M. R. DELGADO, JUAN LERMA, RAFAEL MARTÍN DEL RÍO, AND JOSÉ M. SOLÍS

Departamento de Investigación
Centro Ramón y Cajal
Madrid, Spain

I. INTRODUCTION

The study of local neurochemical events is essential for the understanding of epileptic phenomena, kindling, behavioral activities, and other basic aspects of brain functions. For many years our group has been interested in these problems (*1, 5, 6, 10, 11, 24, 38*) and has tried to develop suitable technologies for long-term investigation of the regional neurochemistry of the awake brain (*4, 7, 9, 33*).

Establishment of correlations between regional chemistry of the unanesthetized brain and general behavioral expression has attracted the interest of many investigators and the concept of neurohumoral coding of brain functions is well established (*29*). This coding may be related to ag-

IN VIVO PERFUSION AND RELEASE
OF NEUROACTIVE SUBSTANCES

ISBN 0-12-083350-6

gressive behavior (*32, 36*), brain excitability (*34*), motor conditioning (*2*), sleep (*13, 26*), and other normal and abnormal behavioral manifestations.

It is doubtful, however, that a specific behavior is dependent on activity of a specific neurohumor, and as indicated by Kety (*20*), most of these proposed relations are based on indirect pharmacological experiments in which analyses were usually performed in homogenates of the whole brain. These experiments cannot be repeated in the same preparation, their chemical correlations with ongoing behavior have a temporal delay, brain death may introduce artifacts, and information about local chemistry is lost within the cerebral pool.

To minimize these problems, several devices have been developed which permit local brain perfusions:

1. Cortical cup: As originally described by MacIntosh and Oborin (*23*), a small cup (0.3–3.0 cm^2) is anchored to an opening in the skull and filled with artificial cerebrospinal fluid (CSF) which is circulated to collect substances released by the cerebral cortex.
2. Push–pull cannula: As originally described by Gaddum (*15*), it is formed by two parallel or concentric tubings permanently implanted in the brain, permitting local injection and collection of fluids. For further details and references, see Myers (*28*), and chapters in this book.
3. Chemitrode: As originally described by Delgado *et al.* (*12*), it is formed by an array of electrical contacts cemented to a push–pull cannula permanently implanted in the brain, permitting long-term, 2-way (in and out) chemical and electrical communication with discrete areas of the unanesthetized brain. For further details and references, see Delgado (*7*), Myers (*28*), and chapters in this book.
4. Dialytrode: As originally described by Delgado (*8*), it consists of a chemitrode with its terminal tip closed by a porous membrane which forms a barrier for microorganisms and cells, while permitting the passage of fluids and chemicals. The electrical contacts also permit recording and stimulation. For further details and experimental results, see Delgado *et al.* (*9*). Modifications of this technique have been described by Kovacs *et al.* (*21*), Ungerstedt *et al.* (*35*), and in this book.

While the advantages of long-term studies of local electrical and chemical phenomena inside the brain of awake animals are obvious, technical difficulties have limited the use of these methods.

The purposes of this chapter are (1) to describe our improved dialytrode system; (2) to discuss problems involved in long-term perfusion of the unanesthetized brain; (3) to present data concerning profiles of amino acids collected from specific brain structures in the cat; and (4) to demonstrate

GABA release in the substantia nigra evoked by electrical stimulation of the caudate nucleus in the awake cat.

II. METHODS

A. Construction of Dialytrodes

A piece of 18-ga (1.2 mm o.d.) or 19-ga (1.0 mm o.d.) stainless-steel tubing long enough to reach a predetermined brain structure (e.g., 26 mm for the cat amygdala) was prepared with one end cut at a 60° angle and polished with a very fine emery sanding wheel. The membrane (see later) was cemented to the end of the tubing with cyanoacrylate glue, providing a permeable exchange surface of about 1.2 mm^2. The other tubing end was threaded for 2 mm to receive a matching metallic screw between perfusions and was cemented inside one of the lateral holes of a 7-pin Winchester female subminiature connector (7RME). When performing perfusions, the screw cap was withdrawn and a finer (25 ga) stainless-steel tubing was screwed in with its tip about 0.5 mm from the membrane, as shown in Fig. 1. A silastic "O" ring provided watertight fitting. In addition, an electrode assembly with six contacts 3 mm apart, made of 36-ga stainless-steel wire and insulated with quadruple teflon, was cemented alongside the cannula. The upper ends of the contacts were soldered to the Winchester connector. The seventh contact of the connector was soldered to the dialytrode cannula and served as ground. The unit was sterilized with ethylene oxide.

The dialytrode is characterized by the closing of the push–pull tip with a membrane having mechanical resistance, biological tolerance, and adequate permeability. The original dialytrode (*8, 9*) terminated in a 5 × 1-mm polysulfone bag which had tested biocompatibility (*17*) but was brittle, difficult to prepare, and had an undesirably high static electrical charge. During the past few years, different membrane materials, thicknesses, porous sizes, and extents of membrane surface and shape have been tested. Experimental materials with biological tolerance included polysulfone, cellulose, acetate, silastic, polycarbonate, and polyester. It was important to attain maximum permeability with minimum total size and porous size, as well as easy handling and tight cementation at the cannula tip. After many trials, we chose a polyester, nonhydroscopic membrane, 10 μm thick, with a very smooth surface, capillar pore size 0.2 μm, pore density of 3 × $10^8/cm^2$, and with low absorption and adsorption characteristics (Nucleopore Corp., Pleasanton, California). This membrane becomes wet or dry rapidly, eliminating the "sponge" effect of cellulose membranes without

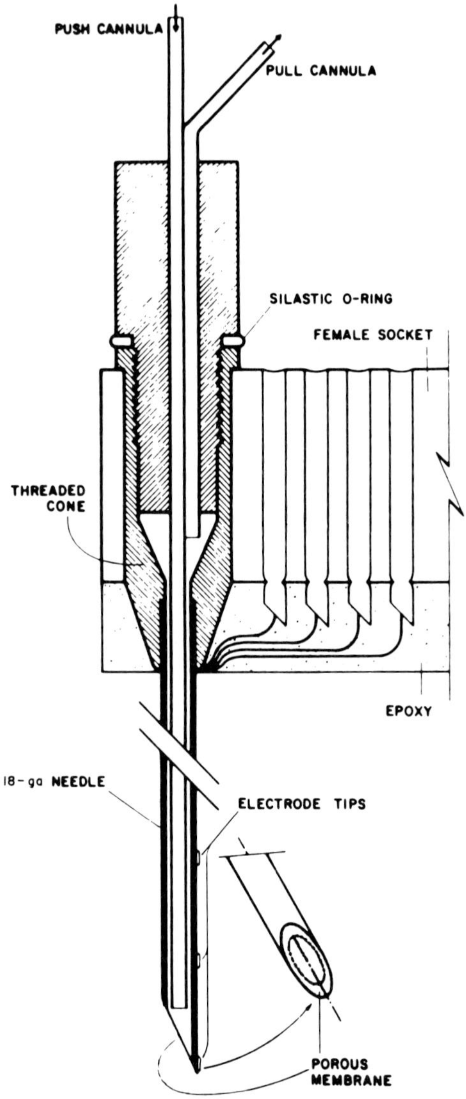

Fig. 1. Diagram of a dialytrode: the outer cannula is permanently implanted in the brain, being closed by a permeable polyester membrane with a 1.2-mm^2 surface. The inner cannula ends 0.5 mm from the membrane. Arrays of electrodes are cemented along the outer cannula. The whole device ends in a Winchester socket.

retaining solvents or substances, and greatly reducing artifacts and temporal delays. The small pore size avoids leukocytic infiltration of the membrane (*21*).

B. Surgical Procedures

After receiving pentothal intravenously and local anesthesia of the pharynx with procaine, cats were intubated and general anesthesia was maintained with a mixture of fluothene, nitrous oxide, and oxygen (Boc Fluothec-3 open system instrument). Each animal was placed in a Kopf stereotaxic instrument and, with aseptic precautions, 3-mm burr holes were drilled in selected points of the skull. A 10 mm-long guide, attached to the micromanipulator, was introduced inside the dialytrode tubing and used to insert the device slowly into the brain. The implanted dialytrode, with its socket, was then attached to the skull with dental cement. Four dialytrodes were usually implanted, for example, in the right caudate nucleus, right substantia nigra, and in both sides of the amygdala. The wound was closed with sutures and a few hours later the cat was awake. One week after surgery experiments began.

In this study 17 cats were used, weighing 2.0–3.4 kg. The implants have been well tolerated and in some animals, dialytrodes have remained in working order for over a year. In a series of acute experiments, 16 guinea pigs were used, as explained later.

C. Perfusion and Recording Procedures

In vivo studies were conducted in unanesthetized cats fitted with a specially designed torso suit and loosely confined to a hammock (Fig. 2). Animals were comfortable throughout the experiment, as shown by their placidity, frequent purring, and normal responses to intermittent petting.

Simultaneous perfusions of the four implanted dialytrodes were performed with a Gilson peristaltic pump, model Minipuls 2, through polyethylene tubing (.018 ga.) The liquid was pulled from a 1.5-ml "feed-in" tube reservoir, circulated through the dialytrode, and pushed by the pump to be collected in a 1.5-ml tube. In some experiments, the pump was used to circulate liquids continuously at a slow speed such as 10 μl/min. In other cases, as explained later, the pump was stopped for a predetermined time to allow diffusion of substances in and out of the dialytrode membrane, after which the pump was activated to collect the total amount of intradialytrode liquid (about 20 μl). Pressures of perfusion tubes were monitored continuously, using differential pressure transducers (National Semiconductors,

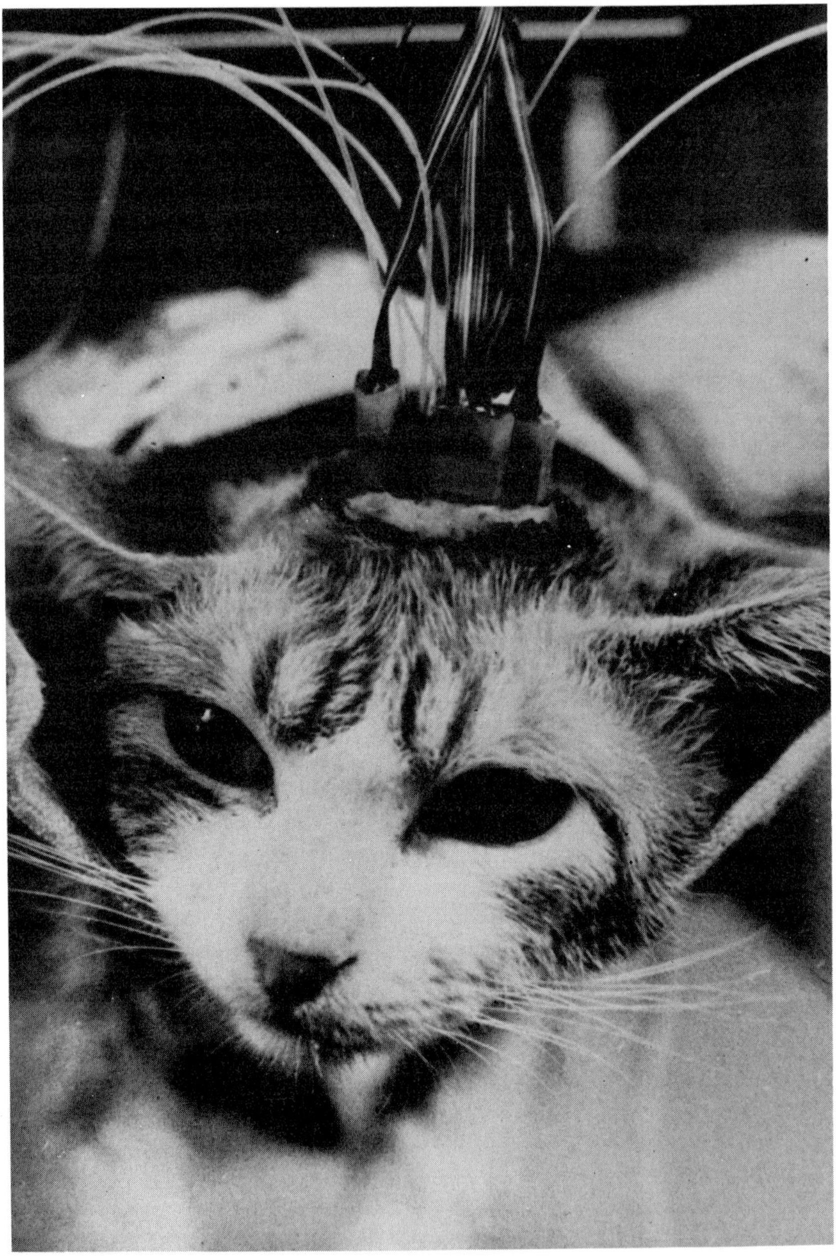

Fig. 2. Brain perfusions in the awake cat were performed with the animal restrained in a specially designed torso suit. All animals were comfortable throughout the experiment as shown by their frequent purring and response to petting.

LX1604D) and an electronic instrument of our own design which provided direct readings, giving a resolution of ± 1 mm Hg. The standard perfusion fluid was sterile Ringer or physiological saline. Collected perfusates were evaporized in a Savant Speed Vacuum concentrator and the amino acid content was determined by a Beckman Automatic Aminoacid Analyzer, model 121MB.

Electrical brain activity was recorded with an 8-channel Grass Polygraph, model 78D. Electrical stimulations were applied with a Grass instrument, model S48, and monitored with a Tektronix oscilloscope, model 5113.

III. FINDINGS

A. Optimization of the Experimental Procedures

The dialytrode is a *closed* system and perfusate recovery should be 100% when pressures are equal on both sides of the membrane. The dialytrode, however, should actually be recognized as a system *open* through the porosity of its membrane and fluids and solutes flow in and out, depending on gradients of pressure and liquid concentrations. To obtain reliable recovery rates, connections between dialytrodes and tubings must be hermetically sealed. The screwed-in attachment with the silastic ring at the dialytrode terminal has proved important, especially for *in vivo* experiments in which the animal moves and sometimes shakes its head. While peristaltic action of the pump did not modify perfusion pressure (oscillations were below 1 mm Hg), spontaneous movements of the animal could alter the perfusions, and continuous electronic monitoring of intradialytrode pressure was important to insure experimental reliability and consistency of results.

1. *IN VITRO* EXPERIMENTS

To evaluate some of the physical characteristics of the dialytrode system, different experiments were performed while circulating saline through the inside of the dialytrode with its tip immersed in a beaker containing 1.0 ml of saline.

a. *Perfusions: Pushing or Pulling* A pump was used to circulate fluids through the push–pull cannula of the dialytrode and results of injecting or withdrawing liquid in the same unit and at the same speed and pressure were compared. In our experiments, the two procedures yielded similar results, which was expected since hydraulic pressure inside the dialytrode system was the same in each case. The decisive factors were the inside resistance and especially the intradialytrode pressure, as determined by the

TABLE I

In Vitro Experiments to Evaluate the Passage of Fluids through the Dialytrode Membrane at Negative and Positive Pressures[a]

Pressure (mm Hg)	Total pump flow	Amount in bath	Vial collection
−20	355 ± 2	−189.9 ± 64.5	554.0 ± 45.0
0	360 ± 2	+2.3 ± 10.0	361.9 ± 14.2
+20	355 ± 28	+124.8 ± 31.6	221.0 ± 29.1

[a] The dialytrode was filled with saline and immersed in a saline bath. Perfusion rate was 12 μl/min for a total of 30 min. Intradialytrode pressure was measured electronically and established by lowering or raising the inflow vial. Values are expressed in microliters.

height of the free end of the system which was the feed-in vial. In most of our *in vivo* studies, circulation of fluids was performed with the pump pulling liquid through the dialytrode.

b. Intradialytrode Pressure Since permeability of the membrane is related to the differential pressure on its two sides, the flow of fluids in our experimental conditions was tested at positive and negative intradialytrode pressures while the dialytrode was filled with saline and immersed in a vial also filled with saline. By raising or lowering the inflow vial, pressures were adjusted to different levels and measured by the electronic sensors. Results of three sets of 10 experiments each are shown in Table I. The total pump flow was similar in all cases, although there was some variability when positive pressure was used.

At zero pressure, the amount of liquid delivered by the pump (360 μl in 30 min) was fully collected in the vial without gains or losses in the bath.

When the intradialytrode pressure was negative (−20 mm Hg), about 190 μl were sucked from the bath and the liquid collected in the vial increased by a corresponding amount, whereas when the intradialytrode pressure was positive (+20 mm Hg), about 125 μl were injected into the bath, and the amount of collected liquid decreased proportionally. This experiment showed that, as expected, with positive pressures, liquids flow at exchange rates related to the existing pressure.

These findings, however, have limited validity for *in vivo* studies because when a dialytrode is implanted within the brain it may be influenced by the pressures and hydraulic characteristics of the cranial cavity. When the dialytrode was immersed *in vitro* in a bath under negative intradialytrode pressure, liquid was continuously collected even in the absence of the pump, whereas there was no collection at all when the dialytrode was implanted *in vivo* in the brain.

c. Diffusion of [^{14}C]Urea To evaluate the chemical microenvironment at the tip of the dialytrode, the usual procedure has been to circulate fluids continuously at low speeds of a few microliters per minute (9). It is assumed that the passage of chemicals through the membrane is rather constant through time and therefore longer perfusions should yield larger amounts of collected substances.

To determine the diffusion rate in and out of the dialytrode, two experiments were performed. The first of these was *passage from bath to dialytrode.* The bath where the dialytrode was immersed was filled with a solution of 40 μ*M* of [^{14}C]urea and the dialytrode and connecting tubings were filled with saline. In order to study passive diffusion in a static situation, the pump was stopped and after periods of 5, 10, 15, 20, 25, and 30 min the dialytrode was flushed to determine the amount of collected [^{14}C]urea. A scintillation counter was used for this purpose. Results are presented in the interrupted line of Fig. 3. In the first 5 min there were almost 250 counts/μl,

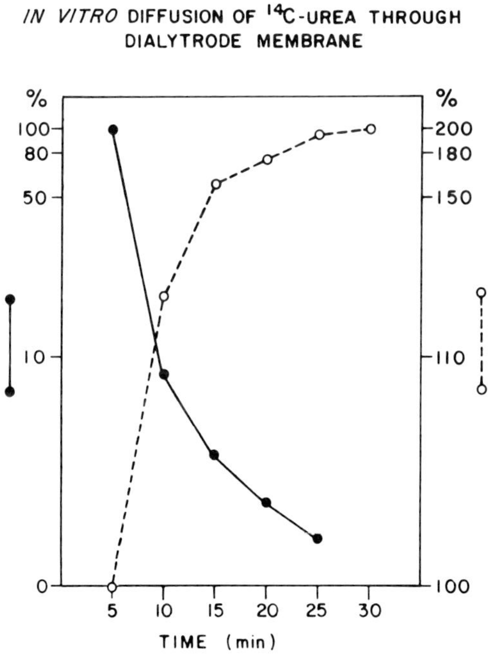

Fig. 3. The interrupted line shows the passage of [^{14}C]urea from bath to dialytrode. In the first 5 min there were 250 counts/μl (= 100%). In other experiments, collection time was increased to 10, 15, 20, 25, and 30 min. As shown by the graph, efficiency of collection diminished through time. The continuous line shows the passage of [^{14}C]urea from dialytrode to bath, demonstrating that the initial 5-min period was more effective, followed by an exponential decline.

while in the total of 30 min the count did not reach 500, demonstrating that diffusion was faster in the first 5 min than in the following 25 min. We concluded that 5 min was an acceptable time with the system static to allow the diffusion of [^{14}C]urea from the outside to inside the dialytrode. The second experiment was *passage from dialytrode to bath*. The inverse experiment was performed, filling the inside of the dialytrode with a solution of 40 μM of [^{14}C]urea and placing it for periods of 5, 10, 15, 20, and 25 min in different saline baths without changing the intradialytrode fluid and then counting the amount of [^{14}C]urea in each bath. Results are shown in the solid line of Fig. 3. During the first 5 min, most [^{14}C]urea diffused out with an exponential decline in the successive periods. From the above tests the conclusion was drawn that the initial period of 5 min was sufficient and effective for the passive diffusion of [^{14}C]urea in and out of the dialytrode. It may be assumed that chemicals with molecules similar to those of [^{14}C]urea diffuse in a similar way, but this possibility must be tested experimentally.

To explain the lack of temporal linearity in the exchange of chemicals through the dialytrode, it should be clarified that its total internal volume is about 15 μl, in a 25 mm-long tubing, of which only about 1.0 μl is at the tip close to the membrane. The remaining volume occupies capillary spaces with very low diffusion rates, representing a minor contribution to the exchange of chemicals.

The exact intradialytrode tip volume which easily and precisely equilibrates with the outer bath is not known and could be from 0.5 to 2.0 μl. The exact amount is not critical and our study shows that circulation of 5 μl in 10 sec every 5 min was suitable for the collection of chemicals exchanged through the dialytrode membrane, diminishing the dilution factor of the fluids inside the dialytrode. Washing out the whole system after a total experimental time of 15–30 min was in agreement with the work of Meeker and Myers (*25*).

The above-described *in vitro* experiments provided some information about dialytrode permeability and rates of liquid exchange, but ratios between external and internal pressures, as well as metabolic processes, blood circulation, and the physiological activities of the *in vivo* cerebral tissue are very different from the characteristics of a saline bath.

2. *IN VIVO* EXPERIMENTS

a. *Injection of Fluids* Some experiments may require the injection of liquids, including drugs, through the dialytrode membrane into a brain structure. The amount of injection per unit of time should be related to the differential pressure between the interior or the dialytrode and the cerebral tissue. The latter is difficult to modify, but the intradialytrode pressure may be adjusted at different levels simply by changing the height of the inflow vial.

Injection rates were tested in four experiments with the dialytrode implanted in the amygdala. Intradialytrode pressure was measured electronically, as explained in Section II, and it was varied by placing the inflow vial at different heights above the animal's head while the dialytrode exit was closed by stopping the pump. The amount of liquid injected during 5 min was measured by the displacement of a small bubble of air traveling along the calibrated inflow tubing attached to a vertical millimetric scale. With 30 mm HG of intradialytrode pressure, 3.2 μl ± 0.08 SD were injected in 5 min at a rate of 0.64 μl/min. With 70 mm Hg of intradialytrode pressure, 7.9 μl ± 0.6 were injected in 5 min at a rate of 1.6 μl/min. Other pressure and injection values are shown in Fig. 4. Results were reliable in different animals and it was concluded that predetermined amounts of liquids can be injected into the brain through the dialytrode membrane. The combined use of dialytrodes with the osmotic minipump, as described by Girgis *et al.* (*16*), could be a simple brain injection method. The advantage of dialysis was lost when injecting volumes of fluid, but in some experiments it may be necessary to inject a known volume in a determined time. The dialytrode technology has, therefore, a dual use and can be employed in

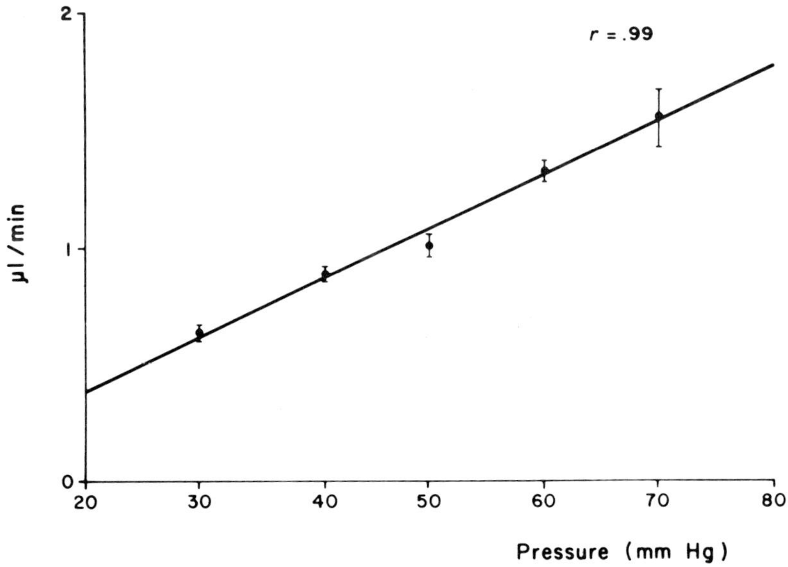

Fig. 4. The amount of fluid injected into the *in vivo* cat brain through the dialytrode membrane was proportional to the intradialytrode pressure.

different kinds of investigations as (1) a dialysis system to collect or to deliver chemicals passively, or (2) an open system for direct injections.

b. Passage of [^{14}C]Urea from Brain to Dialytrode To evaluate the possible rates of diffusion and collection of chemicals from the brain, two experiments were performed in a total of 16 guinea pigs. In each animal, anesthetized with nembutal, a 25-ga stainless-steel cannula was implanted in the center of the thalamic nuclei. Then 10 μl of [^{14}C]urea plus 1.0 μl of Neutral Red were slowly injected through the cannula. In the first experiment, groups of four guinea pigs were decapitated 1.5, 2.5, and 3.5 hr, respectively, after the intracerebral injection. The brain of each animal was removed and sectioned coronally in 5-mm blocks and dye-stained area, which weighed about 10 mg, was dissected, immersed in a 5% sulfosalycilic acid solution, and reduced to pulp by sonication. The amount of [^{14}C]urea remaining in the brain sample (per 5 mm of tissue) after the different injection times was measured in the scintillation counter and values are shown in Fig. 5. The decreasing values of radioactivity content could be expected because [^{14}C]urea was progressively being removed from the injected site by radial diffusion through the tissue.

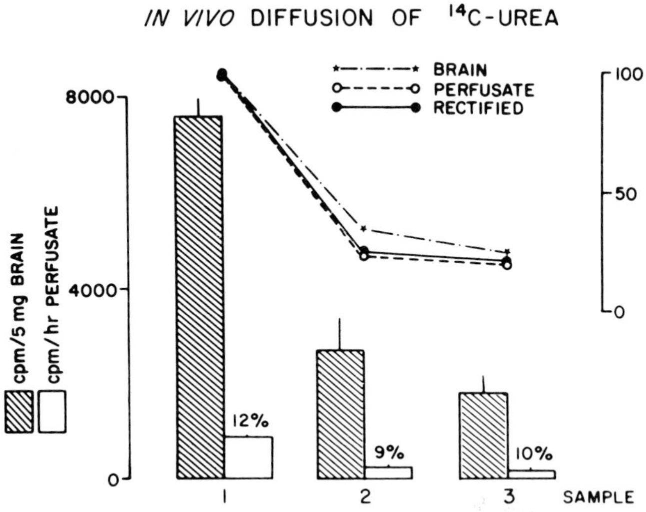

Fig. 5. In guinea pigs, 10 μl of [^{14}C]urea were injected into the thalamus and the brain was removed 1.5 (sample 1), 2.5 (sample 2), and 3.5 (sample 3) hr after injection to evaluate the progressive removal of [^{14}C]urea from the injected site, as shown in the hatched column. In another series of guinea pigs, the experiment was repeated in the presence of implanted dialytrodes to measure the collection of existing [^{14}C]urea, as shown in the white column. The experiment shows the proportionality between existing intracerebral and dialytrode-collected [^{14}C]urea.

In the second experiment with four anesthetized guinea pigs, a dialytrode with a laterally attached 25-ga stainless-steel cannula terminating at its tip was implanted in the center of the thalamic nuclei. Then 10 μl of [^{14}C]urea were injected into the thalamus through the lateral cannula and perfusion via the dialytrode started immediately, circulating 10 μl of fluid every 5 min, and flushing the entire dialytrode at the end of each test period.

The initial fluid sample (first 60 min) was discarded to avoid possible artifacts of [^{14}C]urea uptake due to increased local pressure during its injection. The next sample, number 1, was collected between the first and second hours of injection, and the counts per minute represented 12% of the existing [^{14}C]urea in the brain (Fig. 5). Sample 2 was collected between 2 and 3 hr after injection and the counts per minute represented 9% of the intracerebral [^{14}C]urea. Sample 3, collected between 3 and 4 hr after injection, represented 10% of the intracerebral [^{14}C]urea. The decline in the amount of [^{14}C]urea present within the brain and the dialytrode is shown in the upper part of Fig. 5. With the initial amount considered as 100%, the remaining value in the brain was 35.9% between hours 2 and 3 and 23.8% between hours 3 and 4, while in the perfusate, the remaining value was 26.8% in sample 2 and 20.6% in sample 3. The decline curve appeared slightly different between brain and perfusate, probably due to the fact that in each of the samples, some of the [^{14}C]urea from the brain had been removed by the dialytrode. Correcting the figures for this amount of removed [^{14}C]urea, the "rectified" (solid line) curve was obtained, showing a perfect coincidence of declines of [^{14}C]urea in both brain and perfusate. Then the mean recovery by the dialytrode was 12.5 ± 0.8% (SD) of the tissue content.

Data from Yaksh and Yamamura (*41*) indicate that in the rat, intracarotid injections of [^{14}C]urea result in the appearance of 0.31% of the injected substance in the whole brain 10 min after injection. In the perfusate, [^{14}C]urea appears abruptly and disappears in a single-phase exponential fashion. Their data indicated the integrity of the blood–brain barrier. The amount of urea collected by the push–pull cannula was proportional to the amount present in the brain. Our results with injection of [^{14}C]urea and its collection by the dialytrode are in basic agreement with these findings, supporting the conclusion that levels detected in the perfusate closely parallel changes observed in the brain tissue being perfused.

c. *Changes in Perfusion Pressure* It could be expected that by applying negative pressure, more fluids or chemicals would be extracted from the brain. The cranial space, however, is a closed system and in over 10 experiments using continuous perfusion at 5 μl/min for 30 min, intradialytrode pressures up to −50 mm Hg did not modify the amount of collected fluid or chemicals. It was therefore concluded that zero intra-dialytrode pressure was appropriate for neurochemical studies with dialytrodes.

d. Tissue Damage The relative magnitude of local tissue damage may be reflected by the concentration of proteins in the perfusate which, in the experiments of Yaksh and Yamamura (*41*), was 75 μg/ml when perfusing the caudal thalamus of rats. This level of proteins decayed asymptotically with time. Histological examinations indicated a layer of destroyed cells approximately 0.2–0.6 mm thick along the penetration tract. Although initial tissue damage depends on the diameter of the cannulae and may be similar with push–pull units and with dialytrodes, accumulative tissue damage near the cannula tip is evident using push–pull models because the internal cannula must be reintroduced for each experiment.

After completion of our experiments, each cat with dialytrodes was anesthetized with nembutal intraperitoneally and perfused through the heart with saline and 10% formaline. The brain was removed and after fixation, the hemispheres were included in paraffin cut in 20-μm sections and stained to identify the location of electrodes and to evaluate local histology. One example of a dialytrode tract in a cat 7 months after implantation and after many perfusions is shown in Fig. 6, demonstrating the clean walls and the integrity of neurons close to the penetration site.

One of the main problems in the push–pull method is the occlusion of the system, particularly at the cannula tip. Most investigators discard experimental data in which the amount collected does not reach a certain percentage of the inflow volume (3–10% variation, according to different studies). These "unsuccessful experiments" represent a technical handicap, a waste of time and material, and they interfere with long-term experiments because it is difficult to maintain the implanted cannula functioning for months. These problems are solved with the dialytrode technology.

B. Neurobiological Applications

Autonomic functions, somatic activities, and behavioral manifestations are related to local dynamic processes which involve different areas of the brain and many chemical substances. If we kill the experimental animal and extract the brain, we may have static information but cannot capture the temporal development of chemical changes or their functional correlations. Dialytrode technology permits the simultaneous study of several areas of the awake brain and repetition of experiments in the same animal. In this way we may investigate, for example, the local profiles of amino acids, catecholamines, peptides, and other substances in the caudate nucleus, substantia nigra, amygdala, and hypothalamus before, during, and following

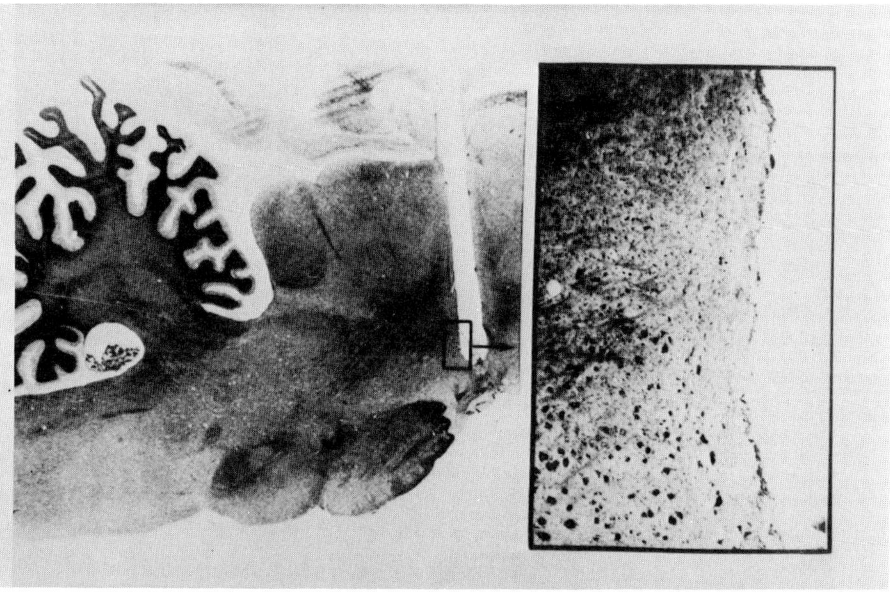

Fig. 6. A dialytrode was implanted for 7 months in the substantia nigra of a cat. The insert shows a detail of the limiting wall and the neuronal normality of the brain (Klüver–Barrera stain).

after-discharges evoked by intracerebral stimulation, or we may design other experiments to explore pharmacological, behavioral, and pathological problems. As shown many years ago, it is possible to investigate the local synthesis and release of catecholamines (*33*) and the local effects of anesthetics and psychoactive drugs (*4, 10, 38*).

1. PROFILE OF AMINO ACIDS IN EXTRACELLULAR SPACE

In two cats with dialytrodes implanted in the substantia nigra, both amygdalas, and the head of the caudate nucleus, 26 experiments were performed to determine the relative amounts of eight amino acids present in the extracellular spaces, and some of these results are presented in Fig. 7. Glutamine was the most abundant substance and aspartate was the least. Variability from day to day and also between animals was very small, as shown by the standard deviations, indicating constancy of the profiles. Differences in amino acid content in substantia nigra and amygdala were significant with respect to taurine, glutamate, glutamine, and glycine. Content of the other four amino acids was similar in both structures.

The amino acid profile for the caudate nucleus was similar to that of the substantia nigra, but more experiments are necessary in order to perform a statistical evaluation of these data.

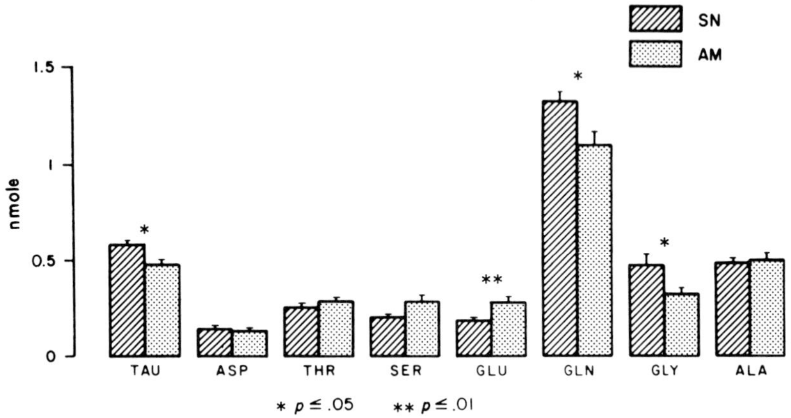

Fig. 7. Profile of the amount of amino acids detected by perfusion with dialytrodes in substantia nigra (SN) and amygdala (AM). Values were obtained in 26 experiments performed in two cats. Observe the small standard error, indicating reliability of results. See also the significant differences between taurine (TAU), glutamine (GLN), glutamate (GLU), and glycine (GLY).

An important negative result was that GABA was always *absent* in our perfusates. The fact that GABA was undetectable in spite of its known high intracellular content indicates that dialytrode implantation does not alter neuronal membranes.

The temporal reliability of our results is indicated by the fact that in one cat with dialytrodes implanted for more than 1 year, as shown in Fig. 8,

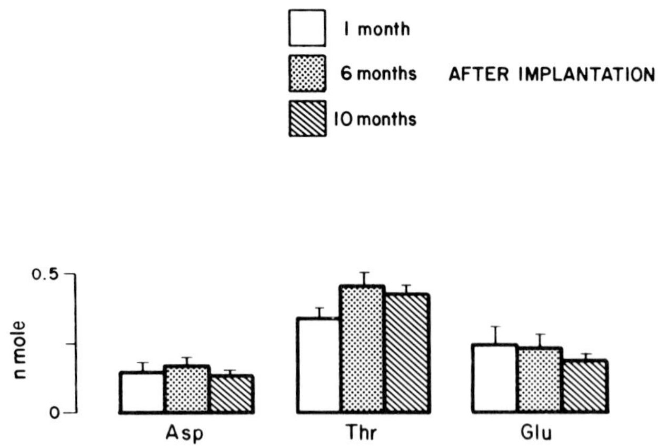

Fig. 8. Values of aspartate (Asp), threonine (Thr), and glutamate (Glu) obtained in the substantia nigra of a cat in perfusions performed 1, 6, and 10 months after dialytrode implantation. Results were reliable through time.

values for aspartate, threonine, and glutamate were similar during different months. These values are also comparable with those presented in Fig. 7.

2. CORRELATION ANALYSIS OF SPONTANEOUS AMINO ACID CHANGES

As shown in Figs. 7 and 8, the amount of amino acids present in brain structures was reliable in different animals and through time. Some small spontaneous oscillations occurred, however, and simultaneous perfusions of the amygdala and substantia nigra were performed in two cats (a total of 26 experiments) to determine whether these oscillations were correlated in both structures. Results are shown in Table II where 0 represents no correlation and the + and − signs represent significant postive and negative correlations ($p < .05$). Taurine variations in the substantia nigra were not significantly correlated with variations of taurine and glutamate in the amygdala, but they were *negatively* correlated with amygdala changes of aspartate, threonine, serine, glutamine, glycine, and alanine.

All these amino acids of the amygdala correlated *positively* with aspartate changes in the substantia nigra. Other correlations may be found in the data of Table II. The fact that glutamine was only 5 times higher than glutamate was surprising, but it should be emphasized that variations in the glutamine were not correlated with variations in glutamate, and therefore a possible breakdown of glutamine inside the dialytrode perfusion system was unlikely. Future work will determine possible correlations of different brain structures in relation to normal and abnormal functional states of the brain, including the effects of drug administration.

TABLE II

Correlation between Spontaneous Variation in the Amount of Amino Acids Collected in the Perfusions of Right Substantia Nigra and Right Amygdala[a]

Right amygdala	Right substantia nigra: Tau	Asp	Thr	Ser	Glu	Gln	Gly	Ala
Tau	0	0	0	0	0	0	0	0
Asp	−	+	0	+	0	0	0	0
Thr	−	+	+	+	0	0	+	+
Ser	−	+	+	+	0	0	+	+
Glu	0	0	0	0	0	0	0	0
Gln	−	+	+	+	0	0	+	+
Gly	−	+	+	+	0	0	+	+
Ala	−	+	+	+	0	0	+	+

[a] Observed in the absence of correlation among several amino acids (e.g., glutamate) and the existence of negative (e.g., taurine substantia nigra/amygdala) and positive (e.g., aspartate substantia nigra/amygdala) correlations.

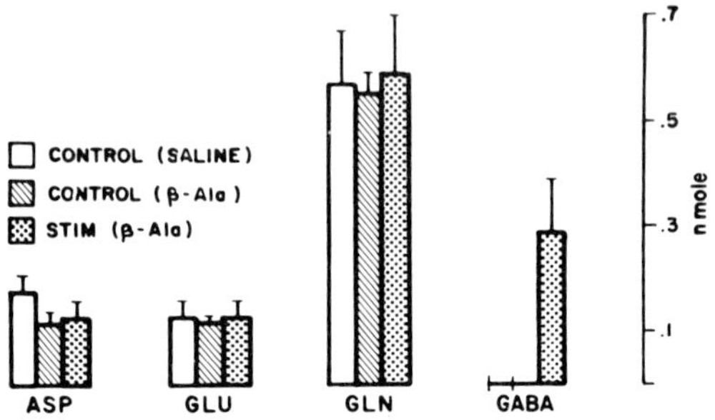

Fig. 9. GABA was undetectable in controls (saline and β-alanine). Electrical stimulation of the caudate nucleus produced a considerable release of GABA in the substantia nigra without changing the amounts of other amino acids.

3. GABA RELEASE FROM SUBSTANTIA NIGRA

Two cats were prepared with dialytrodes implanted in the right caudate nucleus and substantia nigra. Two weeks after surgery, spontaneous intracerebral EEG was recorded and perfusion experiments were begun, obtaining amino acid profiles similar to those in our other series of results in 17 cats and without ever detecting any GABA. Perfusions were then performed with saline containing 0.1 *M* β-alanine which should flow out through the dialytrode membrane to the surrounding cerebral tissue, blocking possible GABA reuptake by glial mechanisms. The presence of GABA, however, was still undetectable, as shown in Fig. 9. Electrical stimulation was then applied to the caudate nucleus using constant current, cathodal, 300 Hz, 0.5-msec pulse duration, and 500- to 700-μA intensity, delivered in trains of 100 msec (30 pulses) every 2 sec, lasting for the entire perfusion period of 30 min. As shown in Fig. 9, caudate nucleus stimulation evoked a clear GABA peak in the substantia nigra.

Specificity of GABA release determined by caudate stimulation was supported by another series of experiments perfusing the substantia nigra with (a) saline, (b) saline + β-alanine, and (c) saline + β-alanine while the caudate nucleus was electrically stimulated. In the three experiments, the amount of collected aspartate, glutamate, and glutamine did not change, proving once more the reliability of our results. GABA was undetectable in experiments (a) and (b), whereas when the caudate nucleus was stimulated (c), there was a spectacular increase of GABA in the substantia nigra perfusate. This finding is more significant considering that glutamate and GABA are present in similar amounts in the substantia nigra (*27*).

During these experiments, the electrical activity of the substantia nigra was continuously monitored and periods of wakefulness and sleep could be identified in the EEG coinciding with observable eye opening and closing.

Behavior of the animal and EEG cycles were similar during controls and during β-alanine perfusions. Electrical stimulation of the caudate nucleus produced a tremor in the ipsilateral forelimb and ear starting a few minutes after onset of stimulation and lasting for the rest of the 30-min period, disappearing 1 or 2 min after cessation of stimulation.

IV. PERSPECTIVES AND DISCUSSION

As discussed earlier, the dialytrode is a closed system characterized by the closing of the push–pull cannula with a permeable membrane which represents a considerable improvement over open push–pull cannulae.

Three types of dialytrodes have been described in the literature. The original device (*8*) had some difficulties related to the construction and use of the polysulfone membrane. In the unit of Kovacs *et al.* (*21*), the parallel cannulae were less efficient than the concentric systems, and cementing of the polycarbonate membrane at the cannulae tips facing each other represented a double triangular surface with some mechanical and biological drawbacks. The dialysis tubing and nylon thread introduced through two parallel cannulae as described by Ungerstedt *et al.* (*35*) and Zetterström *et al.* (*42*), with an exposed permeable tubing about 2.0 mm long, may be reliable and efficient, but our present dialytrode has the following advantages: it is constructed with concentric cannulae, the inner one being removable and the outer one being closed by a commercially available membrane which is small (1.2 mm^2), thin, strong, reliable, highly permeable, nonabsorbent, and easy to cement.

The most convincing demonstration of any technology is its successful use, and over 2 years' experience with our improved dialytrodes supports the following conclusions:

1. The dialytrode has no occlusion problems.

2. The technique is suitable for acute, anesthetized preparations and also for long-term experiments with awake animals. Some of our chronic preparations have been studied for more than 1 year, permitting repeated controls and experiments.

3. In chronic preparations, the initial brain reaction due to surgical trauma becomes stabilized, assuring functional reliability.

4. The dialytrode allows for controlled collection efficiency. Our perfusate collection procedure consisted of stopping the pump for 5 min circulation of 5 μl of fluid, repetition of this cycle six times, and flushing the dialytrode 30 min later in order to recover all liquid inside the dialytrode. This procedure was important because the exchange of chemicals through the membrane involves only the very few microliters which are at the dialytrode tip. The remaining intradialytrode liquid occupies capillary spaces

with much lower diffusion rates and its contribution to the collection of chemicals is negligible. In agreement with most investigators, slow perfusion speed increases the efficiency of collection, and stopping perfusion for 5 min provides optimal results.

It is generally agreed that with chemitrodes as well as with dialytrodes, the uptake is better at slower rates of perfusion. Zetterström *et al.* (*42*), for example, reported that *in vitro* experiments with a modified (hollow fiber) dialytrode yielded higher purine concentrations in the outflow if the flow rate was 2 instead of 5 μl/min. We have obtained similar results with amino acids working *in vivo* (*22*).

5. The dialytrode is a barrier for mechanical changes. Constancy of perfusion speed is very important in push–pull perfusions (*40*), and interruptions as brief as 1 min may produce long-lasting local biochemical changes (*41*). This occurs with chemitrodes because the volume of the liquid bubble at the tip may change according to perfusion speed and pressure, altering the mechanical and physiological characteristics of the area under study. Variability of results may be very high, and the amount of acetylcholine released by the brain ranges from 0.1 to 200 μg/ml (*40*), a variability which cannot be explained by differences between animals or brain structures and which probably depends on some limitation in the chemitrode technology. The dialytrode, however, represents a barrier for mechanical changes, being an important factor of reliability, and interruptions in perfusion do not affect collectability.

The efficiency of the push–pull system improves with increased tip protrusion, reaching a plateau around 0.65 mm. When the inner cannula extends beyond 1.0 mm, there is (especially with high perfusion rates) a marked increase in unacceptable experiments (e.g., 5 out of 8 in Yaksh and Yamamura's data). Variations in efficiency related to tip protrusion may be an important source of artifacts if the tip of the inner cannula moves during the experiment. With concentric chemitrodes, reintroduction of the inner cannula for each experiment signifies that its protrusion and functioning do not remain constant. In contrast, the inner cannula of the dialytrode is introduced inside of the brain within the outer cannula, 0.5 mm from the membrane, and small variations in its position have no functional significance.

One advantage of our methodology is the possibility of implanting several dialytrodes and perfusing simultaneously several cerebral areas in the awake animal. In this way, static and fuctional correlations may be established. The present chapter described a typical experiment in which the amounts of eight amino acids present in the substantia nigra and amygdala were evaluated and correlated. Glutamate was unrelated with changes of other amino acids, indicating a local functional independence perhaps related to its role as a putative neurotransmitter. Threonine, serine, glutamine, glycine, and alanine levels in the amygdala were correlated negatively or positively with amino acids in the substantia nigra, except for glutamate and glutamine. Analysis of these correlations could be of great interest for the evaluation of pharmacological experiments and behavioral activities.

Another important application is the *in vivo* determination of the release of neurotransmitters, as shown by the collection of GABA in the substantia nigra after caudate nucleus stimulation. In our experiments, the fact that GABA was undetectable in controls and appeared in the substantia nigra after electrical stimulation of the caudate nucleus provides a strong support for its role as a neurotransmitter, meeting the difficult criterion of reliable *in vivo* collectability (*14, 31*). Our results are in agreement with the data of Canzek *et al.* (*3*) reporting the absence of GABA detection (<0.5 pmol/5min) in the optic tectum of the pigeon, probably due to the high efficiency of reuptake mechanisms and GABA increase, determined by electrical stimulation of the midbrain nucleus isthmi. The fact that in normal conditions GABA is not detectable in extracellular fluid suggests that it is rapidly removed by glial and/or neuronal reuptake. This is probably also true for other amino acid neurotransmitters which can only be detected in the presence of uptake inhibitors. Most studies about GABA release have been performed in acute anesthetized animals, using sometimes local preloading of the tissue with GABA precursors (*3, 18, 19. 27, 30, 37, 39*). The methodology described here avoids the above-mentioned problems because the animals may be unmedicated and experiments can be repeated indefinitely with reliability of results.

ACKNOWLEDGMENTS

The histological and technical help of Drs. E. Garrido and D. Muñoz, the editorial assistance of C. S. Delgado, and the support of the Fondo de Investigaciones Sanitaria are warmly acknowledged. A modified version of some of this material has appeared in the *Journal of Neurochemistry*, **42** (1984) 1218–1228.

REFERENCES

1. Allikmets, L., Delgado, J. M. R., and Richards, S. A. Intramesencephalic injection of imipramine, promazine and chlorprothixene in awake monkeys. *Int. J. Neuropharm.* **7** (1968) 185–193.
2. Brust-Carmona, H., Prado-Alcalá, R., Grinberg-Zylberbaum, J., Alvarez-Leefmans, J., and Zarco Coronado, I. Modulatory effects of acetylcholine and catecholamines in the caudate

nucleus during motor conditioning. *In* "Neurohumoral Coding of Brain Function," (R. D. Myers and R. R. Drucker-Colín, eds.), 1974, pp. 171–187. Plenum, New York.
3. Canzek, V., Wolfensberger, M., Amsler, U., and Cuénod, M. *In vivo* release of glutamate and aspartate following optic nerve stimulation. *Nature (London)* **293** (1981) 572–574.
4. DeFeudis, F. V., Delgado, J. M. R., and Roth, R. H. Content, synthesis and collectability of amino acids in various structures of the brains of rhesus monkeys. *Brain Res.* **18** (1970) 15–23.
5. Delgado, J. M. R. Cerebral structures involved in transmission and elaboration of noxious stimulation. *J. Neurophysiol.* **18** (1955) 261–275.
5. Delgado, J. M. R. Pharmacology of spontaneous and conditioned behavior in the monkey. *In* "Pharmacology of Conditioning, Learning, and Retention," (M. Ya. Mickhel'son and V. G. Longo, eds.) 1965 pp. 133–156. Pergamon, Oxford.
7. Delgado, J. M. R., Intracerebral perfusion in awake monkeys. *Arch. Int. Pharmacodyn.* **161** (1966) 442–462.
8. Delgado, J. M. R. Telecommunication in brain research. *In* "Telemetric Methods in Pharmacology" (Proc. 4th Int. Congr. Pharmacol.), Vol. V, 1970 pp. 270–278. Schwabe, Basel.
9. Delgado, J. M. R., DeFeudis, F. V., Roth, R. H., Ryugo, D. K., and Mitruka, B. M. Dialytrode for long term intracerebral perfusion in awake monkeys. *Arch. Int. Pharmacodyn.* **198** (1972) 9–21.
10. Delgado, J. M. R., and Kitahata, L. M. Reversible depression of hippocampus by local injection of anesthetics in monkeys. *EEG Clin. Neurophysiol.* **22** (1967) 453–464.
11. Delgado, J. M. R., and Rubinstein, L. Intracerebral release of neurohumors in unanesthetized monkeys. *Arch. Int. Pharmacodyn.* **150** (1964) 530–546.
12. Delgado, J. M. R., Simhadri, P., and Apelbaum, J. Chronic implantation of chemitrodes in the monkey brain. *Proc. XXII Int. Congr. Union Physiol. Sci.* **2** (1962) 1090(abstr.).
13. Drucker-Colín, R. R. Endogenous sleep peptides. *In* "Psychopharmacology of Sleep," (D. Wheatley, ed.), 1981, pp. 53–72. Raven, New York.
14. Fagg, G. E., and Lane, J. D. The uptake and release of putative amino acid neurotransmitters. *Neuroscience* **4** (1979) 1015–1036.
15. Gaddum, J. H. Push–pull cannulae. *J. Physiol. (London)* **155** (1961) 1–2P.
16. Girgis, M., Kent, J., Kohlhardt, S., Rasko, J., and Stobo, P. Combined use of the chemitrode with osmotic minipumps for experimental brain research. *Brain Res. Bull.* **7** (1981) 719–721.
17. Imai, Y., Kuo, Y-S., Watanabe, A., and Masuhara, E. Evaluation of polysulfone as a potential biomedical material. *J. Bioeng.* **2** (1978) 103–107.
18. Iversen, L. L., Mitchell, J. F., and Srinivasan, V. The release of gamma-aminobutyric acid during inhibition in the cat visual cortex. *J. Physiol. (London)* **212** (1971) 519–534.
19. Jasper, H. H., and Koyama, I. Rate of release of amino acids from the cerebral cortex in the cat as affected by brain stem and thalamic stimulation. *Can. J. Physiol. Pharmacol.* **47** (1969) 889–905.
20. Kety, S. S. The central physiological and pharmacological effects of the biogenic amines and their correlations with behavior. *In* "The Neurosciences," (G. C. Quarton, T. Melnechuk, and F. O. Schmitt, eds.), 1967, pp. 444–451. Rockefeller Univ. Press, New York.
21. Kovacs, D. A., Zoll, J. G., and Erickson, C. K. Improved intracerebral chemitrode for chemical and electrical studies of the brain. *Pharmacol. Biochem. Behav.* **4** (1976) 621–625.
22. Lerma, J., Solís, J. M., Martín del Río, R., and Delgado, J. M. R. Chronic dialytrode perfusion: amino acid profiles of brain structures. *Neuroscience* (Suppl.) **7** (1982) S131 (abstr.).

23. MacIntosh, F. C., and Oborin, P. E. Release of acetylcholine from intact cerebral cortex. *Proc XIX Int. Congr. Union Physiol. Sci.* (1963) 580–581 (abstr.).
24. MacLean, P. D., and Delgado, J. M. R. Electrical and chemical stimulation of frontotemporal portion of limbic system in the waking animal. *EEG Clin. Neurophysiol.* **5** (1953) 91–100.
25. Meeker, R., and Myers, R. D. *In vivo* [^{14}C]amino acid profiles in discrete hypothalamic regions during push–pull perfusion in the unrestrained rat. *Neuroscience* **4** (1979) 495–506.
26. Monnier, M., and Schoenenberger, G. A. Neuro-humoral coding of sleep by the physiological sleep factor delta. *In* "Neurohumoral Coding of Brain Function," (R. D. Myers and R. R. Drucker-Colín, eds.), 1974, pp. 207–232. Plenum, New York.
27. Moroni, F., Cheney, D. L., and Costa, E. β-Endorphin inhibits ACh turnover in nuclei of rat brain. *Nature (London)* **267** (1977) 267–268.
28. Myers, R. D. "Handbook of Drug and Chemical Stimulation of the Brain. Behavioral, Pharmacological and Physiological Aspects," 759 pp. Van Nostrand-Reinhold, New York.
29. Myers, R. D., and Drucker-Colín, R. R. (eds.). "Neurohumoral Coding of Brain Function," 480 pp. Plenum, New York.
30. Obata, K., and Takeda, K. Release of gamma-aminobutyric acid into fourth ventricle induced by stimulation of the cat's cerebellum. *J. Neurochem.* **16** (1969) 1043–1047.
31. Orrego, F. Criteria for the identification of central neurotransmitters, and their application to studies with some nerve tissue preparations *in vitro*. *Neuroscience* **4** (1979) 1037–1057.
32. Reis, D. J. The chemical coding of aggression in brain. *In* "Neurohumoral Coding of Brain Function," (R. D. Myers and R. R. Drucker-Colín, eds.), 1974, pp. 125–150. Plenum, New York.
33. Roth, R. H., Allikmets, L., and Delgado, J. M. R. Synthesis and release of noradrenaline and dopamine from discrete areas of the monkey brain. *Arch. Int. Pharmacodyn.* **181** (1969) 273–282.
34. Tapia, R. The role of β-aminobutyric acid metabolism in the regulation of cerebral excitability. *In* "Neurohumoral Coding of Brain Function," (R. D. Myers and R. R Drucker-Colín, eds.), 1974, pp. 3–26. Plenum, New York.
35. Ungerstedt, U., Forster, C. H., Herrera-Marschitz, M., Hoffman, I., Jungnelius, U., Tossman, U., and Zetterström, T. Brain dialysis. A new *in vivo* technique for studying neurotransmitter release and metabolism. *Neurosci. Lett.* (Suppl.) **10** (1982) S493 (abstr.).
36. Valzelli, L. Aggression and violence: a biological essay of the distinction. *In* "Aggression and Violence: A Psychobiological and Clinical Approach," (L. Valzelli and L. Morgese, eds.), Edizioni Centro Culturale y Congressi Saint Vincent, 1981, pp. 39–60. Saint Vincent, Italy.
37. Van der Heyden, J. A. M., Venema, K., and Korf, S. *In vivo* release of endogenous GABA from rat substantia nigra measured by a novel method. *J. Neurochem.* **32** (1979) 469–476.
38. Vas, C. J., Delgado, J. M. R., and Glaser, G. H. A comparative study of effects of anticholinergic drugs on epileptic activity from amygdala and frontal cortex. *Neurology* **19** (1969) 234–241.
39. Vellucci, S. V., and Webster, R. A. Studies on GABA release *in vivo* using a simple method for perfusion of the fourth ventricle of the rat. *Neuropharmacology* **19** (1980) 1099–1104.
40. Wieraszko, A. Release of acetylcholine from the brain *in vivo:* some comments on estimation methods and their application. *Acta Neurobiol. Exp.* **40** (1980) 687–707.
41. Yaksh, T. L., and Yamamura, H. I. Factors affecting performance of the push–pull cannula in brain. *J. Appl. Physiol.* **37** (1974) 428–434.
42. Zetterström, T., Vernet, L., Ungerstedt, U., Tossman, U., Jonzon, B., and Fredholm, B. B. Purine levels in the intact rat brain. Studies with an implanted perfused hollow fibre. *Neurosci. Lett.* **29** (1982) 111–115.

8

In Vivo Brain Dialysis of Extracellular Nontransmitter and Putative Transmitter Amino Acids

ANDERS HAMBERGER, CLAES-HENRIC BERTHOLD,* INGEMAR JACOBSON, BIRGITTA KARLSSON, ANDERS LEHMANN, BRITTA NYSTRÖM, AND MATS SANDBERG

Institute of Neurobiology and
**Department of Anatomy*
University of Göteborg
Göteborg, Sweden

I. INTRODUCTION

The microenvironment of the cells in the central nervous system (CNS) serves as a communication channel between neurons and in glia–neuronal interactions. This microenvironment is determined by the cells in the brain parenchyma, by the blood, and by the cerebrospinal fluid (CSF). The specific transport-barrier functions and the uptake and secretion properties of the

IN VIVO PERFUSION AND RELEASE
OF NEUROACTIVE SUBSTANCES

ISBN 0-12-083350-6

CNS cells make homeostasis of the extracellular fluid highly unpredictable. Although the precision of analytical neurochemistry cannot match that of morphology or electrophysiology, the development of "probes" for collection of brain fluid *in vivo* opens the possibility to a more dynamic, on-line neurochemistry, especially as the sensitivity of many analytical techniques has improved in later years.

An early step in the dialysis approach to neurochemistry and neuropharmacology was taken by Bito and collaborators in 1966 (*1*). In order to test their assumption that the concentration of a given amino acid in the cerebrospinal fluid is a steady-state condition determined by the rates of exchange between it and both the blood plasma and the CNS parenchyma, Bito and co-workers had to find a means to study the CNS parenchyma. This was measured in an *in vivo* dialysate collected from a sac which was filled with dextran in saline and implanted into the cerebral cortex of the dog, between its surface and the lateral ventricle. The size of the dialysis sac was 9 × 8–12 mm and it was made from a piece of tubing which was tied off at both ends with silk sutures. Such sacs were kept in the brain for 10 weeks, after which they were removed and their content analyzed. During the 10 weeks, a thin capsule developed around the sac. This capsule comprised a few layers of sparse, spindle-shaped cells and had a fibrillary, collagen-like appearance. The brain parenchyma itself exhibited proliferation of both capillaries and glial cells peripheral to the capsule.

However, the development of the chronically implanted dialytrode, described by Delgado and co-workers in 1972 (*4*), was of pioneering importance, as their system allows continuous analysis of a brain dialysate from a region with a volume of a few cubic millimeters. In addition, the dialytrode is implanted with standard stereotactic equipment and is combined with electrodes for the recording of electrical activity in its vicinity. The later developments of the dialytrode by Delgado's group provide refined precision and accuracy (*11*). Taking advantage of the availability of very thin dialysis tubings, less than a third of a millimeter in outer diameter, Ungerstedt and co-workers (*22*) presented new technical solutions for brain dialysis.

The main advantages with the brain dialysis systems vs for example, a free-diffusion push–pull cannula perfusion are (1) it is a closed system—no net transport of water occurs to or from the tissue, (2) it is made of soft material which makes the tube an "integrated" part of the brain, and (3) it can be precalibrated in media containing, for example, amino acids of known concentrations. Consequently it provides data for the calculation of absolute concentrations in the extracellular fluid.

This chapter describes the application of these techniques in the analysis of specific regions of the rabbit brain. The aim is to obtain insight into certain aspects of amino acid transmitter physiology, to characterize metabolically the gliosis reaction which develops with time around the dialysis tubing, and to study the homeostasis of the extracellular fluid in the CNS during changes in total body amino acids as they occur, for example, in liver failure.

II. METHODS

The technique involves analysis of dialysates collected *in vivo* in a continuous perfusion system. A thin dialysis tubing is implanted in a desired region of the brain parenchyma. Samples of a few microliters in size are analyzed for endogenous amino acids by means of liquid chromatography according to Lindroth and Mopper (*12*).

A. Dialysis Probe

The dialysis sampling probes consist either of a straight piece of dialyzing tubing (10 × 0.3 mm o.d., acrylic copolymer, Hollow Fiber H1×50, 50,000 MW cut off, Amicon Corporation, or Cuprophan B4AH, 3000 MW cut off, Cobe Laboratories, Inc.) or of the tubing in a loop arrangement. In the latter, two apposed stainless-steel cannulae serve as inlet and outlet. The straight piece (5–10 mm long) is glued between nylon tubings and the inlet and outlet are usually on opposite sides of the skull (Fig. 1).

B. Surgical Procedures

For the loop-type probe surgical procedures do not differ from those of electrode implantation. A holder is fastened on the skull surface with steel screws and dental cement. The straight tubings require a somewhat more complicated technique (Fig. 1). In the present studies on the hippocampus of 1.5–2 kg rabbits, the skull bone was exposed for bilateral bone trepanations (ϕ 3.5 mm) at a level 4 mm behind the coronal suture and 18 mm lateral of the sagittal suture. The meninges were coagulated, and stainless-steel screws with a 0.7 mm i.d. piece of annula in the center were aligned while being screwed into the bone with a simple sliding caliper device. This setup is prepared for the correct insertion of a 100–120 mm long, 0.3–0.5 mm thick steel guide from one side of the skull to the other. The guide then

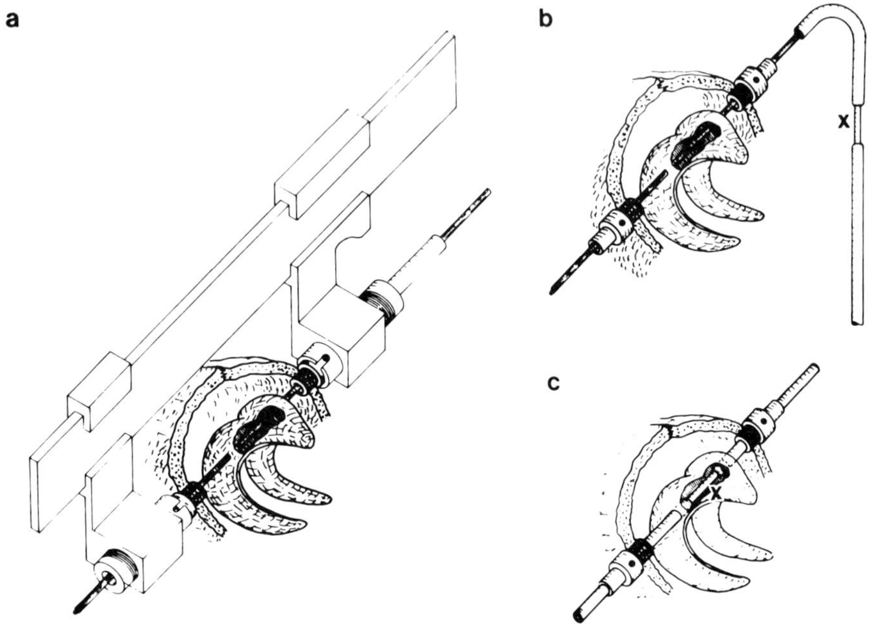

Fig. 1. Sketch of implantation of dialysis tubing in the rabbit hippocampus. (a) Insertion of screws in trepanized holes and stainless-steel guide (ϕ 0.5 mm) through the anterior part of hippocampus. (b) Nylon tubing glued onto guide. Dialysis tubing (X) glued between the pieces of nylon tubings. (c) Dialysis tubing (X) pulled into position in the hippocampus.

is used to pull the 10-mm nylon dialysis tubing (X in Fig. 1), previously glued to it, until reaching the desired position in the frontal part of the hippocampus. The connecting nylon tubings are fastened onto the cannula–steel screw fittings with cyanoacrylate. The screw fittings are then secured in the skull bone with dental cement.

C. Perfusion-Dialysis Procedure

The cannulae on each side serve as inlet and outlet for the perfusion fluid, Krebs–Ringer bicarbonate solution, which is delivered at a rate of 2.5 μl/min with a precision pump (Bioinvent AB, Lidingö, Sweden). Experiments are done from the day after implantation of the dialysis tube, at which time the animals are unanesthetized and moving freely. The connections are sealed between experiments. The perfusate is collected usually in 10-min fractions. Small, Micro-Fuge (Beckman) tubes are fastened at the outlet tube, the end of which is slightly widened (by pressing the heated end of the tube against a flat surface) to ensure a tight fitting of the tube.

III. FINDINGS

A. Optimization of Experimental Procedures

1. *IN VITRO* TESTS

Transport of amino acids into the dialysis tubing occurs mainly as a result of concentration driving forces. Some of the basic relationships have been examined *in vitro*, the dialysis tubing being bathed in media with known concentrations of amino acids. These experiments revealed a nonlinear, inverse relationship between perfusion rate through the tubing and recovery (concentration dialysate/bathing medium × 100) of amino acids (Fig. 2).

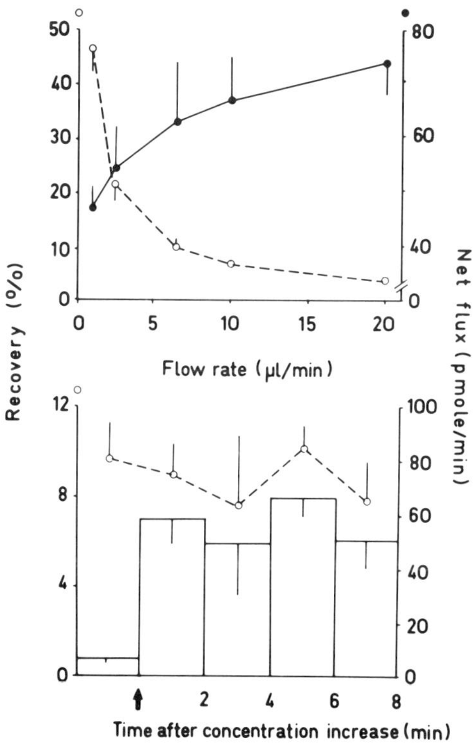

Fig. 2. Top: Effect of flow rate in the dialysis tube on [^{14}C]glutamate recovery and net flux in a model experiment. Five-minute fractions were collected and assayed for radioactivity. The concentration of glutamate was 100 µ*M* (---). Radioactivity ratio inside/outside × 100 (recovery); (——), net flux of radioactivity into the dialysis tube; *N* = 4. Means ± SD. Bottom: Effect on the recovery of a sudden increase of [^{14}C]glutamate in the external solution. External concentration increased from 10 µ*M* to 100 µ*M* (arrow). Two-minute fractions. Flow rate 6.5 µl/min. Open circles indicate net flux into the probe. Dotted lines indicate the recovery; *N* = 3. Means ± SD.

TABLE I

Transport Characteristics—Cuprophan B4AH Dialysis Tubing[a]

Amino acid	Recovery: Perfusion rate (μl/min) 1	2.5	20	200	Net inflow: Perfusion rate (μl/min) 1	2.5	20	200
Asp	54	22	4	1	100	100	150	250
Glu	57	21	9	5	100	100	360	1400
Gln	52	21	3	0.4	100	100	130	100
Tau	61	33	4	0.8	80	100	120	150
Ala	59	26	5	1.6	90	100	160	370
Val	48	20	3	0.7	100	100	150	220
Phe	39	19	3	0.5	100	100	150	170
Ileu	41	17	4	0.8	100	100	170	300
Leu	40	17	4	0.5	100	100	150	200

[a] 0.3 mm o.d., length 6–7 mm. Recovery (dialysate/medium × 100) and net inflow (recovery × vol/min) at different perfusion rates assayed *in vitro*. Net inflow at 2.5 μl/min set to 100.

The net flow of amino acids into the dialysis tubing increased with increasing flow rate at the same time as recovery decreased. The recovery was almost linearly related to the fiber length in the range studied (4–20 mm). The response to a quick change in the concentration of amino acids was fully achieved in the first fraction when 2-min fractions were collected and the perfusion rate was 6 μl/min. The recovery was independent of external concentrations of amino acids in the range 10^{-6}–10^{-3} *M*. The properties of the dialysis tubing were tested in KRB medium and in CSF. The recovery factors varied somewhat among amino acids and were around 40% for a 10-mm dialysis tubing perfused at 2.5 μl/min.

By using the recovery percentage at a given perfusion rate for a specific amino acid (Table I), the extracellular concentration is calculated (e.g., for taurine in a 2.5 μl/min perfusion experiment, extracellular concentration = concentration in perfusate/0.33).

2. CALCULATION OF AMINO ACID CONCENTRATIONS IN THE EXTRACELLULAR FLUID

The amino acid concentrations in the dialysates from the implanted tubings were suitable for the calculation of their concentrations in the extracellular space of the brain parenchyma. This presumption implies that no damaged cells are present that could leak amino acids, that no clogging of the fiber occurs in the brain, and that the extracellular fluid around the tubing is in a steady state. Light and electron microscopic examinations

TABLE II

Comparisons between the Levels of Free Amino Acids in Plasma, Cerebrospinal Fluid (CSF) and Extracellular Fluid in the Hippocampus and in the Olfactory Bulb of the Rabbit[a]

		Extracelluar fluid		
Amino acid	Plasma	Hippocampus	Olfactory bulb	CSF
Taurine	43	6	11	6
Phosphoethanolamine	20	5	4	11
Glutamic acid	46	4	2	11
Glutamine	868	267	266	578
Alanine	382	15	10	39
Valine	191	12	7	15
Leucine	81	9	—	8
Lysine	137	21	—	8

[a] Micromoles per liter.

indicated very little brain cell damage, although small bleedings were occasionally observed. The steady-state situation was tested by increasing the perfusion rate for 1 hr to increase the net efflux of amino acids from the brain. Upon return to the original perfusion rate, the concentration of amino acids in the dialysate was the same as before the high-speed perfusion. The cell-response findings, in terms of amino acid increments in the extracellular fluid during perfusion with K^+ or veratridine (see later) with subsequent return to basal amino acid levels, also speak in favor of a reasonable steady-state situation. The calculated concentration in the extracellular fluid was lower than the CSF levels for a number of amino acids, whereas others were found to be similar in the two compartments (Table II). Again, this provides evidence against the possibility of clogging, although this problem cannot be completely ruled out. The amino acid concentration in the dialysate was steady over several days, making it most unlikely that clogging occurs.

3. BASAL LEVELS OF AMINO ACIDS

The levels of free amino acids in the extracellular space of the rabbit hippocampus (Table II) were calculated from the concentrations in the dialysate during perfusion at 2.5 μl/min. Corresponding values for the CSF are also shown. The concentrations of taurine, valine, and leucine were similar in the extracellular fluid and CSF, while glutamate, glutamine, alanine, and lysine concentrations in the extracellular fluid were approximately 50% of those in the CSF. The levels in the extracellular fluid apparently decreased

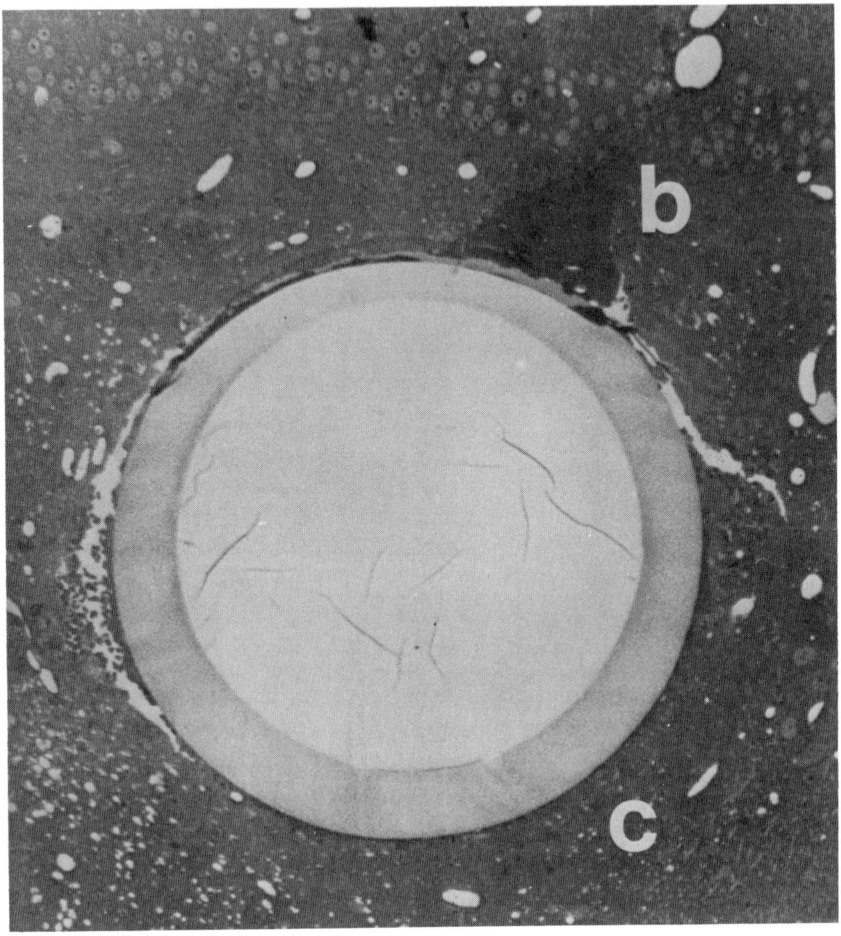

Fig. 3. (a) Low-power photomicrograph of the Cuprophan dialysis tubing (ϕ 0.3 mm) in the hippocampus 3 days after implantation (b and c; regions shown in Figs. 3b and c).

slightly during continuous perfusion for a few hours on the day after implantation. At that time, the levels had stabilized and were highly reproducible during perfusion recordings over the subsequent 3–4 days. The only exception was glutamate which tended to increase on the second and third day, probably because of uncontrolled glutamine breakdown.

Table II also illustrates the amino acid concentrations in the extracellular fluid of the olfactory bulb while being perfused at 6.5 μl/min with a loop-type fiber during the day of implantation and in the anesthetized animal. The results agree fairly well with those from the hippocampus. As the con-

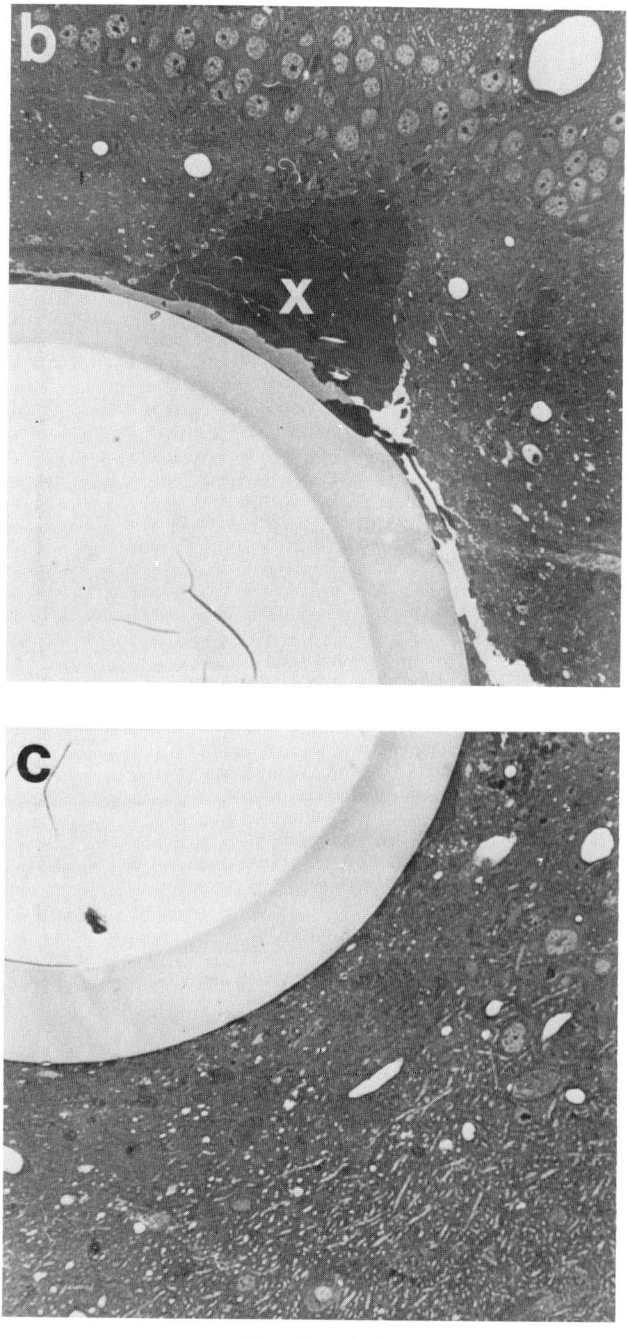

Figs. 3B and C.

centrations from different regions measured at different times agree, and as the extracellular fluid had a characteristic pattern of amino acids differing from that in the CSF, it is confirmative that the calculated data are a true representation of amino acids in the extracellular fluid.

4. TISSUE DAMAGE

In a number of animals, the tubing had been implanted "chronically" (up to 4 weeks) in order to check whether a gliosis reaction would develop around the tubing. In such a case, amino acid changes might be correlated with morphological changes in the parenchyma surrounding the tubing. Under "bacteria-free" conditions the brain parenchyma was in close apposition to the tubing (Fig. 3), with no nonneuronal cells present except for a few erythrocytes (up to 8 days after implantation). However, in spite of a rigorous condition of sterility during the implantation surgery, bacterial growth inside the tubing could not always be avoided without treating the rabbits with chloromycetin (50 mg iv × 2 daily). In cases of chronic implantation and insufficient sterility, the cells immediately surrounding the fiber had the appearance of macrophages and leukocytes. Outside this region, a striking gliosis developed in 7–9 days, as revealed by immunohistochemical staining for the presence of the glia marker protein S-100. Presently, the effect of mitosis inhibitors are being tested to see whether it might be possible to suppress the proliferation of nonneuronal cells. The percentage of successful perfusions is now over 95%.

B. Neurobiological Applications

1. TISSUE/EXTRACELLULAR CONCENTRATION RATIOS OF AMINO ACIDS

The concentration ratios between free amino acids extracted from the hippocampus tissue and amino acids in the extracellular fluid are given in Table III. Amino acids from total hippocampus were measured in 70% ethanol extracts of dissected, weighed, and homogenized tissue samples. Since the extracellular space in the CNS is in the range of 10% of the volume, and since the concentration of almost all amino acids in the extracellular fluid is less than 10% of that in total tissue, the contribution of extracellular amino acids to the total free acids is less than 1% and, consequently, negligible.

A ranking of amino acids according to the intracellular/extracellular concentration ratio (Table III) agrees well with that of *in vitro* studies on tissue/medium ratios (*8*), although the absolute numbers seen here are higher than in tissue slice experiments. The ratios were particularly high for the transmitter amino acids GABA and glutamate, reflecting the efficient sodium-dependent uptake systems in both nerve terminals and glia for the removal of

TABLE III

Intra-Extracellular Concentration Ratios for Amino Acids During Conditions Close to Steady-State *in Vivo* Rabbit Hippocampus

Amino acid	Intracellular/ extracellular
Taurine	287
Phosphoethanolamine	304
Glutamic acid	2694
Glutamine	18
Alanine	153
GABA	9000
Valine	11
Leucine	12
Lysine	7

neuroactive compounds from the extracellular space. This is demonstrated in Fig. 4 where the effect of nipecotic acid is seen when present in the medium perfusing the hippocampus. Nipecotic acid is one of the most potent inhibitors of GABA uptake by both neuronal and glial cells (*7, 19*). With 0.5 m*M* nipecotic acid in the medium, the GABA level in the dialysate increased from hardly measurable to a level half of that for glutamate, while at 2 m*M* nipecotic acid, GABA was 10–20 times the control. Glutamate was

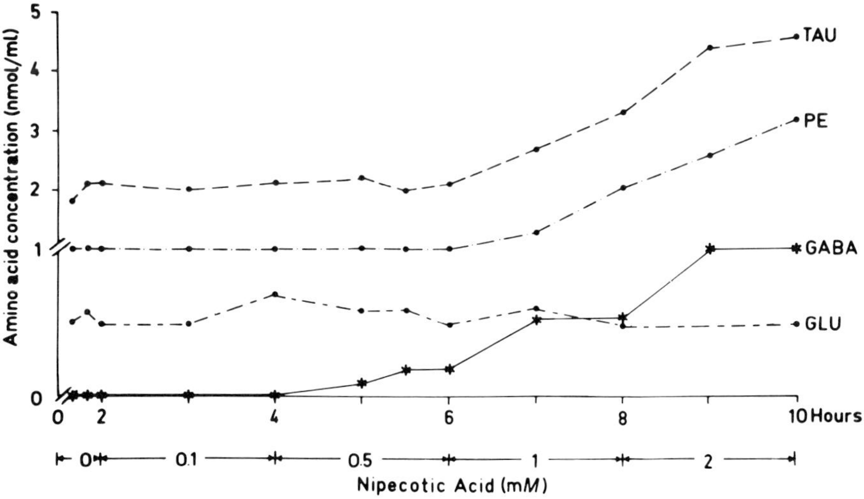

Fig. 4. Effect of increasing concentrations of nipecotic acid in the perfusion medium on the extracellular concentration of GABA, glutamate, phosphoethanolamine, and taurine.

unaffected, but both taurine and phosphoethanolamine levels increased at 1 and 2 m*M* nipecotic acid. The reasons for the latter increases are presently unknown by the authors. The effect on GABA transport agrees well with the results obtained in tissue slice experiments by Szerb (*21*).

2. INDUCED RELEASE OF AMINO ACIDS

Release of amino acids from the intracellular to the extracellular compartment was achieved chemically by perfusion through the dialysis tubing with media containing 56 or 80 m*M* K^+ or 100 μ*M* veratridine, and electrically by stimulation of nerve tracts terminating in the perfused region or near the dialysis tubing.

Perfusion of the hippocampus via the dialysis tubing with modified KRB, containing 56 or 80 m*M* K^+, caused an increase in endogenous glutamate (2–5 ×), GABA (0–10 ×), taurine (7–10 ×), and phosphoethanolamine (4–6 ×). Alanine also increased slightly, while the concentrations of most other amino acids were unaffected. The quantitatively dominating effect by K^+, however, was the decrease in glutamine concentration to approximately 50% of the control. Generally, 80 m*M* K^+ was at least 50% more powerful than 56 m*M* K^+ in releasing amino acids. However, the reaction pattern was similar at the two concentrations. Testing the Ca^{2+} dependence of the release is obviously connected with difficulties. Perfusion with Ca^{2+}-free media for 30–60 min decreased the calculated extracellular Ca^{2+} from 1.2 to 0.75 m*M*. Free calcium was measured in the perfusate with ion-selective elctrodes. Calibration and calculations were done as for amino acids (see previously). The Ca^{2+} could apparently be further decreased by perfusion with EGTA-containing media. So far a significant reduction in the evoked release of taurine has been observed after a decrease in extracellular Ca^{2+}. When 1 m*M* nipecotic acid was added to the perfusion medium, starting 120 min before pulsing with 80 m*M* K^+, the depolarization-induced efflux of GABA increased by over five times (Fig. 5).

Veratridine (100 μ*M*) perfusion of the rabbit olfactory bulb increased significantly the extracellular concentrations of GABA (40 ×), aspartate (2 ×), glutamate (2 ×), and taurine (2 ×). Phosphoethanolamine and alanine were virtually unaffected, while glutamine concentration again decreased by approximately 30%. Tetrodotoxin at 2 μ*M* completely blocked the effects in GABA, glutamate, and aspartate. The decrease in glutamine, which was also inhibited by tetrodotoxin, suggests its close coupling to the transmitter amino acids, particularly glutamate and GABA (*25*).

A close look at the time course of veratridine effects revealed that the response of GABA was rapid at first (maximal after 2 min) and then declined, while the responses of glutamate and aspartate were sustained (same level at 30 min compared with 5 min after start of veratridine perfusion). At the other

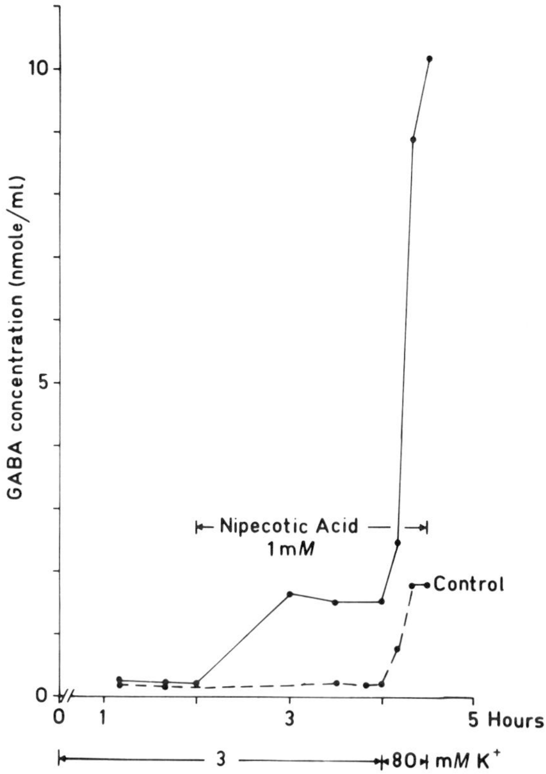

Fig. 5. Effect of 1 m*M* nipecotic acid in the perfusion medium on endogenous GABA before and during release evoked by 80 m*M* K^+ in the medium.

extreme, the response of taurine was negligible at 5 min while still increasing at 30 min after the start of veratridine perfusion. This "delayed response" of taurine was also seen in the hippocampus during K^+ depolarization.

A comparison of veratridine-induced release *in vivo* and *in vitro* with olfactory bulb slices (0.4 mm) in a perfusion system (0.1 ml/min) is shown in Fig. 6. The basal efflux was normalized to glycine for comparison of *in vitro* with *in vivo* levels. At 5 min, GABA release was considerable both *in vivo* and *in vitro*. At 30 min, the increase *in vivo* had declined and a fairly good correlation was seen between the *in vivo* and *in vitro* situations. However, with the exception of GABA, amino acid release *in vivo* was considerably more modest than in the *in vitro* situation, most likely due to the efficient reuptake systems in the living brain.

Electrical stimulation was used with the dialysis sampling probe im-

Basal efflux of amino acids in arbitrary units (Gly = 100)		GLY	TAU	GLU	ASP	GABA
	In vitro	100	44	9	4	6
	In vivo	100	53	12	2	1

Veratridine induced efflux of amino acids

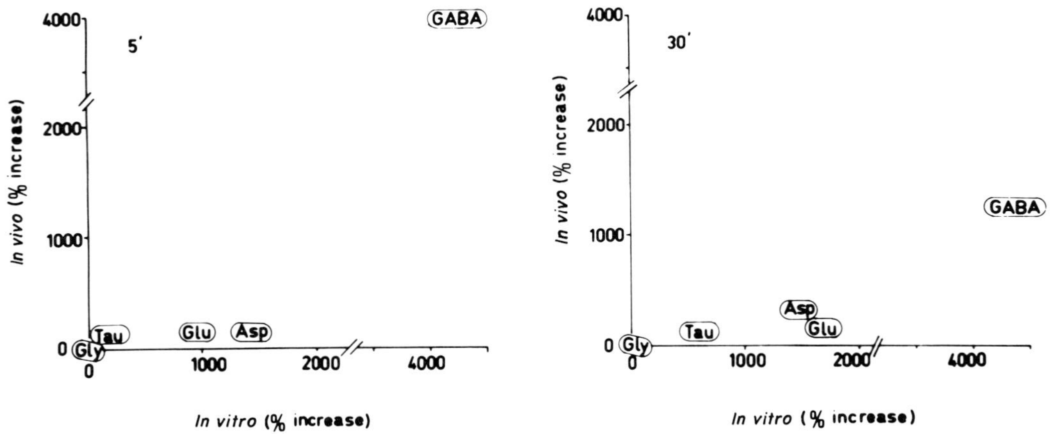

Fig. 6. *In vivo–in vitro* correlation of veratridine (100 μ*M*) induced release of endogenous glycine, taurine, glutamate, aspartate, and GABA at 5 min (left) and at 30 min (right) after start of veratridine perfusion. Increases expressed as evoked portions in percentage of basal levels. Basal levels were normalized to the glycine concentration for comparison *in vivo* and *in vitro* (top).

planted in the dorsolateral geniculate nucleus of the cat (*18*). Local stimulation (50 Hz, 2 mA, delivered as 500 msec-long impulse trains at 100 Hz, 1 impulse train/sec for 5–10 min) caused a four- to five fold increase in aspartate, GABA, and glutamate levels and a two fold increase in taurine. Glutamine behaved also in an inverse manner here, decreasing in concentration in response to stimulation (Fig. 7). Other amino acids were unaffected. Stimulation of the optic nerve or in the visual cortex caused an increase in concentration for a number of amino acids as well as those previously mentioned. The effects were also quite variable from one animal to the other.

3. KAINIC ACID

The original view of kainic acid as a pure glutamate agonist, acting on postsynaptic receptors, has been somewhat modified in later years. Unbalanced ion fluxes, depletion of high-energy phosphates, and neuronal cell death are some of the events in kainic acid neurotoxicity (*13*). Focal injections of kainic acid in the hippocampus induce motor manifestations, including seizures, via its "distant" effects (*10, 20*). Furthermore, analysis of various brain regions after treatment has revealed a concentration reduction in a number of transmitters due to extensive nerve cell death (*15*).

Perfusion of the hippocampus with kainic acid at 1.0 m*M* in the dialysis tubing induced epileptiform activity in the animal (9). Glutamate, taurine, and phosphoethanolamine concentrations increased selectively and significantly during perfusion with 0.1 m*M* kainic acid. Kainic acid (1.0 m*M*) with time, however, increased amino acid concentrations in the perfusate in an unselective way (Fig. 8). In contrast to K^+ and veratridine, kainic acid had no decreasing effect on the glutamine levels, a fact which may support a glial origin for the released glutamate, in accordance with the work of Krespan *et al.* (6).

4. THE GLUTAMINE-GLUTAMATE SYSTEM

As indicated, glutamine was the dominant amino acid compound in the dialysates from all regions studied to date. This is hardly surprising as glutamine accounts for 65% of the total amino acid content in the CSF. Glutamine, being nonneuroactive per se, is a precursor of both glutamic acid and GABA in those nerve terminals rich in glutaminase (*2, 17*). Glutamine synthetase, on the other hand, is essentially a glial enzyme (*16*). Local perfusion of the hippocampus with inhibitors, first, of glutamine synthesis (methionine sulfoximine, MSO), and second, of glutaminase (6-diazo-5-oxo-L-norleucine, DON) would provide information on the consequences of changing the conditions of glutamine availability and of utilization, respectively.

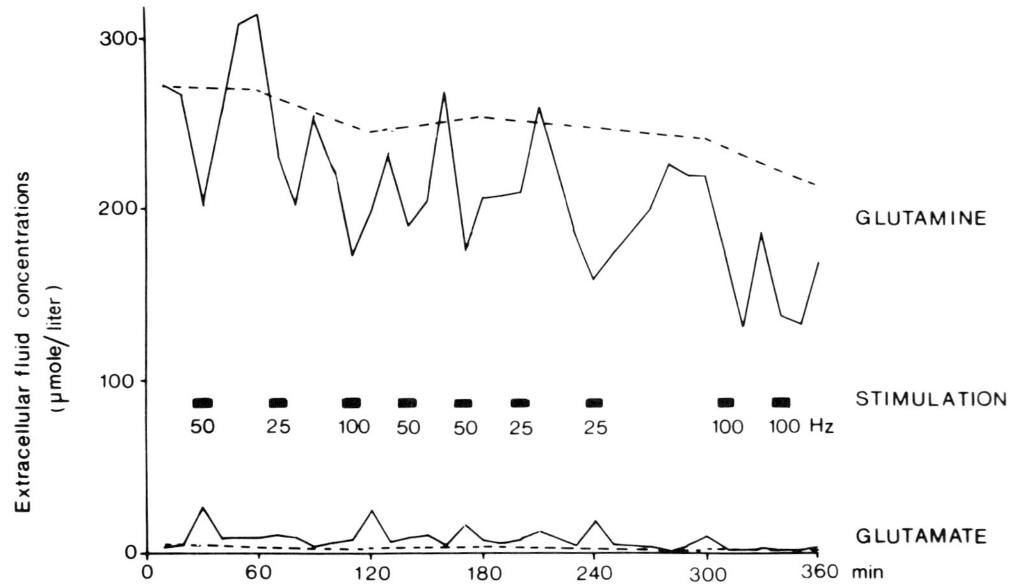

Fig. 7. Effect of repeated, local, electrical stimulation in the dorsolateral geniculate nucleus of the cat on extracellular levels of endogenous glutamate and glutamine. (——), Amino acid levels during electrical stimulation; (---), control levels.

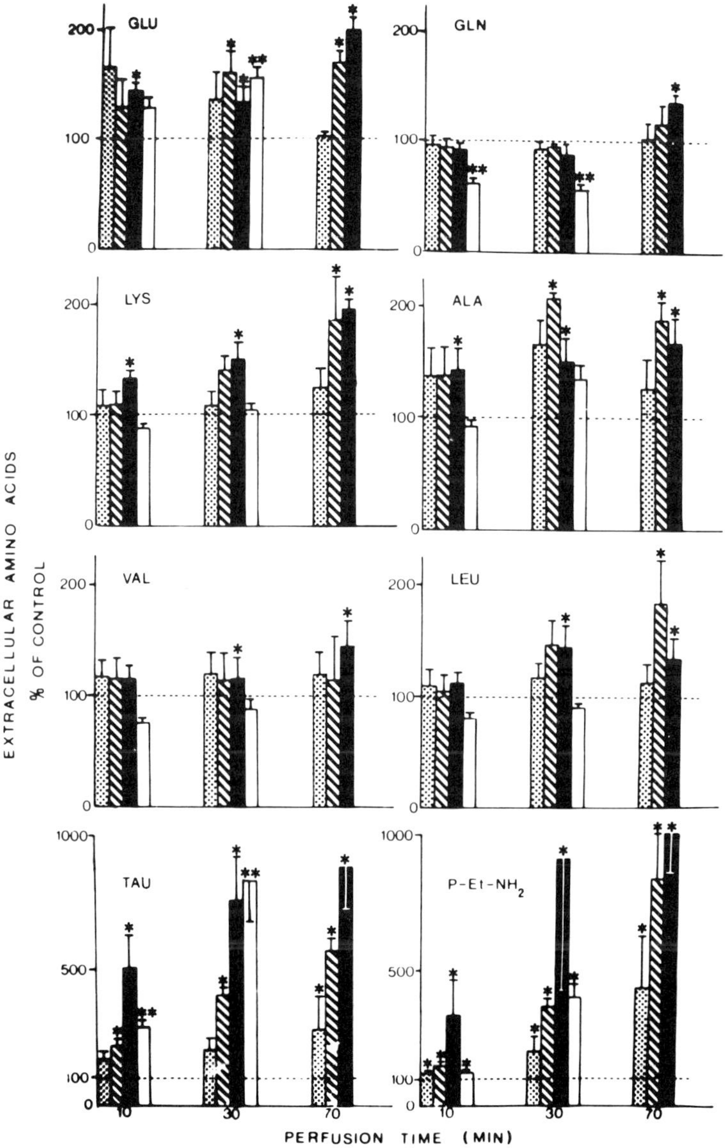

Fig. 8. Effects of kainic acid (dotted, 0.1 m*M;* striped, 0.5 m*M;* and black, 1 m*M*) or K^+ (unfilled, 56 m*M*) on the concentration of endogenous amino acids in the extracellular fluid of the rabbit hippocampus. The effects are shown as percentage of baseline levels (---) at 10, 30, and 70 min after the beginning of kainic acid or K^+ perfusion. *, $p < .05$; **, $p < .01$.

Perfusion with MSO at 2 m*M* for 1 hr decreased glutamine by 80% and glutamate by 40% in the extracellular fluid. On the other hand, alanine levels increased by 200% while other amino acids were unaffected. DON (10 m*M*) in the perfusion medium had no effect on glutamine concentration but decreased glutamate in a similar way to MSO. Alanine also increased after DON treatment (by 200%). Thus, although both MSO and DON decreased the glutamate levels significantly, they were unable to inhibit the K^+-evoked increase of glutamate. This correlation suggests that glucose plays an important role as the direct precursor of glutamate and may even compensate for a reduced availability of glutamine.

5. EXPERIMENTAL HEPATIC ENCEPHALOPATHY

Several types of liver damage induce morphological (gliosis) and functional excitation, coma) changes in the CNS (*3*). One of the causative factors is ammonia which increases severalfold in all body fluids, including those of the brain. Ammonia is detoxicated only by glutamine formation in the brain and, furthermore, ammonia inhibits the breakdown of glutamine. Consequently, liver failure results in a disturbance in the precursor system for glutamate and GABA.

Experimental acute liver failure was produced with galactosamine intravenously (*14*), and the effects on amino acids were monitored in the hippocampal extracellular fluid, in the blood plasma, and eventually, in the hippocampus after the death of the animal. Virtually all plasma amino acids increased 20–45 hr after galactosamine injection. Serine, asparagine, glutamine, methionine, tyrosine, ornithine, and lysine were particularly elevated. Although amino acids in the extracellular fluid also increased, the change was considerably more modest than in plasma. Analysis of the hippocampal tissue showed a greater increase in amino acids than was found in the extracellular fluid. These results show that an induced increase in amino acids in the brain affects intracellular more than extracellular levels (Fig. 9).

IV. PERSPECTIVES

The potentials and advantages of techniques for *in vivo* studies of neuroactive substances are obvious, and they open a new field of physiological neurochemistry. The biochemical synaptology as a response to physiological stimulation may appear an ideal approach to transmitter identification. The gap in time resolution to the real events is, however, of many orders of magnitude. This, together with an almost similar gap in size between probe and synapse, limits the role of dialysis techniques to describing excitation-

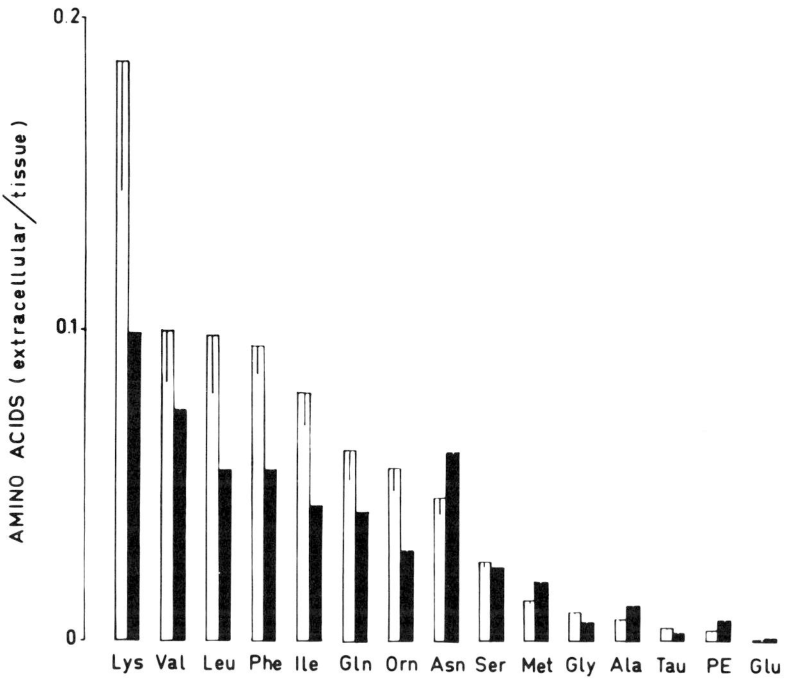

Fig. 9. Concentration ratio of extracellular/intracellular amino acids in the hippocampus of the rabbit. Unfilled bars represent control animals, while black bars represent animals which had received 6.75 mmol/kg of galactosamine 45 hr before the experiment.

related biochemical changes in defined CNS regions. The drawback in comparison with, for example, electrodes for intracellular recording is obvious. To date, exact implantations and physiological stimulations have been only in the visual system in our laboratory (*18*). Upon stimulation of either the optic nerve or the visual cortex in the cat, amino acids such as alanine, valine, aspartate, glutamate, GABA, and taurine, and even serine accumulated in the extracellular fluid of the lateral geniculate body. This and other preliminary findings have led us to conclude that the presynaptic signal most likely is contaminated by active uptake phenomena, metabolic changes causing amino acid fluxes in the excited postsynaptic neuron (+ glia?), as well as excitation of secondary nerve tracts. Technically, a combination and uptake inhibitors may be the solution, but the number of potential substances of importance in a given region would require a considerable "conditioning cocktail." A certain amount of progress with inhibitors of GABA uptake is given in Section III. These limitations refer to endogenous amino acids which are the only group of neuroactive substances we have studied so far. The use of radioactive amino acid isotopes gives only an apparent solution, as different uptake pools and metabolism may simply add to the confusion.

A number of advantages of the dialysis techniques are seen once the limitations are recognized. The effects of conditions or drugs on the nervous system, previously reported as an increase or decrease in all or single free amino acids extracted from a dissected region, may now be extended to separate analyses of the intra- and extracellular compartments. A 1% change in total glutamate in an area, for example, is deleterious if it reflects a change in the extracellular fluid, but harmless for the intracellular compartments. The metabolic pathways of the brain are more easily and economically studied, since a radiolabeled precursor can be employed at maximal specific radioactivity for a long time without the usual waste of 99% or so in *in vivo* experiments. In addition, ion fluxes are also available for analysis without the use of implanted intracerebral electrodes. Experimental foci of different types can be induced. Epileptic foci, for example, can be induced by perfusion with penicillin, kainic acid, or other agents, providing an idea of the innumerable neuropharmacological applications that exist. The absence of a blood–brain barrier between the dialysis membrane and the brain parenchyma allows easier testing of many substances. Furthermore, the passage of administered drugs from blood to brain may also be followed continuously. Since the dialysis systems are easily combined with electrodes for EEG recording, the response from local application of a drug is conveniently recorded.

ACKNOWLEDGMENTS

This work was supported by grants from the Swedish Medical Research Council (12X-00164) and from Axel and Margret Axelson Johnsons Foundation. The skillful secretarial work of Ms. Gull Grönstedt also is gratefully acknowledged.

REFERENCES

1. Bito, L., Davson, H., Levin, E., Murray, M., and Snider, N. The concentrations of free amino acids and other electrolytes in cerebrospinal fluid, *in vivo* dialysate of brain and blood plasma of the dog. *J. Neurochem.* **13** (1966) 1057–1067.
2. Bradford, H. F., and Ward, H. K. Glutamine as a metabolic substrate for isolated nerve-endings: inhibition by ammonium ions. *Biochem. Soc. Trans.* **3** (1975) 1223–1226.
3. Conn, H. O., and Lieberthal, M. M. (eds.). *In* "The Hepatic Coma Syndromes and Lactulose," 1979. Williams & Wilkins, Baltimore, Maryland.
4. Delgado, J. M. R., De Feudis, F. V., Roth, R. H., Ryngo, D. K., and Mitruka, B. M.

Dialytrode for long-term intracerebral perfusion in awake monkeys. *Arch. Int. Pharmacodyn.* **198** (1972) 9–21.

5. Hamberger, A., Jacobson, I., Molin, S.-O., Nyström, B., Sandberg, M., and Ungerstedt, U. Metabolic and transmitter compartments for glutamate. *In* "Neurotransmitter Interaction and Compartmentation," (H Bradford, ed.). 1982, pp. 359–378. Plenum, New York.
6. Krespan, B., Berl, S., and Nicklas, W. J. Alteration in neuronal-glial metabolism of glutamate by the neurotoxin kainic acid. *J. Neurochem.* **38** (1982) 509–518.
7. Krogsgaard-Larsen, P., and Johnston, G. A. R. Inhibition of GABA uptake in rat brain slices by nipecotic acid, various isoxazoles and related compounds. *J. Neurochem.* **25** (1975) 797–802.
8. Lajtha, A. Transport as control mechanism of cerebral metabolite levels. *Prog. Brain Res.* **29** (1968) 201–218.
9. Lehmann, A., Isacsson, H., and Hamberger, A. Effects of *in vivo* administration of kainic acid on the extracellular amino acid pools in the rabbit hippocampus. *J. Neurochem.* **40** 1983 1314–1320.
10. Lenique, P. M., Wepierre, J., and Cohen, Y. Protection by 4-aminohex-5-enoic acid (gamma-vinyl GABA) and hypobaric hypoxia against kainic acid neurotoxicity. *Psychopharmacology* **66** (1979) 51–53.
11. Lerma, J., Martin del Rio, R., Solis, J. M., and Delgado, J. M. R. Dynamics of brain amino acids determined by dialytrodes. *Neurosci. Lett.* (Suppl.) **10** (1982) 290.
12. Lindroth, P., and Mopper, K. High-performance liquid chromatographic determination of subpicomole amounts of amino acids by precolumn fluorescence derivatization with O-phthaldialdehyde, *Anal.Chem.* **51** (1979) 1667–1674.
13. McGeer, P. L., McGeer, E. G., and Hattori, T. Kainic acid as a tool in neurobiology. *In* "Kainic Acid as a Tool in Neurobiology," (E. G. McGeer, J. W. Olney, and P. L. McGeer, eds.), 1978, 123–138. Raven, New York.
14. Miller, D. J., Hickman, R., Fratter, R., Terblanche, J., and Saunders, S. J. An animal model of fulminant hepatic failure: a feasibility study. *Gastroenterology* **71** (1976) 109–113.
15. Nicklas, W. J., Duvoisin, R. C., and Berl, S. Amino acids in rat neostriatum: Alteration by kainic acid lesion. *Brain Res.* **167** (1980) 107–117.
16. Norenberg, M. D., and Martínez-Hernández, A. Fine structural localization of glutamine synthetase in astrocytes of rat brain. *Brain Res.* **161** (1979) 303–310.
17. Salganicoff, L., and De Robertis, E. Subcellular distribution of the enzymes of the glutamic acid, glutamine and γ-aminobutyric acid cycles in rat brain. *J. Neurochem.* **12** (1965) 287–309.
18. Sandberg, M. An approach to the identification of neurotransmitters in the optic nerve-evoked release of amino acids and related compounds. Thesis, University of Göteborg, 1982. Göteborg, Sweden.
19. Schousboe, A., Krogsgaard-Larsen, P., Svenneby, G., and Hertz, L. Inhibition of the high-affinity, net uptake of GABA into cultured astrocytes by β-proline, nipecotic acid and other compounds. *Brain Res.* **153** (1978) 623–626.
20. Schwarcz, R., Zaczek, R., and Coyle, J. T. Microinjection of kainic acid into the rat hippocampus. *Eur. J. Pharmacol.* **50** (1978) 209–220.
21. Szerb, J. C. Effect of nipecotic acid, a γ-aminobutyric acid transport inhibitor, on the turnover and release of γ-aminobutyric acid in rat cortical slices. *J. Neurochem.* **39** (1982) 850–858.
22. Ungerstedt, U., Herrera-Marschitz, M., Jungelins, U., Ståhle, L., Tossman, U., and Zetterström, T. Dopamine synaptic mechanisms reflected in studies combining behavioural recordings and brain dialysis. *Adv. Dopamine Res.* **37** (1982) 219–231.

9

Voltammetry Measurement *in Vivo* of Neurotransmitter Release in the Freely Moving Rat

PETER J. KNOTT,* CHRISTOPHER D. ANDREWS, AND KATHYRNE J. MUELLER

Department of Pharmacology
Marshall University School of Medicine
Huntington, West Virginia

I. INTRODUCTION

The concept of neurohumoral transmission is fundamental to our understanding of changes of brain function during both spontaneous and drug-induced behavioral states. Despite general acceptance among neuroscientists that neuronal communication is chemically mediated and that demonstration of release is an important criterion for establishing a substance as a neurohumoral agent, comparatively few approaches have been developed for the measurement of neurotransmitter release from brain tissue *in*

*Present address: Departments of Psychiatry and Pharmacology, The Mount Sinai Medical Center, One Gustave L. Levy Place, New York, New York 10029.

ISBN 0-12-083350-6

vivo. Moreover, very few methods are available which allow the monitoring of neurotransmitter release from discrete brain regions in the conscious, behaviorally unrestrained animal. Ventricular perfusion, while feasible in larger conscious animals, presents considerable difficulty in the rat, with collectable outflow being successfully obtained in only a small number of experiments (*31, 32*). Other complications of ventricular perfusion are cerebral hemorrhage and increased intracranial pressure which appears if the outflow rate drops below the inflow rate (*31*). Additionally, measurement of neuroactive substances will tend to reflect only release from structures bordering the ventricular system. Cortical perfusion, while possible in the larger unanesthetized animals such as the rhesus monkey (*2*), is generally unsuitable for smaller animals and, of course, only provides information on release of neuroactive substances from the cortical surface. The use of push–pull cannulae offers the advantage of perfusing discrete portions of brain tissue (*13*), and versions of this approach have been used to study neurotransmitter release in unanesthetized animals. Furthermore, the development of extremely sensitive and specific analytical procedures such as GC-MS, radioenzymatic assay, and high-performance liquid chromatography (HPLC) has facilitated the measurement of amines and their metabolites in the small volumes of perfusate collected by this method. For example, push–pull perfusion and analysis by HPLC have enabled the measurement of hypothalamic norepinephrine release in the conscious rat (*29, 37*), and a cannula incorporating a dialysis membrane has been used to measure caudate dopamine release in rotating rats (*41*). Use of push–pull cannulae is technically difficult in the rat and occlusion of the outflow may result in significant tissue damage (*31*).

In vivo voltammetry (or *in vivo* electrochemistry), a completely different approach to the measurement of neuroactive substances and their metabolites, is based on established electroanalytical techniques and has evolved in the past decade, pioneered by the groups of Adams (*17, 21*) and Lane (*24, 25*). With this methodology, electroactive substances located extraneuronally in brain tissue may be oxidized at a miniature electrode (usually of graphite paste or carbon fiber) by the application of a potential difference between the electrode and the tissue surrounding it. The neurotransmitters dopamine (DA), norepinephrine (NE), and 5-hydroxytryptamine (5HT) and their metabolites dihydroxyphenylacetic acid (DOPAC), homovanillic acid (HVA), and 5-hydroxyindoleacetic acid (5HIAA) are electrooxidizable whereas a number of other neurotransmitters are not (e.g., acetylcholine, γ-aminobutyric acid, glutamic acid). Optimal oxidation occurs at characteristic potentials for individual substances, and the current generated by passage of electrons into the working electrode may be measured and is proportional to the concentration of molecular species oxidizing at the electrode surface. The potential is applied relative to a standard reference electrode (usually silver–silver chloride) which just makes contact with the brain surface. It is common practice to use a third auxiliary electrode which functions by feedback to rigidly control the applied potential (*21*). Variants of this method have now been used in numerous laboratories. Thus, electrochemical measurement *in vivo* of either DA release or changes in the extraneuronal concentration of DOPAC have been measured reflecting altered striatal dopaminergic activity (*4, 9, 10, 14–18, 22, 24–27, 36, 39, 40*). Similarly, altered serotonin release or extraneuronal changes of 5HIAA concentration have been measured by voltammetric techniques in the striatum (*5, 6, 7, 25, 28*), in the hippocampus (*19, 20*), and in the spinal cord (*35*). *In vivo* voltammetry lacks some of the methodological problems seen with perfusion techniques which are dependent on the successful flow and collection of the perfusate. It also enables the monitoring of extraneuronal molecular concentrations of substances (providing they are electroactive) at smaller surfaces which range from 8 to 250 μm in diameter. Voltammetric electrodes may be placed stereotaxically at precise loci. In addition, electrical connections allowing free movement of the animal are more easily effected than are fluid inflow–outflow lines. *In vivo* electrochemistry allows either frequent sampling and therefore a better time resolution (every 30 sec with chronoamperometry) or the measurement of extraneuronal concentrations of neuroactive substances chronically over periods of several weeks. The major advantage that perfusion techniques have over *in vivo* electrochemical methods is that they allow accurate identification of the substance being measured. Whereas neurotransmitters may be measured both quantitatively and qualitatively in perfusion fluids with considerable accuracy using advanced analytical methods currently available, some controversey surrounds the identity of substances which are detected by voltammetry *in vivo*. For example, when voltammetric measurements are obtained from the rat striatum with carbon-paste electrodes, significant contributions to DA oxidation current may be produced by DOPAC (*14*) or by ascorbic acid (*3, 15, 34*). Various modifications in electrode construction and pretreatment have culminated in the successful resolution of DOPAC (*14, 15*) and ascorbic acid (*12*), and the elimination of ascorbic acid contribution because the electrode tip is surrounded with a dialysis membrane containing ascorbic acid oxidase (*33*). Improved catecholamine specificity with carbon-paste electrodes may be achieved by the addition of stearic acid which repels acidic moieties such as ascorbic acid and DOPAC from the electrode surface (*40*).

In the studies described here we have initially evaluated the specificity of the stearate-modified electrodes in detecting DA in the presence of ascorbic acid and also determined oxidation potentials of several neurotransmitters and metabolites because electrode surface changes may produce shifts of the voltammetric peaks. These studies were followed by investigations of the striatal voltammetric responses to administration of drugs generally accepted to influence DA release and metabolism in parallel with locomotor activity.

II. METHODS

A. Electrodes

Working electrodes were constructed from Teflon-coated silver wire (250 μm diameter). The end of each was packed with carbon paste to a depth of about 0.5 mm. The carbon paste (140 mg stearate, 0.9 g silicone oil, 2.1 g Ultra F carbon powder) was prepared with added stearic acid which enhances the selectivity for DA (*40*). Each reference electrode was formed from chloridized silver wire in a small conical well (disposable plastic pipette tip which was cut to about 1 cm in length) plugged with cotton and filled with a solution of 10% gelatin in 3 *M* sodium chloride (see Fig. 1).

B. Surgical Procedures

Male Sprague–Dawley rats were housed for 1 week in an environmentally controlled room (22°C, lights on 0600 hr: off 1800 hr) before surgical implantation of the voltammetric electrodes. Routinely four working electrodes were implanted bilaterally in each rat brain: two in the striatum [stereotaxic coordinates: A, 8.00 mm, L, 2.5 mm, H, 0.0 mm (*23*)] and two in the nucleus accumbens, although in the studies described here only results from striatal recordings are discussed. Electrodes were placed under Nembutal anesthesia (60 mg/kg). Additionally a silver–silver chloride reference electrode and an auxiliary electrode (stainless-steel screw) were placed in burr holes to make contact with the brain surface. Electrodes were soldered to gold-plated connecting pins in a Teflon pedestal connector (Plastic Products, Roanoke, Virginia). Two additional steel screws were placed into the skull to form an anchor for the pedestal and electrode assembly which was surrounded by cranioplastic cement. At least 48 hr were allowed for recovery before obtaining voltammetric recordings. At the end of each study rats were anesthetized and perfused with 10% formal saline. Fixed brain specimens were sectioned and stained to verify accurate electrode placement.

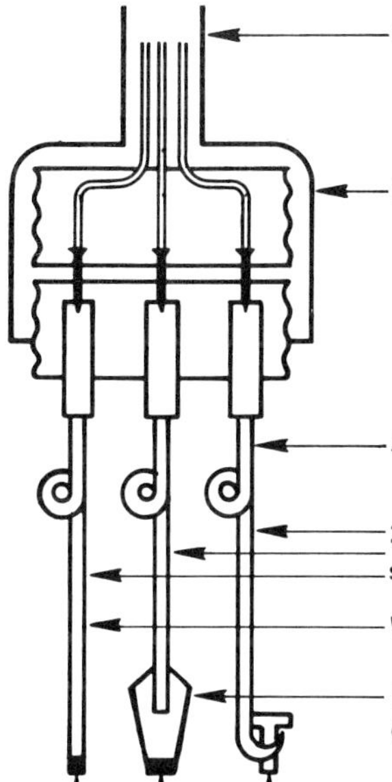

Fig. 1. All three electrodes are formed from 250-μm Teflon-coated silver wire in the following manner. (a) Working electrode: The wire is straightened by slightly stretching. About 2 mm of insulation is stripped from one end and the Teflon sleeve pulled down over the other end to form a well (0.5–1.0 mm depth), after which a tight loop is made near the bare end which is ultimately soldered to a gold-plated connector pin. The loop prevents the Teflon coating from sliding after the electrode is made. The well is packed by tamping the wire repeatedly into the carbon paste. Surplus paste is removed by wiping. Finally, each electrode surface is polished by twisting the end on a piece of Teflon tape stretched across the rim of a petri dish. (b) Reference electrode: Silver wire is bared (2.0 mm) at each end and tightly looped as above. One end is chloridized by immersing in 1 *N* hydrochloric acid and passing an anodal current between this and a copper cathode (E=3.0 V), which gives a pale gray coating of AgCl. The chloridized end is then pushed into a shortened 200-μl disposable pipette tip, plugged with cotton, and filled with 10% gelatin in 3 *M* sodium chloride solution. The wire is fixed in place with a bead of cranioplastic cement at the wider end. (c) Auxiliary electrode: Teflon-coated silver wire (about 4.0 cm in length) is bared for 2.0 mm at each end. One end is wrapped around a stainless-steel screw fixed in a midline burr hole and just makes contact with the brain surface.

C. Recording Procedures

The methodology used was essentially similar to that described in earlier studies (*8, 22, 24*). A potential difference was applied between each of the working electrodes and the tissue surrounding them, starting at −200 mV and scanning up to +500 mV at a constant rate (10 mV/sec). The generated current from the oxidation of electroactive substances at the electrode surface was recorded (after conversion to a measurable voltage) either in relation to the applied voltage (on an X-Y recorder) or against time using a strip chart recorder. It appears most unlikely that the applied potential modifies neuronal firing since the ongoing behavior of the animal is not altered by the recording procedure. With our voltammetry controller (see later), we have the additional facility of being able to process the current output in a semidifferentiated form (i.e., we are recording the rate of change of the generated current) which improves peak resolution from the background current.

1. AUTOMATED CONTROL OF ELECTROCHEMICAL MEASUREMENTS

We have previously used custom-built instrumentation for performing the timing and electrode selection (multiplexing) functions but found the system to be inflexible and not readily adapted for storage of digitalized data. The *in vivo* voltammetric technique is still rapidly developing and a system with greater flexibility is a high priority. Others have described computer-controlled instrumentation (*8, 27*) but since these systems require mainframe computers, we have built a system based on the versatile and comparatively inexpensive Apple II+ microcomputer. A block diagram of the system is shown in Fig. 2. Timing functions of the Apple II+ are controlled by a clock calendar card (Mountain Hardware) which connects to the multiplexer through an 8-bit parallel interface card. This allows the reference electrode and any of four working electrodes to be connected appropriately to the voltammetry controller (Bioanalytical Systems DCV5) at any predetermined interval. The microcomputer was programmed to switch on the chart recorder (Houston Omniscribe fitted with a remote control for the chart drive), followed by connection of the electrodes, to initiate voltage scans of the voltammetry controller and finally to stop the chart drive after recording from the working electrodes. With this system, consecutive scans were obtained from each working electrode at 12-min intervals. In addition to supplying the output from the DCV5 voltammetry controller to the chart recorder for hard copies of the voltammograms, we were able to collect data on disc following processing of the output with a 10-bit analog-digital converter. Thus, in addition to measuring voltammetric peak heights from the Y-T recordings we could also integrate areas under these peaks. A full description of the construction of this system may be obtained from the authors.

2. CONCURRENT BEHAVIORAL AND ELECTROCHEMICAL RECORDING FROM THE RAT

Rats were placed in a sound-attenuated environmentally controlled chamber (Fig. 3) and connections from the electrodes were made through

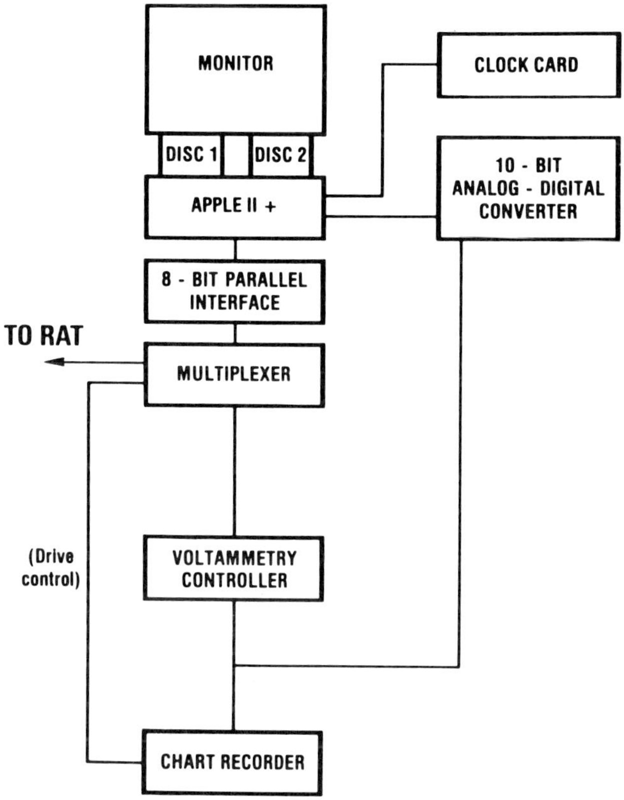

Fig. 2. Block diagram of microcomputer-controlled voltammetric equipment. The equipment was situated outside the environmental chamber which housed the rat during recording. Automated connection of electrodes, the voltage scanning produced by the DCV5 voltammetry controller, and on–off switching of the chart recorder were all regulated by the Apple II+ microcomputer. In addition, data could be collected and stored on disc following analog-digital conversion.

the pedestal to a multichannel slip ring (*1*) which connected to the microcomputer-controlled voltammetry equipment and recorder situated outside the chamber. The recording cage was placed in a beam-type animal activity recorder (Columbus Instruments, Optovarimax) for monitoring the rats' locomotor activity. The counter for the activity monitor was also located outside the environmental chamber. Additional facility for remote observation of the animals' behavior was provided by a video monitor and recorder outside the chamber which received input from the TV camera (Panasonic) situated about 3 ft from the rat and located inside the chamber.

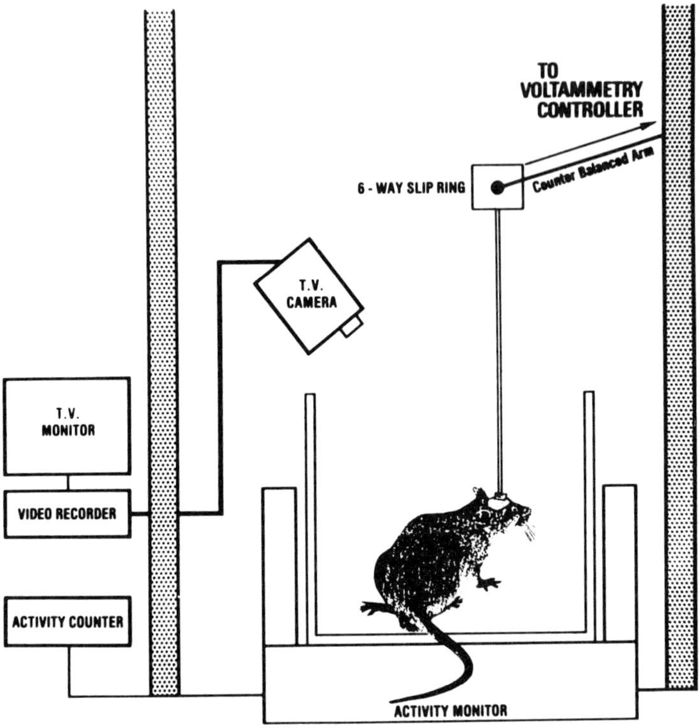

Fig. 3. Electrochemical recording and behavioral monitoring of the rat.

III. FINDINGS

A. Optimization of the Experimental Procedures

1. STUDIES *IN VITRO*

Electrode specificity: Preliminary investigations were made *in vitro* to evaluate the viability of stearate-modified electrodes for measurement of brain DA *in vivo*. In these studies unmodified carbon-paste electrodes were compared with those prepared from the stearic acid–carbon paste mixture.

Figure 4 shows linear sweep voltammograms using semidifferential output of solutions of DA (100 μm) and of ascorbic acid (1 m*M*) obtained with the modified electrode. With mixtures of DA (100 μm) and abscorbic acid (1 m*M*) using the unmodified electrode (Fig 4b) only a single composite peak was obtained, whereas addition of stearic acid to the electrode paste gave two peaks. The oxidation potentials for peaks 1 and 2 in the mixture corresponded with voltammetric peaks obtained with single solutions of DA and

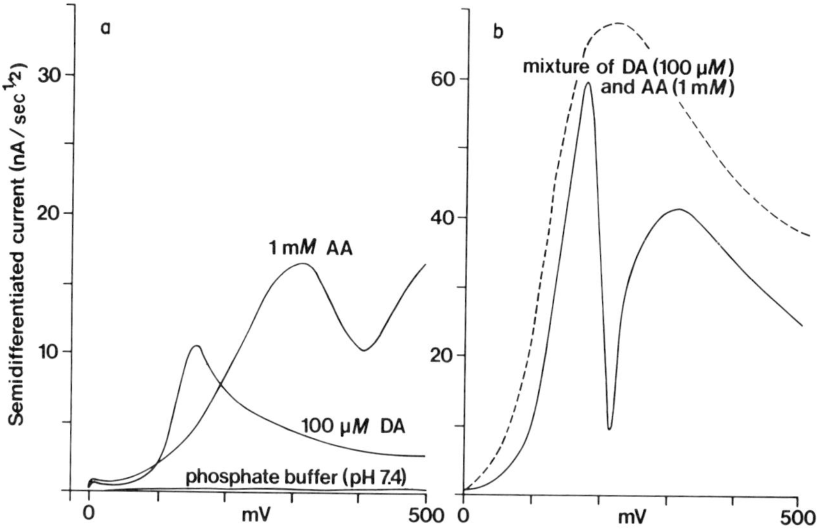

Fig. 4. Linear sweep voltammograms *in vitro* of dopamine (DA) and ascorbic acid (AA). (a) Linear sweep voltammogram of a solution of DA (10 μ*M*) and of AA (1 m*M*) seen with the stearate-modified electrode. (b) Linear sweep voltammogram of a mixture of DA (100 μ*M*) and AA (1 m*M*) seen with the stearate-modified electrode (———) and with a carbon–silicon oil electrode without added stearate (---).

ascorbic acid, respectively. We have also found that if the concentration of ascorbic acid in the mixture was reduced from 1 m*M* to below approximately 200 μm [i.e., about the concentration found in the rat brain (*30*)], then the peak corresponding to ascorbic acid oxidation progressively diminished until it produced only a small increase in background oxidation current and only the peak apparently due to DA remained.

In other studies *in vitro* we investigated the responsiveness of the stearate-modified electrodes to other electroactive amines and metabolites of importance to striatal neuronal function. Table I summarizes the responses recorded *in vitro* of DA, its acid metabolites DOPAC and HVA, and also of 5HT and its acid metabolite 5HIAA alone in 0.1 *M* phosphate-buffered 0.9% saline (pH 7.4) and in buffer containing 1 m*M* ascorbic acid. The responses of DA and, to a lesser extent, DOPAC and HVA were potentiated in the presence of ascorbic acid. This has been explained by rapid oxidation of DA followed by reduction in the presence of an excess of a second readily oxidizable species (i.e., ascorbic acid). Cycling apparently occurs with larger surfaced electrodes or in situations where the oxidizing potential is applied for a comparatively long duration, as with linear sweep voltammetry, but may be minimal with small (8 μm) carbon-fiber electrodes when using chronoamperometry (*11*). There appeared to be little augmentation of

TABLE I

Summary of Responses *in Vitro*[a]

	In pH 7.4 buffer			In buffer containing 1 m*M* AA		
Compound	Concentration	Peak (mV)	nA/sec$^{1/2}$ [b]	Peak (mV)	nA/sec$^{1/2}$ [b]	Response
DA	100 μ*M*	151	9.2	91	57.4	6.2X
DOPAC	100 μ*M*	202	2.3	184	8.1	?[c]
HVA	100 μ*M*	382	2.9	410	13.2	4.6X
AA	1 m*M*	179	5.5	164	23.1	4.2X[d]
5HT	100 μ*M*	315	8.4	314	9.7	1.2X
5HIAA	100 μ*M*	365	8.8	—[e]		
Creatinine	1 m*M*	—[f]				

[a] Summary of responses recorded *in vitro* to a variety of compounds both in 0.1 *M* phosphate buffer (pH 7.4) and in buffer containing 1 m*M* ascorbic acid (AA). The responses to DA and to a lesser extent its metabolites (DOPAC and HVA) were potentiated in the presence of ascorbic acid. For example, the response to DA was potentiated 6.2-fold. Creatinine was also tested because 5HT used in these studies was only available as creatinine phosphate salt. Values are means obtained from at least 4 electrodes.

[b] nA/sec$^{1/2}$ = semidifferentiated current.

[c] DOPAC and ascorbic acid peaks merged but appeared to be additive.

[d] The response to ascorbic acid recorded in 100 μ*M* DA was potentiated.

[e] Not tested.

[f] Not electroactive in this range.

the 5HT peak oxidation current produced by the presence of ascorbic acid. We conclude from these *in vitro* experiments that the stearate-modified electrodes are able to differentiate between DA and ascorbic acid, but when ascorbic acid concentrations are increased, there is a significant potentiation of the voltammetric response to DA. However, it may be relevant that the concentrations of ascorbic acid used in these *in vitro* studies are considerably higher than those reported for rat brain tissue (*30*), that extraneuronal concentrations of ascorbic acid may not fluctuate appreciably (*38*), and that administration of large doses of ascorbic acid to rats (1 g/kg) only raised its brain concentration by about 20% (Mueller, Andrews, Veneziano, and Knott, unpublished). Therefore, the potentiation of DA voltammetric responses by ascorbic acid in brain may be of minimal importance.

2. STUDIES *IN VIVO*

Linear sweep voltammetry in the striatum: Figure 5 shows a single voltammogram from a striatal electrode in a conscious rat. In earlier studies, voltammograms were obtained using a scan rate of 10 mV/sec over a range of 0–500 mV. More recently, we found that scanning from −200 to +500 mV improved the separation of the peak identified from *in vitro* studies as DA. Subsequently we have routinely adopted these conditions, obtaining volt-

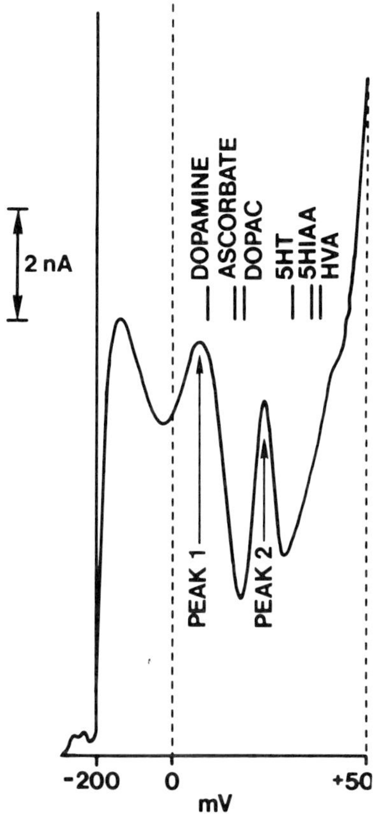

Fig. 5. Linear sweep voltammogram from the rat striatum. The recording was obtained with stearate-modified electrodes from a conscious freely moving rat by scanning from −200 mV to +500 mV. Peak 1 appeared to reflect dopamine oxidation based on its response to pharmacological manipulations (see Figs. 6–8). Peak 2 may result from oxidation of 5-hydroxyindoles but awaits identification.

ammograms at 0.2-hr intervals for several hours. Peak oxidation potential *in vivo* showed some variation, but the mean positions were as follows: peak 1, 74.6 + 4.1 mV; peak 2, 222.8 + 2.1 mV (N=16). Figure 4 also shows for comparison the peak positions for DA, ascorbic acid, DOPAC, 5HT, 5HIAA, and HVA that we obtained from *in vitro* studies.

B. Neurobiological Applications

A method which allows the measurement of certain neurotransmitters from discrete brain regions during ongoing behavior or during concurrent physiological changes would obviously provide an immensely powerful tool for understanding central neural control mechanisms. In our previous work we have examined the changes of striatal electrochemical signals in relation to tail pinch-induced gnawing, licking, and biting (a DA-mediated behavior) and found a remarkable parallelism between striatal signal increases and the provoked behavior (*10, 18, 22*). Obviously, if the changes of electrochemical oxidation current at peak 1 reflect altered DA release, then this should also be modified in an appropriate direction by drugs which either increase or decrease DA release. We describe here the results of such experiments in which amphetamine, which is believed to release DA, and γ-butyrolactone, which decreases nigral activity, were investigated. Furthermore, inhibition of monoamine oxidase also would be expected to increase the peak 1 signal if it reflected extracellular DA but to decrease this peak if it resulted from the acid metabolite DOPAC.

1. EFFECTS OF AMPHETAMINE ADMINISTRATION

Figure 6 shows a series of voltammograms obtained at 0.2-hr intervals in an individual animal from a striatal electrode over a 6-hr period before and following the administration of amphetamine (2.0 mg/kg, ip) 1 hr after starting the recording. Studies *in vitro* show that amphetamine is not elec-

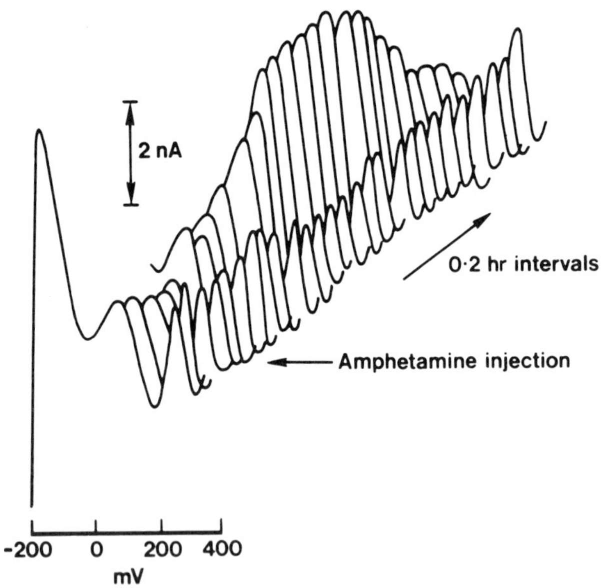

Fig. 6. Effect of amphetamine on striatal oxidation peaks. Consecutive linear sweep voltammograms obtained at 0.2-hr intervals from the rat striatum over a 6-hr period are shown here in sequence. Amphetamine (2 mg/kg, ip) was injected at 1 hr and produced a large increase of peak 1.

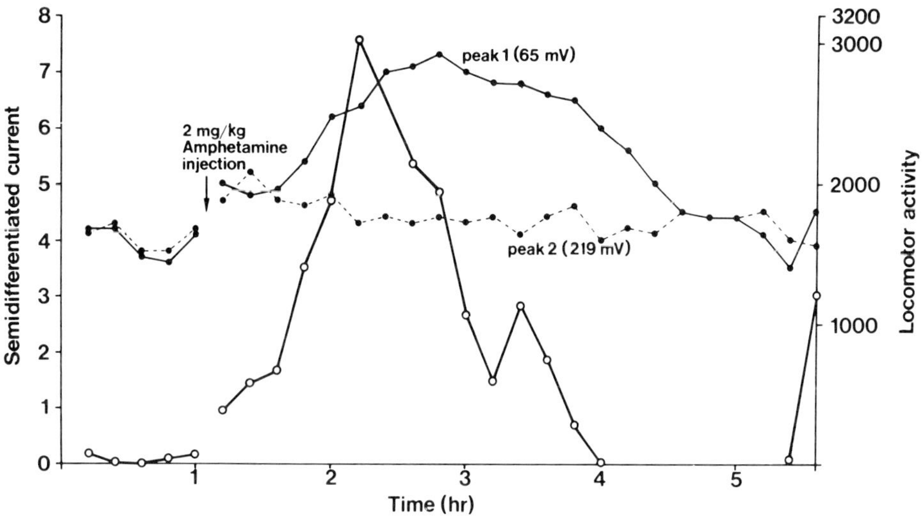

Fig. 7. Effect of amphetamine on striatal voltammetric signal and locomotor activity. Amphetamine was injected 1 hr after the start of recording. The semidifferentiated oxidation current of peaks 1 and 2 from a striatal electrode obtained at 0.2-hr intervals is plotted against time. General locomotor counts are also shown (○——○).

troactive per se. The peak occurring at 75 mV, which we believe to reflect extraneuraonal DA oxidation, was considerably increased following amphetamine injection to about 190% of the basal values. The other characteristically sharp peak shown in this series occurred at approximately +230 mV and was unchanged following amphetamine. Figure 7 shows data derived from the same experiment together with changes of locomotor activity occurring after amphetamine administration. The increase in the height of peak 1 broadly paralleled the increase in locomotor activity which we have substantiated in many other experiments.

2. EFFECTS OF γ-BUTYROLACTONE

γ-Butyrolactone (GBL) (250 mg/kg, ip) injection was found to reduce the magnitude of peak 1 which returned to pre-injection values after several hours. Figure 8 shows the changes in an individual rat and is one of several experiments in which similar changes were observed. This is also consistent with another study using 1-hydroxy-3-aminopyrrolidone-2 (HA-966) which, like GBL, reduces dopaminergic activity and has been demonstrated to reduce striatal DA release measured by differential pulse voltammetry (4). We also observed that the decrease in the height of this striatal oxidation peak was always accompanied by a complete suppression of general locomotor activity. Typically, peak 2 showed a rapid increase up to about 50

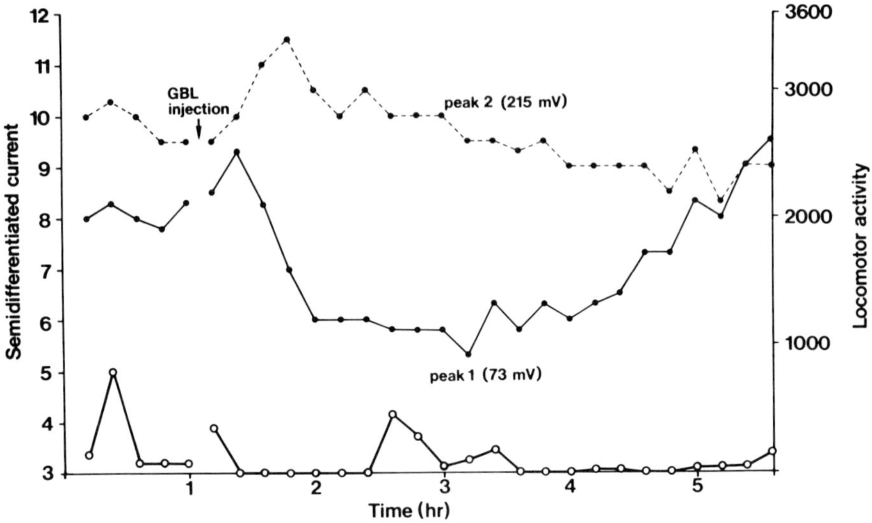

Fig. 8. Effect of γ-butyrolactone on striatal voltammetric signal. GBL (250 mg/kg, ip) was injected 1 hr after the start of recording. Values of peaks 1 and 2 obtained from semidifferential linear sweep voltammograms are plotted at 0.2-hr intervals together with general locomotor activity (○——○).

min after injection followed by a progressive decline over the next few hours.

3. EFFECTS OF MONOAMINE OXIDASE INHIBITION

The monoamine oxidase inhibitor pargyline (75 mg/kg, ip) caused a gradual increase in peak 1, which is thought to reflect extraneuronal DA concentration, and reached 83% above pre-injection levels 5 hr after injection (Fig. 9). The increase of peak 1 following monoamine oxidase inhibition is

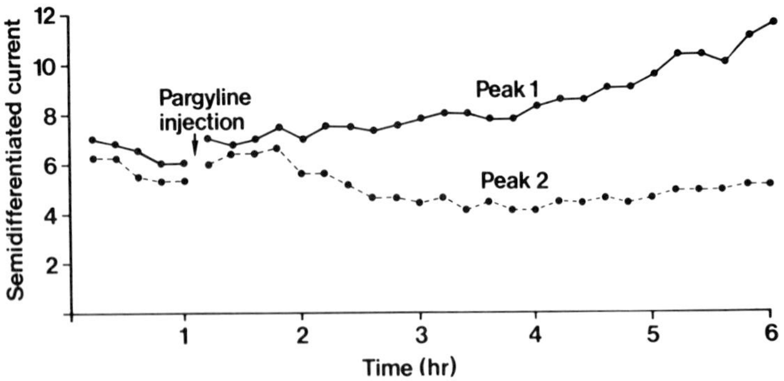

Fig. 9. Effect of monoamine oxidase inhibition. Pargyline (75 mg/kg, ip) was injected 1 hr after the start of recording. Values of peaks 1 and 2 are plotted at 0.2-hr intervals.

consistent with the peak being produced by amine. Peak 2, however, declined to a minimum 25% below pre-injection values after 2 hr. It seems probable that this second peak represents, at least in part, a monoamine acid metabolite because it is reduced following inhibition of monoamine oxidase.

IV. PERSPECTIVES AND DISCUSSION

The ability to relate release of neuroactive substances to changes of behavior, physiological processes, and endocrine function has always been an attractive objective. Early interest in the electrochemical approach to the study of central neurotransmitters was stimulated by the discoveries that voltammetric signals recorded from the brain changed in response to electrical stimulation of brain nuclei (*9, 22, 35, 39*), to administration of drugs (*4, 9, 17, 22, 28*), and to altered sensory input (*10, 19, 22, 26*). The optimistic view was that the technique would provide a rapid and simple method to measure neurotransmitter release in the conscious animal. It is now realized that the voltammetric signals recorded from the brain probably reflect the oxidation of several substances at a given potential, with some not obviously related to neurotransmitter function. Accordingly, considerable effort is being made to overcome electrode selectivity problems by developing electrodes that have increased specificity for neuroactive substances.

The problem of the interference of ascorbic acid in the electrochemical detection of DA has already been mentioned. Some workers have attempted to remove ascorbic acid by utilizing the enzyme ascorbic acid oxidase. Using an "ascorbic acid eliminator" electrode, Adams and co-workers were still able to detect release of electroactive species from rat caudate slices (*33*), which they suggest may reflect extraneuronal changes of DA or DOPAC. Injection of ascorbic acid oxidase into the vicinity of unmodified carbon-paste electrodes located in the rat striatum or nucleus accumbens caused a large reduction in peak oxidation current, suggesting the remaining current reflected either DA or DOPAC (*3*). However, the potentiation of DA voltammetric signals in the presence of ascorbic acid suggests that when ascorbic acid is removed enzymatically, then the signal attributable to DA also will be decreased. This casts some doubt on the conclusions drawn from ascorbic acid oxidase injection that the contribution of DA to the early oxidation peak in normal brain tissue is minor (*3*). With the stearate modification our *in vitro* studies confirm the ability to separate DA from DOPAC and ascorbate voltammetric signals (*40*), although the potentiation of DA responses by ascorbic acid occurs *in vitro* and is likely to occur *in vivo* also. If extraneuronal ascorbic acid concentrations remain fairly constant, as has been suggested (*38*), then it may be that changes of peak 1 in our studies will reflect release of DA.

The identity of peak 2 occurring in the present studies at about 230 mV still remains unclear. We are currently investigating the components of this peak observed when voltammograms are obtained from the striatum with stearate-modified electrodes. In the absence of ascorbic acid *in vitro,* the 5-hydroxyindoles 5HT and 5HIAA oxidize at 315 and 354 mV, respectively, whereas DOPAC and HVA oxidize at 202 and 382 mV, respectively. Conceivably, in the presence of ascorbic acid and in brain tissue, a shift in the oxidation peaks to a more negative potential could mean that one or more of these substances contribute to peak 2. In some of our studies we have observed a small reduction of peak 2 following monoamine oxidase inhibition with pargyline, which suggests that it may be in part due to an acid metabolite. Certainly the sharpness of peak 2 indicates that if it results from more than one substance, then the oxidation potentials are very similar. Other workers have advanced compelling evidence that it is possible to measure an oxidation peak at a higher potential than the catecholamine peak, which appears to reflect serotonergic activity in the hippocampus (*19, 20*).

In conclusion, *in vivo* voltammetry offers a unique approach for the measurement of extraneuronal concentrations of substances in the brain of the freely moving animal. Variants of electrochemical methodology and modifications to electrode construction are under investigation both in our laboratory and elsewhere for improved analytical specificity in the measurement of substances of relevance to neuronal function. We are cautiously optimistic that methodological advances of *in vivo* voltammetry will ultimately provide an immensely powerful tool for investigating the relationship of neurotransmitter release with brain function.

ACKNOWLEDGMENTS

The research was supported by the National Institutes of Health (MH 35543-02 to P. J. K. and N50660-01A1 to K. J. M.).

REFERENCES

1. Andrews, C. D., and Hutson, P. H. A reliable multichannel commutator for making electrical connections with conscious, freely moving rats. *J. Neurosci. Meth.* **5** (1982) 73–76.
2. Beleslin, D. B., and Myers, R. D. A technique for the repeated perfusion or withdrawal of fluid from the exposed cerebral cortex of a conscious animal. *Physiol. Behav.* **5** (1970) 1173–1175.

3. Brazell, M. P., and Marsden, C. A. Intracerebral injection of ascorbate oxidase—effect on *in vivo* electrochemical recordings. *Brain Res.* **249** (1982) 167–172.
4. Broxterman, J. J., and Mos, J. Depamine hypoactivity measured by *in vivo* voltammetry. *Eur. J. Pharmacol.* **68** (1980) 389–391.
5. Cespuglio, R., Faradji, H., Riou, F., Buda, M., Gonon, F., Pujol, J. F., and Jouvet, M. Differential pulse voltammetry in brain tissue II. Detection of 5-hydroxyindolacetic acid in the rat striatum. *Brain Res.* **223** (1981) 299–311.
6. Cespuglio, R., Faradji, H., Ponchon, J. L., Buda, M., Riou, F., Gonon, F., Pujol, J. F., and Jouvet, M. Differential pulse voltammetry in brain tissue I. Detection of 5-hydroxyindoles in the rat striatum. *Brain Res.* **223** (1981) 287–298.
7. Cespuglio, R., Riou, F., Buda, M., Faradji, H., Gonon, F., and Jouvet, M. Mésure *in vivo* par voltametric impulsionnelle differentielle du 5-HIAA dans le striatum du Rat. *C. R. Acad. Sci. (Paris)* **190** (1980) 901–906.
8. Cheng, H. Y., White, W., and Adams, R. N. Microprocessor controlled apparatus for *in vivo* electrochemical measurement. *Anal. Chem.* **52** (1980) 2455–2488.
9. Conti, J. D., Strope, E., Adams, R. N., and Marsden, C. A. Voltammetry in brain tissue: chronic recording of stimulated dopamine and 5-hydroxytryptamine release. *Life Sci.* **23** (1978) 2705–2715.
10. Curzon, G., Hutson, P. H., and Knott, P. J. Voltammetry *in vivo:* effect of stressful manipulations and drugs on the caudate nucleus of the rat. *Br. J. Pharmacol.* **66** (1979) 127–128P.
11. Dayton, M. A., Ewing, A. G., and Wightman, R. M. Response of microvoltammetric electrodes to homogenous catalytic and slow heterogenous charge-transfer reactions. *Anal. Chem.* **52** (1980) 2392–2396.
12. Falat, L., and Cheng, H. Y. Voltammetric differentiation of ascorbic acid and dopamine at an electrochemically treated graphite/epoxy electrode. *Anal. Chem.* **54** (1980) 2108–2111.
13. Gaddum, J. H. Push–pull cannulae. *J. Physiol. (London)* **155** (1961) 1–2P.
14. Gonon, F., Buda, J., and Cespuglio, R. *In vivo* electrochemical detection of catechols in the neostriatum of anesthetized rats: dopamine of DOPAC? *Nature (London)* **286** (1980) 902–904.
15. Gonon, F., Buda, M., Cespuglio, R., Jouvet, M., and Pujol, J. F. Voltammetry in the striatum of chronic freely moving rats: detection of catechols and ascorbic acid. *Brain Res.* **223** (1981) 69–80.
16. Hefti, F., and Melamed, E. Dopamine release in rat striatum after administration of L-DOPA as studied with *in vivo* electrochemistry. *Brain Res.* **225** (1981) 333–346.
17. Huff, R., Adams, R. N., and Rutledge, C. D. Amphetamine dose-dependent changes of *in vivo* electrochemical signals in rat caudate. *Brain Res.* **173** (1979) 369–372.
18. Hutson, P. H., Knott, P. J., and Curzon, G. Tail pinch-induced gnawing: voltammetric and behavioral effects of fenfluramine. *In* "Central Neurotransmitter Turnover," (C. J. Pycock and P. V. Taberner, eds.), 1981, pp. 151–161. University Park Press, Baltimore, Maryland.
19. Joseph, M. H., and Kennet, G. A. Stress-induced release of 5HT in the hippocampus and its dependence on increased tryptophan availability: an *in vivo* electrochemical study. *Brain Res.* **270** (1983) 251–257.
20. Kennet, G. A., and Joseph, M. H. Does *in vivo* voltammetry in the hippocampus measure 5-HT release? *Brain Res.* **236** (1982) 305–316.
21. Kissinger, P. T., Hart, J. B., and Adams, R. N. Voltammetry in brain tissue—a new neurophysiological measurement. *Brain Res.* **55** (1973) 209–213.
22. Knott, P. J., Hutson, P. H., Scraggs, P. R., and Curzon, G. Electrochemical recording of brain catecholamine and serotonin release during behavioral changes. *In* "Function and

Regulation of Monoamine Enzymes: Basic and Clinical Aspects," (E. Usdin, N. Weiner, and M. B. H. Youdim, eds.), 1981, pp. 771–780. Macmillan, London.
23. König, J. F. R., and Klippel, R. A. "The Rat Brain: A Sterotaxic Atlas of the Forebrain and Lower Parts of the Brain Stem." 1963. Williams & Wilkins, Baltimore, Maryland.
24. Lane, R. F., Hubbard, A. T., and Blaha, C. D. Brain dopaminergic neurons: *in vivo* electrochemical information concerning storage, metabolism and release processes. *Bioelectrochem. Bioenerget.* **5** (1978) 504–525.
25. Lane, R. F., Hubbard, A. T., and Blaha, C. D. Application of semidifferential electroanalysis to studies of neurotransmitters in the central nervous system. *Electroanal. Chem.* **5** (1979) 117–122.
26. Lindsay, W. S., Herndon, J. G., Blakely, R. D., Justice, J. B., and Neill, D. B. Voltammetric recording from neostriatum of behaving rhesus monkey. *Brain Res.* **220** (1981) 391–396.
27. Lindsay, W. S., Kizzort, B. L., and Justice, J. B. Microcomputer controlled multielectrode system for *in vivo* electrochemistry. *Chem. Biomed. Environ. Instrum.* **10** (1980) 311–330.
28. Marsden, C. A., Bennett, G. W., Brazell, M., Sharp, T., and Stolz, J. F. Electrochemical monitoring of 5-hydroxytryptamine release *in vitro* and related *in vivo* measurements of indoleamines. *J. Physiol. (Paris)* **77** (1981) 333–337.
29. McCaleb, M. L., and Myers, R. D. 2-Deoxy-D-glucose and insulin modify release of norepinephrine from rat hypothalamus. *Am J. Physiol.* **242** (1982) 596–603.
30. Milby, K., Oke, A. F., and Adams, R. N. Detailed mapping of ascorbate distribution in rat brain. *Neurosci. Lett.* **28** (1982) 15–20.
31. Myers, R. D. Methods for perfusing different structures of the brain. *Meth. Psychobiol.* **2** (1972) 169–211.
32. Myers, R. D., and Brophy, P. D. Temperature changes in the rat produced by altering the sodium:calcium ratio in the cerebral ventricles. *Neuropharmacology* **11** (1972) 351–361.
33. Nagy, G., Rice, M. E., and Adams, R. N. A new type of enzyme electrode: the ascorbic acid eliminator electrode. *Life Sci.* **31** (1982) 2611–2616.
34. O'Neill, R. D., Grünwald, R. A., Fillenz, M., and Albery, W. J. Linear sweep voltammetry with carbon paste electrodes in the rat striatum. *Neuroscience* **7** (1982) 1945–1954.
35. Rivot, J. P., Chiang, C. Y., and Besson, J. M. Increase of serotonin metabolism within the dorsal horn of the spinal cord during nucleus raphe magnus stimulation as revealed by *in vivo* electrochemical detection. *Brain Res.* **238** (1982) 117–126.
36. Salome, J. D., Lindsay, W. S., Neill, D. B., and Justice, J. B. Behavorial observation and intracerebral electrochemical recording following administration of amphetamine in rats. *Pharmacol. Biochem. Behav.* **17** (1982) 445–450.
37. Salzman, S. K., and Sellers, M. S. Determination of norepinephrine in brain perfusates using high-performance liquid chromatography with electrochemical detection. *J. Chromatog.* **232** (1982) 29–37.
38. Shenk, J. O., Miller, E., Gaddis, R., and Adams, R. N. Homeostatic control of ascorbate concentration in CNS extracellular fluid. *Brain Res.* **253** (1982) 353–356.
39. Wightman, R. M., Strope, E., Plotsky, P., and Adams, R. N. *In vivo* voltammetry: monitoring of dopamine metabolites in CSF following release by electrical stimulation *Brain Res.* **159** (1978) 55–68.
40. Yamamoto, B. K., Lane, R. F., and Freed, C. R. Normal rats trained to circle show asymmetric caudate dopamine release. *Life Sci.* **30** (1982) 2155–2162.
41. Zetterström, T., Herrera-Marschitz, M., and Ungerstedt, U. Simultaneous estimation of dopamine release and rotational behavior induced by D-amphetamine in 6-OHDA denervated rats. *Neurosci. Lett.* (1981) S27.

II

Strategies

10

Dopamine Release and Neuronal Activity in the Two Nigrostriatal Systems

ANDRÉ CHÉRAMY,* RANULFO ROMO,†
AND JACQUES GLOWINSKI

Chaire de Neuropharmacologie
Groupe NB
Collège de France
Paris, France

I. INTRODUCTION

Despite the extraordinary progress made in neuroscience during the past decade, *in vivo* estimations of changes in transmitter release in the brain for various physiological or pharmacological situations have been made in only a few cases. Undoubtedly, studies performed on nigrostriatal dopaminergic neurons have opened new perspectives at a technical and a conceptual level. The first attempts to demonstrate the *in vivo* release of dopamine (DA)

*A. Chéramy is a research fellow of Rhône-Pulenc, Vitry, France.
†R. Romo is an IMSS fellow from Mexico City, Mexico.

ISBN 0-12-083350-6

in the striatum were made about 20 years ago (*28–30, 45–47*). However, successful results were only obtained when new sensitive techniques allowing the fine quantification of DA in superfusates were developed. Since 1966, our group has been contributing to this effort by using a new method based on measurement of the release of [^{3}H]DA continuously synthesized from [^{3}H]tyrosine (*2*). This approach appeared much more accurate than radioenzymatic estimation of unlabeled endogenous DA (*1, 6, 20, 44, 51*). As briefly reviewed in this chapter, experiments can now be performed on animals implanted with several push–pull cannulae which allow simultaneous estimates of the release of the transmitter from nerve terminals and dendrites of DA cells of the two nigrostriatal dopaminergic pathways. Thus, it is possible to elucidate precisely some of the main regulatory processes involved in the control of DA transmission in the basal ganglia.

II. METHODOLOGICAL CONSIDERATIONS

Acute *in vivo* experiments carried out to estimate the release of DA from the caudate nucleus (CN) and the substantia nigra (SN) were usually performed in halothane-anesthetized cats (*6, 24, 26, 36, 40, 41*). In some cases, "encéphale isolé" (*8, 36, 38*) or "gallamine-immobilized" (*2, 3*) preparations were used. Some chronic studies were also performed in the monkey (*6, 19*). Except in early studies where a cup was placed on the dorsal ventricular surface of the CN (*2, 3, 6, 19*), push–pull cannulae were generally used to superfuse simultaneously both CN and SN. In all instances the continuous superfusion of tissues with L[3,5-^{3}H]tyrosine (50 mCi/mmol) allowed the detection of very low amounts of [^{3}H]DA in superfusates. Under these conditions the resting release of newly synthesized [^{3}H]DA (0.5–2 nCi/10 min) was from 25 to 100 times the blank value. Materials, physiological and superfusion procedures, [^{3}H]tyrosine purification, and biochemical analysis have been described in detail elsewhere (*2, 11, 12, 19, 20, 26, 36, 40*).

III. CHANGES IN DOPAMINE RELEASE IN RELATION TO NERVE IMPULSE FLOW

Changes in [^{3}H]DA release observed after several experimental modifications of the activity of DA neurons have confirmed that the amount of DA released from nerve endings in the CN is related, at least partly, to nerve impulse flow. This was expected since messages traveling from dendrites through somata and down axons finally reach nerve terminals from where the neurotransmitter is released.

The influence of action potentials on DA release in the CN was demonstrated in experiments in which either local, nigral, or systematic treatments were applied. A reduction of [^{3}H]DA release was first observed after omission of calcium or addition of tetrodotoxin in the superfusing fluid (*3, 36*). A similar but temporary effect also occurred during a short cooling block of the SN (*36*), whereas this reduction of transmitter release became irreversible following either an electrocoagulation (*36*) of the SN or a frontal hemisection of the brain between the SN and the CN (*3*). In contrast, the depolarization of DA neurons induced either by nigral application of potassium (*22*) or by electrical or mechanical stimulation of the SN (*3, 36*) caused a transient increase in [^{3}H]DA release. Furthermore, halothane anesthesia, which enhances the firing rate of DA neurons (*56*), was also found to increase the release of [^{3}H]DA in the CN (*36*). Subsequent experiments consisted of nigral application of transmitters present in the SN and of their agonists or antagonists known to affect the activity of DA cells. For instance, the nigral application of substance P, which increases the activity of DA neurons, stimulated the release of [^{3}H]DA in the CN, whereas the blockade of substance P transmission with substance P antibodies induced the opposite effect (*7, 9, 32*). In contrast, the reduction of DA cell firing produced by glycine (*16*) was associated with a reduction of the ^{3}H-labeled transmitter release and this effect was blocked by strychnine (*8, 25*). Finally, since the microiontophoretic application of DA and of DA agonists has been shown to inhibit the activity of DA neurons, suggesting the presence of autoreceptors on DA cell bodies or dendrites (*4, 5, 17, 23*), the effects of DA or drugs affecting DA transmission were also investigated. Thus, the nigral application of DA, *d*-amphetamine (a DA releaser), or benztropine (a DA reuptake inhibitor) resulted in a decrease of [^{3}H]DA release from nerve terminals (*7, 11, 24, 38, 42*) (Fig. 1), whereas the inhibition of DA synthesis or the blockage of DA receptors by the local application of α-methylparatyrosine and neuroleptics, respectively, markedly enhanced the release of [^{3}H]DA in the ipsilateral CN (*11, 25, 42*) (Fig. 1). In fact, these latter experiments provided further support for the existence of a dendritic release of DA involved in the self-regulation of the activity of DA cells.

IV. DOPAMINE RELEASE FROM DENDRITES OF THE NIGROSTRIATAL DOPAMINERGIC NEURONS

The first direct indications suggesting that DA could be released from dendrites were obtained in *in vitro* experiments performed on slices of the rat SN (*21, 43*). This led us to look for the existence of this process *in vivo* using experimental conditions identical to those selected in studies of DA release at the CN level. A spontaneous release of newly synthesized [^{3}H]DA

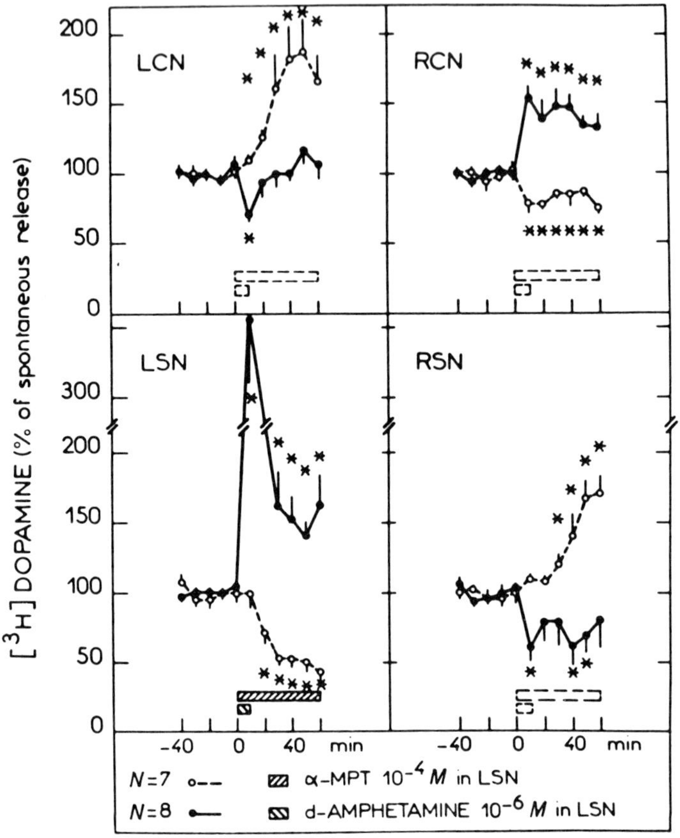

Fig. 1. Effects of unilateral nigral application of α-methylparatyrosine or *d*-amphetamine on the release of [^{3}H]dopamine from the two caudate nuclei and the two substantiae nigrae. Four push–pull cannulae were implanted in the left (LCN) and right (RCN) caudate nuclei and in the left (LSN) and right (RSN) substantiae nigrae in halothane-anesthetized cats. The four structures were superfused with an artificial cerebrospinal fluid containing L-[3,5-^{3}H]tyrosine (50 Ci/mmol, 50 μCi/ml, 1.8 ml/hr). [^{3}H]Dopamine was estimated in 10-min successive superfusate fractions. Either α-methylparatyrosine [α-MpT ○, 10^{-4} *M*, 60 min] or *d*-amphetamine [(●), 10^{-6}*M*, 10 min] was introduced into the medium superfusing the LSN (hatched bar). In each animal and for each cannula, [^{3}H]dopamine in each successive fraction was expressed as a percentage of an average spontaneous release calculated from the 5 fractions collected before the treatment. Data are the mean ± SEM of results obtained with *N* animals. (*), $p < .05$ when compared with corresponding control values obtained in 7 untreated animals (not represented in the figure).

could be detected easily when the SN of the cat was superfused through a push–pull cannula. The amount of [^{3}H]DA released was similar to that observed in the CN and closely dependent on the localization of the push–pull cannula (*10, 37*) (i.e., no release was observed when the cannula was outside the SN). This release was reduced in the absence of calcium and markedly increased under local application of potassium (*22, 37*). In contrast to that observed in the CN, tetrodotoxin stimulated the release of [^{3}H]DA in the SN (*37*). This effect excluded a release of DA from eventual afferent or recurrent DA fibers and suggested that tetrodotoxin-sensitive fast sodium channels were not involved in the spontaneous release of DA from dendrites. It also suggested an inhibitory control of the dendritic release of DA by nigral afferent fibers. In fact, further experiments indicated that several transmitters present in the SN were able to modify the release of DA from dendrites and that important modifications of the DA dendritic release could be induced under treatments affecting the activity of nigral afferent pathways (*10*).

Several studies have been dedicated to the determination of the functional role of DA released from dendrites. As already mentioned, DA is first involved in a self- or lateral inhibition of the activity of the nigral dopaminergic cells (Fig. 1). This effect is mediated by DA autoreceptors which have also been characterized in binding studies using labeled spiroperiodol or apomorphine (*33, 35, 50, 52*). Dopamine receptors associated with an adenylate cyclase and localized on nigral afferent fibers originating from the striatum (*18, 49, 58*) represent a second site of action of DA released from dendrites. These receptors may be distributed on GABAergic terminals since DA has been shown to affect the release of GABA in the SN both *in vitro* (*53*) and *in vivo* (*60*). Finally, electrophysiological as well as binding studies have indicated the presence of DA receptors on nondopaminergic cells in the SN (*16, 33, 50, 52, 57*). Some of these receptors are located on nigrothalamic neurons, since these neurons are activated during the microiontophoretic application of DA and this effect is blocked by neuroleptics (*57*). As discussed more extensively below, evidence for a control of the activity of nigrothalamic neurons by DA released from dendrites has also been obtained in release studies in which we demonstrated that modification of DA transmission in one SN could affect the activity of contralateral DA neurons (*11, 24, 42*).

V. RECIPROCAL CONTROL OF THE ACTIVITY OF THE TWO NIGROSTRIATAL DOPAMINERGIC PATHWAYS

Several circumstances including the delivery of unilateral sensory stimuli (*26, 39*) (Fig. 2) or the unilateral electrical stimulation of the cerebellar dentate nucleus (*41*) induce asymmetric changes in the release of DA from nerve terminals and dendrites of the neurons of the two nigrostriatal DA pathways. A similar pattern of response, which revealed the occurrence of a reciprocal control of the two nigrostriatal DA pathways, was observed during

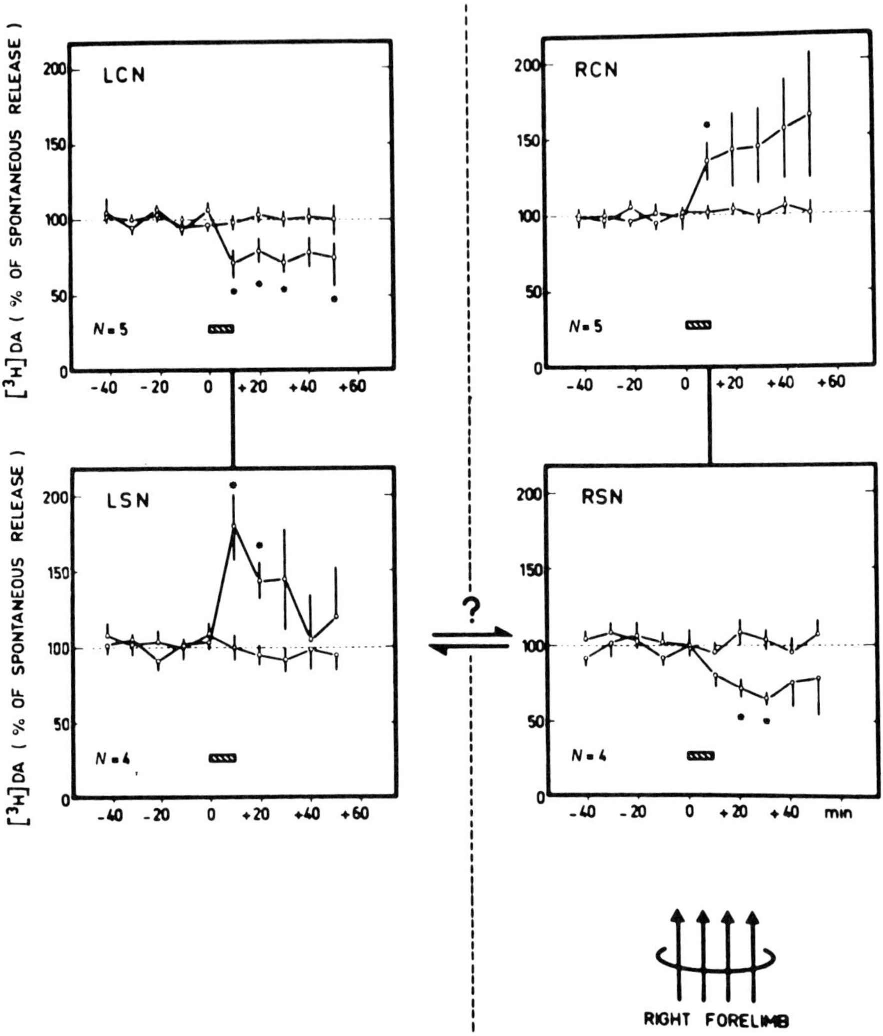

Fig. 2. Effects of unilateral somatic electrical stimulation on the release of [^{3}H]dopamine from the two caudate nuclei and the two substantiae nigrae. Animals were treated as described in Fig. 1 except that the paw of the right forelimb was stimulated (hatched bars) for 10 min using a pair of electrodes (monophasic square pulses, 4–6 V, 0.5 msec, 0.25 Hz). Data are calculated and expressed as in Fig. 1. (*), $p < .05$ when compared with corresponding control value obtained in 5 nonstimulated animals (○).

unilateral pharmacological modification of DA transmission in one SN (*10, 11, 24, 38*). Thus, the application of α-methylparatyrosine in one SN which reduces the release of [^{3}H]DA locally and enhances [^{3}H]amine release in the ipsilateral CN induced opposite responses in contralateral structures (*11, 24*)

Fig. 1). Reverse asymmetric changes in [^{3}H]DA release were observed in both CN and SN when *d*-amphetamine was applied instead of α-methylparatyrosine in one SN (*11, 24*) (Fig. 1). The nigrothalamic neurons are very likely involved in the transfer of messages from one SN to the contralateral DA neurons, since a sagittal section of the thalamic massa intermedia prevented the contralateral effects induced either by a α-methylparatyrosine or

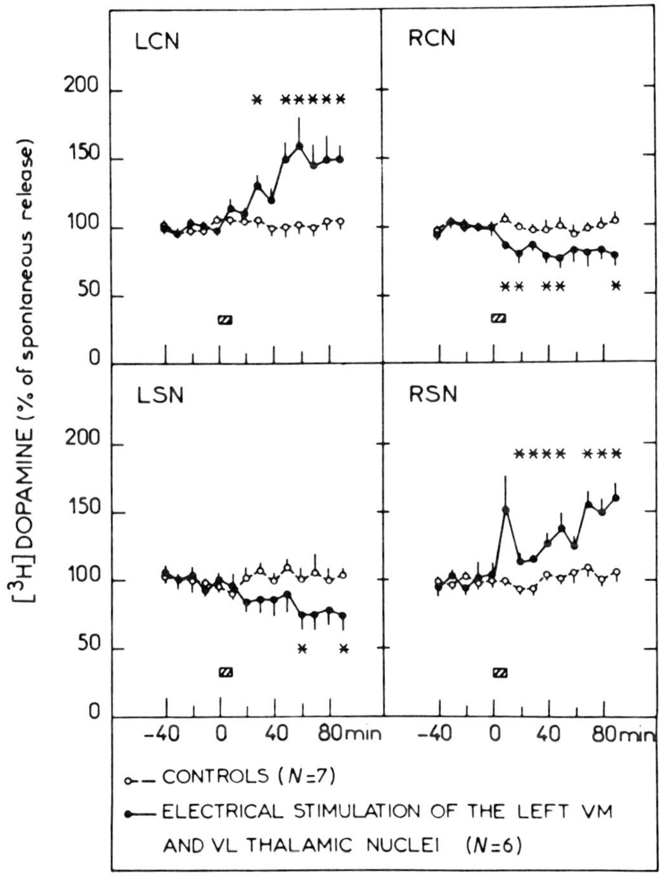

Fig. 3. Effects of the electrical stimulation of the left motor thalamic nuclei on the release of [^{3}H]dopamine in the two caudate nuclei and the two substantiae nigrae. Experiments were carried out as described in Fig. 1 except that the left ventralis medialis (VM) or ventralis lateralis (VL) nuclei were stimulated (hatched bars) for 10 min by passing current between a cathodic monopolar electrode located in the thalamus and a large anodic indifferent electrode inserted in the muscle temporalis on the same side. The stimuli consisted of trains of square pulses (train duration: 100 msec; shock duration: 0.5 msec; shock frequency: 300 Hz) delivered at a frequency of 0.25 Hz and with an intensity of 100 μA. Data are calculated and expressed as in Fig. 1. (*), $p < .05$ when compared with corresponding control values obtained in 7 nonstimulated animals (○).

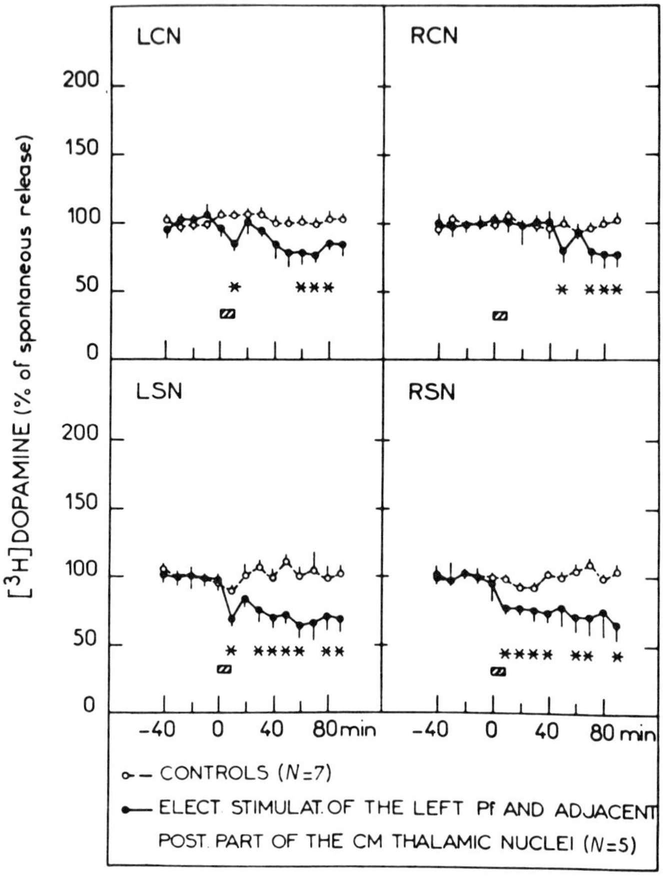

Fig. 4. Effects of the electrical stimulation of the left n. parafascicularis and adjacent part of the n. centrum medianum on the release of [^{3}H]dopamine in the two caudate nuclei and the two substantiae nigrae. Animals were treated as described in Figs. 1 and 3 except that the electrical stimulation was delivered in the most posterior part of intralaminar nuclei. Data are calculated and expressed as in Fig. 1. (*), $p < .05$ when compared with corresponding control values obtained in 7 nonstimulated cats (○).

d-amphetamine, whereas other sections interrupting the corpus callosum or the mesencephalic decussations were ineffective (*11*). This series of observations led us to investigate the effects of either the unilateral electrical stimulation of various thalamic nuclei innervated by the nigrothalamic neurons [which are at least partly GABAergic (*15, 31, 59, 61*)] or of the unilateral application of GABA in these nuclei on DA release from nerve endings and dendrites of ipsi- and contralateral DA neurons (*12, 13, 54*). Both types of treatments made in motor (n. ventralis medialis VM and n. ventralis lateralis VL) as well as in intralaminar (n. centralis lateralis, n. centrum medianum, and n. parafascicularis) thalamic nuclei induced marked changes in [^{3}H]DA release ipsi- and contralaterally, further suggesting that the nigrothalamic neurons were in great part responsible for the bilateral reciprocal regulation of the activity of the two dopaminergic pathways. In particular, an asymmetric pattern of responses intervening in both CN and SN similar to that observed under the unilateral nigral application of α-methylparatyrosine was observed following the electrical stimulation of the VM/VL (*12*) (Fig. 3). Other treatments induced different patterns of responses, symmetrical in most cases (Fig. 4), which were reminiscent of those occurring under unilateral nigral application of potassium or GABAergic agonists or antagonists (*10, 22, 25*) (Fig. 5). These latter results indicated that transmitters other than DA released in the SN could also

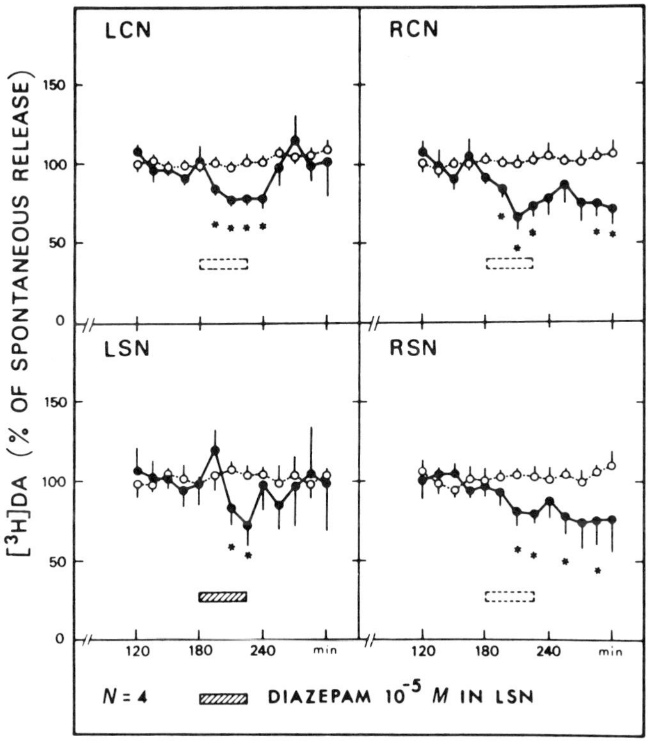

Fig. 5. Effects of the unilateral nigral application of diazepam on the release of [^{3}H]dopamine in the two caudate nuclei and the two substantiae nigrae. Experiments were carried out as described in Fig. 2 except that diazepam [(●), $10^{-5}M$, 30 min] was introduced into the medium superfusing the LSN (hatched bar). Data are calculated and expressed as in Fig. 1. (*), $p < .05$ when compared with corresponding control values obtained in untreated animals (○).

contribute in a different way to the bilateral regulation of the two nigrostriatal DA pathways and that nigrothalamic fibers innervating either motor or intralaminar thalamic nuclei could be involved in these complex regulatory processes.

VI. PRESYNAPTIC REGULATION OF STRIATAL DOPAMINE RELEASE

Several findings suggest that the release of DA from nerve terminals of nigrostriatal DA neurons is not only dependent on nerve activity, but is also under the control of afferents acting at a presynaptic level. Indeed, *in vitro* experiments performed on rat striatal slices indicated that acetylcholine (nicotinic and muscarinic receptors), serotonin, noradrenaline (β-adrenergic receptors), amino acids such as glutamate, GABA, and glycine, and peptides including opiates (δ receptors), angiotensin II, somatostatin, and substance P can influence the release of DA. These effects are mediated by receptors located on DA terminals or on neurons contacting these terminals (*14*). Furthermore, *in vivo* experiments have also shown that several of these transmitters or their agonists may modify the release of DA from nerve terminals when applied locally in the CN of halothane-anesthetized cats (*14*). However, such effects do not necessarily demonstrate that the neurons containing these transmitters are indeed involved in a physiological presynaptic control of DA release as revealed for the presynaptic control of norepinephrine release by cholinergic fibers in the heart (*27, 34*). A first indication for such a physiological presynaptic control was provided by *in vivo* experiments in which we examined the effects of the unilateral electrical stimulation of the motor cortex on DA release in both CN (*40*). In this situation [^{3}H]DA release was enhanced in both CN and the contralateral effect was abolished following a sagittal section of the corpus callosum, suggesting that the corticostriatal glutamatergic fibers control presynaptically the release of DA from dopaminergic fibers. Surprisingly, we also observed that the nigral application of potassium enhanced the release of [^{3}H]DA in the ipsilateral CN despite the physical interruption of nerve impulse flow in DA neurons produced by a complete ipsilateral hemisection made between the SN and the CN (Chesselet and Chéramy, unpublished observation). Such a phenomenon could only be explained by the intervention of a presynaptic control exerted through a polysynaptic neuronal loop which has still to be identified. Finally, more direct evidence for such physiological presynaptic regulation by striatal afferent fibers was provided in experiments in which we investigated more precisely the mechanisms operating to cause the effects induced by the unilateral application of GABA in motor thalamic nuclei (VM/VL) upon the release of [^{3}H]DA in both CN. For this purpose single-unit activity of dopaminergic cells was also recorded in both SN. It could be shown that GABA (10^{-5}*M*) application in the VM/VL reduced the firing rate of DA neurons in both SN while simultaneously enhancing the release of [^{3}H]DA in both CN (*55*). These results clearly demonstrated that changes in DA release from nerve terminals may not always depend on nerve impulse flow and that subtle presynaptic mechanisms are contributing with great efficacy to the physiological modulation of the transmitter release. In fact, in this particular case, a presynaptic facilitatory regulation of DA release mediated by a thalamocorticostriatal or thalamostriatal neuronal loop must be implicated.

VII. CONCLUSION AND PERSPECTIVES

In this chapter, we have attempted to describe briefly some of the main aspects of our investigation of the properties of nigrostriatal DA neurons. This investigation has been made possible by *in vivo* measurement of transmitter release from nerve terminals and dendrites and has focused on analyzing (1) the functional role of DA released from dendrites, (2) the mechanisms contributing to the bilateral asymmetric or symmetric regulatory processes of DA transmission in both CN and SN, and (3) the respective roles of nerve impulse flow and of presynaptic influences in the regulation of DA release from nerve terminals. It is now well established that DA released from dendrites is involved in the control of messages leaving the basal ganglia. If the nigrothalamic neurons are one of the target sites of DA action, it remains to be determined whether other nigral efferent pathways are also influenced by DA. Our analysis of the mechanisms operating in the bilateral regulation of the two nigrostriatal dopaminergic pathways has emphasized the crucial role of the thalamic nuclei. Much has still to be done to better understand the respective roles of motor and intralaminar nuclei in the symmetric vs asymmetric changes in DA release seen in both CN and SN under various conditions. The implication of the cerebral cortex in these processes has to be more precisely determined. One of the most interesting findings of general interest was the demonstration that DA release from nerve terminals may be enhanced when nerve impulse flow is reduced, and vice versa. Such a demonstration was able to be made thanks to the combined determination of the activity of DA cells, through electrophysiological recordings, and of the amount of transmitter released. Undoubtedly, these complementary approaches are absolutely required in order to reach any conclusion concerning changes in DA transmission which may intervene in several physiological or pharmacological situations. Such approaches should be of great value in evaluating (1) the relationship between action potentials and release of transmitter, (2) the importance of the coding of neuronal firing in the release process (*48*), and (3) the role of distinct facilitatory or inhibitory pathways exerting a presynaptic control on DA release. On the other hand, it should also be stressed that improved knowledge of the role of nigrostriatal DA neurons in the basal ganglia is linked to parallel studies on major pathways such as the striatonigral GABAergic and substance P systems, the raphe-striatal or nigral serotonergic neurons, or the corticostriatal glutamatergic neurons. It is also in this direction that our group will concentrate in the future, since *in vivo* release of the corresponding transmitters can now be determined thanks to the push–pull cannula method and the development of sensitive assays.

ACKNOWLEDGMENTS

Part of this work has been performed with the collaboration of Drs. M. J. Besson, B. Bioulac, M. F. Chesselet, M. Desban, P. Feltz, C. Gauchy, G. Godeheu, S. Greenfield, V. Leviel, C. Lubetzki, A. Nieoullon, and T. D. Reisine.

This study was supported by grants from DRET (n. 81,050), INSERM (PRC 120,039), CNRS (ATP), and Rhône-Poulenc S.A.

REFERENCES

1. Bartholini, G., Stadler, H., and Lloyd, K. G. The effect of drugs on the release of striatal neurotransmitters. *In* "Neuropsychopharmacology," (J. R. Boissier, H. Hippius, and P. Pichot, eds.), 1974, pp. 487–492. Excerpta Medica, Amsterdam, and Elsevier, New York.
2. Besson, M. J., Chéramy, A., Feltz, P., and Glowinski, J. Dopamine: spontaneous and drug-induced release from the caudate nucleus in the cat. *Brain Res.* **32** (1971) 407–424.
3. Besson, M. J., Chéramy, A., Gauchy, C., and Glowinski, J. *In vivo* continuous estimation of ^{3}H-dopamine synthesis and release in the cat caudate nucleus: effects of α-methyl-*p*-tyrosine and of transection of the nigro striatal pathway. *Naunyn-Schmiedeberg's Arch. Pharmacol.* **278** (1973) 101–105.
4. Bunney, B. S., Aghajanian, G. K., and Roth, R. H. Comparison of effects of L-dopa, amphetamine and apomorphine on firing rate of rat dopaminergic neurons. *Nature (London), New Biol.* **245** (1973) 123–125.
5. Bunney, B. S., and Aghajanian, G. K. *d*-Amphetamine-induced depression of central dopamine neurons: evidence for mediation by both auto-receptors and striato-nigral feedback pathway. *Naunyn-Schmiedeberg's Arch. Pharmacol.* **304** (1978) 255–261.
6. Chéramy, A., Bioulac, B., Besson, M. J., Vincent, J. D., Glowinski, J., and Gauchy, C. Radioenzymatic estimation of catecholamines released from the caudate nucleus in the cat and in the monkey. *In* "Neuropsychopharmacology," (J. R. Boissier, H. Hippius, and P. Pichot, eds.), 1975, pp. 493–498. Excerpta Medica, Amsterdam, and Elsevier, New York.
7. Chéramy, A., Nieoullon, A., Michelot, R., and Glowinski, J. Effects of intranigral application of dopamine and substance P on the *in vivo* release of newly synthesized ^{3}H-dopamine in the ipsilateral caudate nucleus of the cat. *Neurosci. Lett.* **4** (1977) 105–109.

8. Chéramy, A., Nieoullon, A., and Glowinski, J. Inhibition of dopamine release in the cat caudate nucleus by nigral application of glycine. *Eur. J. Pharmacol.* **47** (1978) 141–147.
9. Chéramy, A., Michelot, R., Leviel, V., Nieoullon, A., Glowinski, J., and Kerdelhue, B. Effects of the immunoneutralization of substance P in the cat substantia nigra on the release of dopamine from dendrites and terminals of dopaminergic neurons. *Brain Res.* **155** (1978) 404–408.
10. Chéramy, A., Leviel, V., and Glowinski J. Dendritic release of dopamine in the substantia nigra. *Nature* (*London*) **289** (1981) 537–542.
11. Chéramy, A., Leviel, V., Daudet, F., Guibert, B., Chesselet, M. F., and Glowinski, J. Involvement of the thalamus in the reciprocal regulation of the two nigrostriatal dopaminergic pathways. *Neuroscience* **6** (1981) 2657–2658.
12. Chéramy, A., Chesselet, M. F., Romo, R., Leviel, V., and Glowinski, J. Effects of unilateral electrical stimulation of various thalamic nuclei on the release of dopamine from dendrites and nerve terminals of neurons of the two nigrostriatal dopaminergic pathways. *Neuroscience* **8** (1983) 767–780.
13. Chesselet, M. F., Chéramy, A., Romo, R., Desban, M., and Glowinski, J. GABA in the thalamic motor nuclei modulates dopamine release from the two dopaminergic nigrostriatal pathways in the cat. *Exp. Brain Res.* **51** (1983) 275–282.
14. Chesselet, M. F., Chéramy, A., Reisine, T., Lubetzki, C., and Glowinski, J. Presynaptic regulation of striatal dopamine release: *in vivo* and *in vitro* studies. *J. Physiol.* (Paris) **78** (1982) 420–425.
15. Di Chiara, G., Porceddu, M. L., Morelli, M., Mulas, M. I., and Gessa, J. L. Evidence for GABAergic projections from the substantia nigra to the ventromedial thalamus and the superior colliculus of the rat. *Brain Res.* **176** (1979) 273–284.
16. Dray, A., and Straughan, D. W. Synaptic mechanisms in the substantia nigra. *J. Pharm. Pharmacol.* **28** (1976) 400–405.
17. Dray, A., Gonye, T. I., and Oakley, N. R. Effects of α-flupenthixol on dopamine and 5-hydroxytryptamine responses of substantia nigra neurons. *Neuropharmacology* **15** (1976) 793–796.
18. Gale, K., Guidotti, A., and Costa, E. Dopamine-sensitive adenylate cyclase location in substantia nigra. Science **195** (1977) 503–505.
19. Gauchy, C., Bioulac, B., Chéramy, A., Besson, M. J., Glowinski, J., and Vincent, J. D. Chronic estimation of dopamine release from the caudate nucleus of the maccaca mulatta. *Brain Res.* **77** (1974) 257–268.
20. Gauchy, C., Tassin, J. P., Glowinski, J., and Chéramy, A. Isolation and radioenzymic estimation of picogram quantities of dopamine and norepinephrine in biological samples. *J. Neurochem.* **26** (1976) 471–480.
21. Geffen, L. B., Jessell, T. M., Cuello, A. C., and Iversen, L. L. Release of dopamine from dendrites in rat substantia nigra. *Nature* (*London*) **260** (1976) 258–260.
22. Greenfield, S., Chéramy, A., Leviel, V., and Glowinski, J. *In vivo* release of acetylcholinesterase in cat substantia nigra and caudate nucleus. *Nature* (*London*) **284** (1980) 355–357.
23. Groves, P. M., Wilson, C. J., Young, S. J., and Rebec, G. V. Self-inhibition by dopaminergic neurons: an alternative to the "neuronal feedback loop" hypothesis of the mode of action of certain psychotropic drugs. *Science* **190** (1975) 522–528.
24. Leviel, V., Chéramy, A., and Glowinski, J. Role of the dendritic release of dopamine in the reciprocal control of the two nigrostriatal dopaminergic pathways. *Nature* (*London*) **280** (1979) 236–239.
25. Leviel, V., Chéramy, A., Nieoullon, A., and Glowinski, J. Symmetric bilateral changes in dopamine release from the caudate nuclei of the cat induced by unilateral nigral application of glycine and GABA-related compounds. *Brain Res.* **175** (1979) 259–270.

26. Leviel, V., Chesselet, M. F., Glowinski, J., and Chéramy, A. Involvement of the thalamus in asymmetric effects of unilateral sensory stimuli on the two nigrostriatal dopaminergic pathways in the cat. *Brain Res.* **223** (1981) 257–272.
27. Lévy, M. N., and Blattberg, B. Effect of vagal stimulation on the overflow of norepinephrine into the coronary sinus during cardiac sympathetic nerve stimulation in the dog. *Circ. Res.* **38** (1976) 81–85.
28. McKenzie, G. M., and Szerb, J. C. The effect of dihydroxyphenylalanine, pheniprazine and dextro-amphetamine on the *in vivo* release of dopamine from the caudate nucleus. *J. Pharmacol. Exp. Ther.* **162** (1968) 302–308.
29. McLennan, H. The release of acetylcholine and 3-hydroxytyramine from the caudate nucleus. *J. Physiol. (London)* **174** (1964) 152–161.
30. McLennan, H. The release of dopamine from the putamen. *Experientia (Basel)* **21** (1965) 725–727.
31. McLeod, N. K., James, A., Kilpatrick, I. C., and Starr, M. S. Evidence for a GABAergic nigro-thalamic pathway in the rat. II. Electrophysiological studies. *Exp. Brain Res.* **40** (1980) 55–61.
32. Michelot, R., Leviel, V., Giorguieff-Chesselet, M. F., Chéramy, A., and Glowinski, J. Effects of the unilateral nigral modulation of substance P transmission on the activity of the two nigrostriatal dopaminergic pathways. *Life Sci.* **24** (1979) 715–724.
33. Murrin, L. C., Gale, K., and Kuhar, M. J. Autoradiographic localization of neuroleptic and dopamine receptors in the caudate-putamen and substantia nigra: effects of lesions. *Eur. J. Pharmacol.* **60** (1979) 229–235.
34. Muscholl, E., Presynaptic muscarine receptors and inhibition of release. *In* "Release of Catecholamines from Adrenergic Neurons," (D. M. Paton, ed.) 1979, pp. 87–110. Pergamon, Oxford.
35. Nagy, J. I., Lee, T., Seeman, P., and Fibiger, H. C. Direct evidence for presynaptic and postsynaptic dopamine receptors in brain. *Nature (London)* **274** (1978) 278–281.
36. Nieoullon, A., Chéramy, A., and Glowinski, J. An adaptation of the push–pull cannula method to study the *in vivo* release of ^{3}H-dopamine synthesized from ^{3}H-tyrosine in cat caudate nucleus: effects of various physical and pharmacological treatments. *J. Neurochem.* **28** (1977) 819–828.
37. Nieoullon, A., Chéramy, A., and Glowinski, J. Release of dopamine *in vivo* from cat substantia nigra. *Nature (London)* **266** (1977) 375–377.
38. Nieoullon, A., Chéramy, A., and Glowinski, J. Interdependence of the nigrostriatal dopaminergic systems on the two sides of the brain in the cat. *Science* **198** (1977) 416–418.
39. Nieoullon, A., Chéramy, A., and Glowinski, J. Nigral and striatal dopamine release under sensory stimuli. *Nature (London)* **269** (1977) 340–342.
40. Nieoullon, A., Chéramy, A., and Glowinski, J. Release of dopamine evoked by electrical stimulation of the motor and visual areas of the cerebral cortex in both caudate nuclei and in the substantia nigra in the cat. *Brain Res.* **145** (1978) 69–84.
41. Nieoullon, A., Chéramy, A., and Glowinski, J. Release of dopamine in both caudate nuclei and both substantiae nigrae in response to unilateral stimulation of cerebellar nuclei in the cat. *Brain Res.* **148** (1978) 143–152.
42. Nieoullon, A., Chéramy, A., Leviel, V., and Glowinski, J. Effects of the unilateral nigral application of dopaminergic drugs on the *in vivo* release of dopamine in the two caudate nuclei of the cat. *Eur. J. Pharmacol.* **53** (1979) 289–296.
43. Paden, C., Wilson, C. J., and Groves, P. M. Amphetamine-induced release of dopamine from the substantia nigra *in vitro*. *Life Sci.* **19** (1976) 1499–1506.
44. Philippu, A., Dietl, H., and Sinha, J. N. Rise in blood pressure increases the release of

endogenous catecholamines in the anterior hypothalamus of the cat. *Naunyn-Schmiedeberg's Arch. Pharmacol.* **310** (1980) 237–240.
45. Portig, P. J., and Vogt, M. Search for substances released on stimulation of the caudate nucleus in the cat. *J. Physiol. (London)* **186** (1966) 131–132P.
46. Portig, P. J., and Vogt, M. Release of dopamine from the cat's caudate nucleus by *d*-tubocurarine. *J. Physiol. (London)* **189** (1967) 42–43P.
47. Portig, P. J., Sharman, D. F., and Vogt, M. Release by tubocurarine of dopamine and homovanillic acid from the superfused caudate nucleus. *J. Physiol. (London)* **194** (1968) 565–572.
48. Poulain, D. A., and Wakerley, J. B. Electrophysiology of hypothalamic magnocellular neurons secreting oxytocin and vasopressin. *Neuroscience* **7** (1982) 773–808.
49. Prémont, J., Thierry, A. M., Tassin, J. P., Glowinski, J., Blanc, G., and Bockaert, J. Is the dopamine-senstive adenylate cyclase in the rat substantia nigra coupled with autoreceptors? *FEBS Lett.* **68** (1976) 99–104.
50. Quik, M., Emson, P. C., and Joyce, E. Dissociation between the presynaptic dopamine senstive adenylate cyclase and [^{3}H[spiperone binding sites in rat substantia nigra. *Brain Res.* **167** (1979) 355–367.
51. Reader, T. A., De Champlain, J., and Jasper, H. Catecholamines released from cerebral cortex in the cat: decrease during sensory stimulation. *Brain Res.* **11** (1976) 95–108.
52. Reisine, T. D., Nagy, J. I., Fibiger, H. C., and Yamamura, H. I. Localization of dopamine receptors in rat brain. *Brain Res.* **169** (1979) 209–214.
53. Reubi, J. C., Iversen, L. L., and Jessell, T. M. Dopamine selectively increases [^{3}H]GABA release from slices of rat substantia nigra *in vitro*. *Nature (London)* **268** (1977) 652–654.
54. Romo, R., Chéramy, A., Desban, M., Godeheu, G., and Glowinski, J. GABA in the intralaminar thalamic nuclei modulates dopamine release from the two dopaminergic nigrostriatal pathways in the cat. *Brain Res. Bull.* **11** (1983) 671–680.
55. Romo, R., Chéramy, A., Godeheu, G., and Glowinski, J. Presynaptic regulation of striatal dopamine release: electrophysiological and *in vivo* release studies. In preparation (1985).
56. Roth, R. H., Walters, J. R., and Aghajanian, G. K. Effect of impulse flow on the release and synthesis of dopamine in the rat striatum. *In* "Frontiers in Catecholamine Research," (E. Usdin and S. Snyder, eds.), 1973, pp. 567–574.
57. Ruffieux, A., and Schultz, W. Dopaminergic activation of reticulata neurons in the substantia nigra. *Nature (London)* **285** (1980) 240–241.
58. Spano, P. F., Di Chiara, G., Tonon, G. C., and Trabucchi, M. A dopamine-stimulated adenylate cyclase in rat substantia nigra. *J. Neurochem.* **27** (1976) 1565–1568.
59. Starr, M. S., and Killpatrick, I. C. Distribution of γ-amino-butyrate following lesion or electrical stimulation of the substantia nigra. *Neuroscience* **6** (1981) 1095–1104.
60. Van Der Heyden, J. A. M., Venema, K., and Korf, J. Biphasic and opposite effects of dopamine and apomorphine on endogenous GABA release in the rat substantia nigra. *J. Neurochem.* **34** (1980) 119–125.
61. Yoshida, M., and Omata, S. Blocking by picrotoxin of nigra-evoked inhibition of neurons of ventro-medial nucleus of the thalamus. *Experientia (Basel)* **35** (1979) 794.

11

Pharmacologically Induced Changes in the Efflux of Metabolites of Dopamine and 5-Hydroxytryptamine from the Brains of Freely Moving Rats

KENNETH E. MOORE AND
JANN A. NIELSEN*

Department of Pharmacology and Toxicology
Michigan State University
East Lansing, Michigan

I. METHODS

A. A Brief Historical Perspective

During the past 30 years investigators have attempted to monitor the activities of the aminergic neurons in the central nervous system using a

*Present address: Program of Pharmacology, Northeastern Ohio University, College of Medicine, Rootstown, Ohio 44272.

ISBN 0-12-083350-6

variety of perfusion techniques. Some of the early efforts involved the measurement of putative neurotransmitters in perfusates of the cerebroventricular cisternal system using techniques developed by Feldberg and co-workers (*5, 9*). With these techniques either the whole ventricular–cisternal system or selected regions of the ventricles could be perfused by introducing artificial cerebrospinal fluid (CSF) through cannulae implanted into the lateral, third, or fourth ventricles and collecting the perfusate from cannulae or catheters inserted into any of these ventricles, the cerebral aqueduct, or the cisterna. Subsequently, Gaddum push–pull cannulae, which are generally employed to perfuse discrete regions of brain tissue, were employed to perfuse the cerebral ventricles (*35, 37*). This chapter is limited to a discussion of studies that have employed cerebroventricular perfusion techniques to monitor the efflux from the brain and into the cerebral ventricles of catecholamines and 5-hydroxytryptamine (5HT) and their metabolites. Other chapters in this volume review efforts to detect the release of these putative amine neurotransmitters using other techniques (e.g., push–pull cannula in tissue, superfusion of cortical and subcortical regions).

For technical reasons early experiments involving the perfusion of the cerebral ventricles were performed in larger experimental animals (dogs, cats) maintained under general anesthesia. A variety of techniques were employed to analyze the perfusates, but in the earliest studies bioassays were used to detect the efflux of putative neurotransmitters. These techniques were successfully employed to quantify the efflux of acetylcholine (*6*), but they were unable to detect dopamine (DA) in cerebroventricular perfusates (*38*). Nevertheless, the O-methylated deaminated metabolite of DA, homovanillic acid (HVA), was identified in the perfusates using a fluorometric assay procedure (*29*). The efflux of HVA fell as the anesthesia deepened, suggesting that HVA entered the cerebral ventricles as a result of neuronal activity (*28*). Furthermore, electrical stimulation of substantia nigra increased the efflux of HVA, suggesting that this metabolite of DA originated from the terminals of nigrostriatal neurons.

Attempts were also made to detect 5HT in the cerebroventricular perfusates using bioassay procedures, but only very small amounts of biologically active materials, which may have been 5HT, could be identified (*13*). Subsequent investigators effectively used bioassay to detect the release of 5HT into cerebroventricular perfusates of cats following either electrical stimulation of raphe nuclei (*2, 19*) or pretreatment with monoamine oxidase inhibitors (*16*). With the use of chemical methods it has been difficult to identify endogenous 5HT in cerebroventricular perfusates, but significant quantities of the major deaminated product of 5HT, 5-hydroxyindoleacetic acid (5HIAA), have been identified in the CSF or in cerebroventricular perfusates using fluorometric assays (*17, 18*).

Radioactive tracer techniques were subsequently employed to detect the release of biogenic amines and their metabolites into cerebroventricular perfusates. Initially, these methods suffered from the lack of specificity since it was not always possible to specifically label endogenous neurotransmitter stores. Early efforts relied on the amine uptake systems to transport the radioactive amines into the desired neuronal terminals. In some instances, however, the lack of specificity of the transport system and/or the use of nontracer doses of the radioactive amines, which overloaded the transport mechanisms, probably resulted in the uptake of a radioactive amine into neurons containing another amine [e.g., formation of artifactual pools of [^{3}H]5HT (*15*); the uptake and release of [^{3}H]norepinephrine (NE) from DA neurons (*10*)]. More specific labeling of intraneuronal amine stores was subsequently achieved by administering radioactive precursors of amines (*4, 14*). Because of the specific localization of synthetic enzymes (e.g., tyrosine hydroxylase, tryptophan hydroxylase, dopamine β-hydroxylase), synthesized radioactive amines appearing in cerebroventricular perfusates must originate from neurons that normally release the amines.

Figure 1 depicts two examples of experiments in which radioactive tracer techniques were employed to detect spontaneous and amphetamine-induced release of DA into cerebroventricular perfusates of anesthetized cats. Figure 1A depicts an experiment in which brain stores of DA were labeled with an intraventricular (i.vent) injection of [^{3}H]DA. After a 2-hr period of washout a pulse of *d*-amphetamine was added to the perfusing CSF, causing a marked increase in the efflux of [^{3}H]DA (top). When the experiment was repeated and an acute electrolytic lesion was made in the ascending nigrostriatal DA neuronal pathway there was an immediate but small decrease in the efflux of [^{3}H]DA (bottom). The acute lesion did, however, markedly attenuate the efflux of [^{3}H]DA induced by *d*-amphetamine. These results suggest that the efflux of [^{3}H]DA evoked by *d*-amphetamine is at least partially dependent upon impulse activity in ascending DA neurons. Figure 1B depicts an experiment showing the ability of an i.vent infusion or a systemic intravenous injection of *d*-amphetamine to increase the efflux of [^{3}H]DA which had been synthesized *in situ* from [^{3}H]tyrosine added to the perfusing CSF.

Similar experiments have been carried out to study the release of 5HT from central neurons. By labeling endogenous stores of 5HT with prior infusions of [^{3}H]tryptophan, it was shown that stimulation of the midbrain raphe increased the efflux of endogenously synthesized [^{3}H]5HT into the cerebroventricular perfusates of anesthetized cats (*11*), while drugs which reduce the firing of raphe units (chlorimipramine, LSD) reduced the efflux of endogenously synthesized 5HT into the lateral cerebral ventricles of rats (*14*).

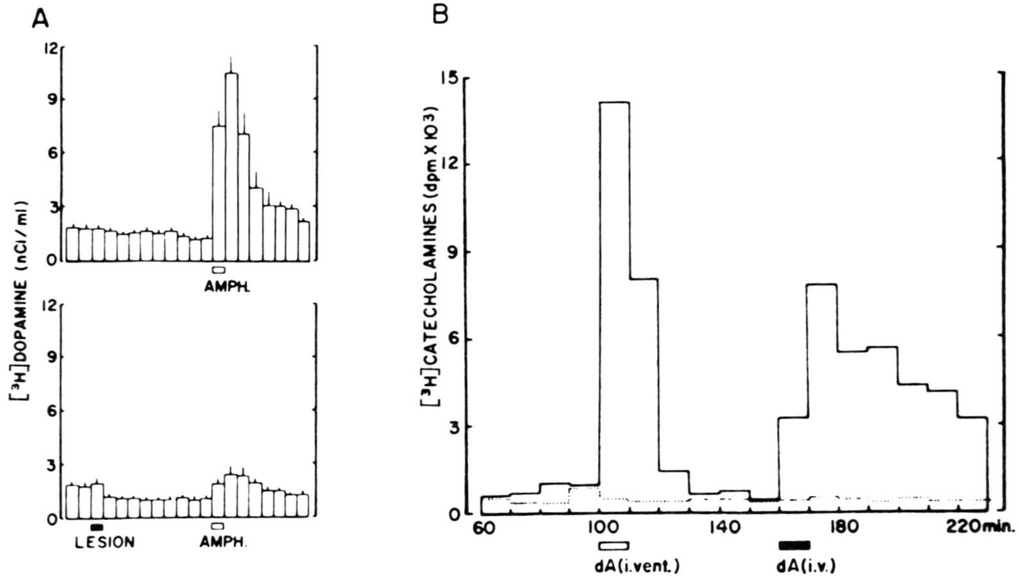

Fig. 1. Effects of *d*-amphetamine on the efflux of [^{3}H]DA into cerebroventricular perfusates of anesthetized cats. (A) Brain stores of DA were labeled with an intracerebroventricular (i.vent) injection of [^{3}H]DA. The ventricles were then perfused for 2 hr prior to the start of the experiment. Each column represents the mean (vertical lines are 1 SE, N=4 of [^{3}H]DA appearing in consecutive 2-min samples of perfusate. The efflux of [^{3}H]DA in response to a 2-min infusion of *d*-amphetamine (AMPH; $1.6 \times 10^{-4} M$) was determined contralateral to (top) and ipsilateral to (bottom) an acute electrolytic lesion (solid bar on abscissa) of the ascending DA neurons [Reprinted from ref. (*39*). © 1973 *American Society for Pharmacology and Experimental Therapeutics*. See ref. (*39*) for further details.] (B) Artificial CSF containing purified [^{3}H]tyrosine (——) was infused into a lateral cerebral ventricle of an anesthetized cat and consecutive 10-min samples of perfusate were collected and analyzed for [^{3}H]DA. An i.vent infusion of *d*-amphetamine (dA; $10^{-5} M$) and an intravenous injection of *d*-amphetamine (2 mg/kg) were made at 100–110 min and at 160 min, respectively. [Reprinted from ref. (*22*). See ref. (*22*) for further details.] A similar experiment was carried out in which an inhibitor of DA synthesis, α-methyltyrosine ($5 \times 10^{-4} M$) (• • •) was added to the perfusing CSF.

More recently, analytical techniques capable of quantifying less than nanogram quantities of biogenic amines and some of their metabolites have been employed to detect these endogenous compounds in CSF and in cerebroventricular perfusates. Radioenzymatic assays (*12, 36*) and high-performance liquid chromatography coupled to electrochemical detection (LCEC; *21, 26, 40*) are two procedures that have been employed with some success to quantify the very small amounts of amines and some of their metabolites in CSF and brain perfusates. The advantages of LCEC in studies of this kind are due to the resolution, selectivity, sensitivity, and simplicity of the technique.

The present chapter describes the application of an *in vivo* technique for monitoring the activities of central DA and 5HT neurons; the technique involves measuring the release of endogenous metabolites of these two amines from brains of freely moving rats. This has been accomplished by perfusing a lateral cerebral ventricle by means of a chronically implanted push–pull cannula, and quantifying the perfusate contents of 3,4-dihydroxyphenylacetic acid (DOPAC), HVA, and 5HIAA using LCEC.

B. Cannulation and Perfusion Techniques

The method of preparing and implanting the push–pull cannula, and the procedure for perfusing the lateral cerebral ventricle employed in the experiments described herein, are based on those developed by Sparber and coworkers (*35, 37*).

The cannula is schematically depicted in Fig. 2. The base is a commercially available stainless-steel injection cannula (David Kopf, Tujunga, California which is modified by trimming the flat portion of the base, and the 25 ga needle tubing (i.d. 0.01 in.; o.d. 0.02 in) is cut so that it extends 6 mm below the bottom of the base. One to three O rings* are fitted into the base to ensure a complete seal between the base and perfusion cap during the perfusion.

The perfusion cap is made by drilling a hole through the center of a socket head stainless-steel screw (1/8 in., 6/32 thread) and securing two pieces of stainless-steel tubing (push and pull tubes) into this hole with Loctite 35 retaining compound (Loctite Corp., Newington, Connecticut). The push tube consists of 33-ga tubing (i.d. 0.004 in.; o.d. 0.008 in) which extends 0.75–1.0 mm past the tip of the base (pull tube) while above the cap the push tubing is reinforced for about 2 cm by cementing 23-ga tubing around the 33-ga tubing. The pull tube (23-ga tubing) extends from about the mid-

*Unless specified otherwise, all parts and materials are obtained from Small Parts, Inc., Miami, Florida.

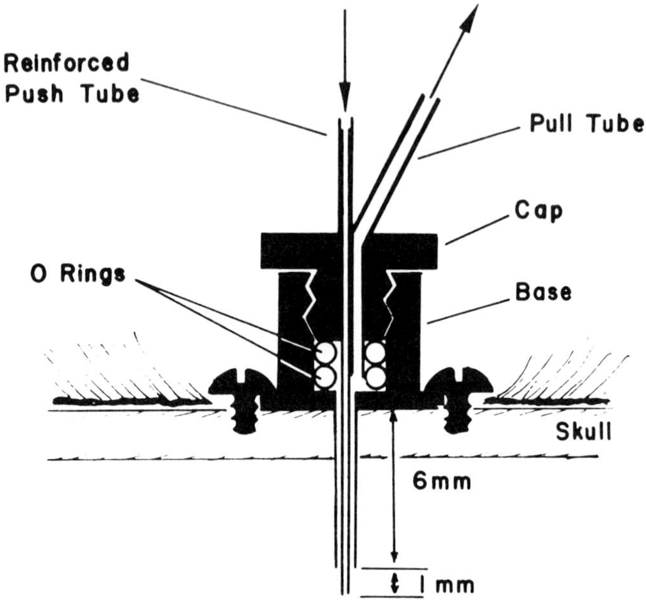

Fig. 2. Schematic diagram (not drawn to scale) of a cross section of the cannula base with the perfusion cap screwed into place. When the ventricle is not being perfused the perfusion cap is replaced by a stylus. [Reprinted from ref. (23).]

dle of the screw to 2 cm above the cap. It is bent at an angle in order to separate it from the reinforced pull tube and thus allow silicone tubing to be slipped over both tubes in the cap for perfusing. The stylus is prepared by cementing 33-ga tubing into a socket head screw and trimming it so that when it is securely screwed into the base it extends approximately 0.5 mm beyond the needle tubing in the base.

Sprague–Dawley rats are anesthetized with Equithesin (3 ml/kg, ip), placed in a stereotaxic frame, and the cannula base with the stylus in place is permanently implanted onto the skull (A 0.0, L 1.6; *27*) so that the tip of the needle base (pull tube) is located in the lateral ventricle. The base is anchored to the clean dry skull with 3 stainless-steel screws (0/80 thread, 3/16 in.) and dental acrylic cement. The stylus is kept in place whenever the ventricles are not being perfused; it is loosened daily so as to prevent it from being permanently stuck in the base. Occasionally, a rat will dislodge the stylus and/or cannula by wedging it between the wire grids on the cage lid. This problem has been rectified by placing a plastic cover over the exposed stylus.

Following cannula placement that rat is housed individually. At least 7 days is allowed to elapse before the brain perfusion experiments are initiated. The animal is perfused in its home cage so as to minimize the possibility of a novel environment influencing the results. The push and pull tubes of the perfusion cap are connected to a 4-channel peristaltic pump (Minipuls II, Gilson Electronics, Middleton, Wisconsin) with Medical-Grade Silastic Tubing (i.d. 0.012 in.; o.d. 0.025 in.; Dow Corning Corp., Midland, Michigan). The push tubing is connected through one channel of the pump to a reservoir containing the artificial CSF perfusion medium (129 m*M* NaCl, 2.5 m*M* $NaHCO_3$, 0.5 m*M* Na_2HPO_4, 3 m*M* KCl, 0.8 m*M* $MgCl_2$, and 1.3 m*M* $CaCl_2$). The solution is filtered (0.22 μm pore, Millipore Corp., Bedford, Massachusetts) and bubbled with 95% O_2 and 5% CO_2 immediately prior to use. The final pH is 7.4.

The pull tube is connected with silicone tubing through a second channel of the pump (in the opposite direction to the push tube) and the end placed over a fraction collector containing tared polyethylene microsample tubes (1.5 ml, Kew Scientific, Columbus, Ohio). Enough tubing (approximately 1 m) is left between the cannula and the pump so as to permit the animal free movement in its cage. The tubing is passed through a spring arrangement over the cage so as to keep it fairly taut during the perfusion sessions. The heavy walls of the silicone tubing prevent crimping when the animal turns.

At the end of each perfusion session the silicone tubing is disconnected, the perfusion cap replaced with the stylus, and the animal returned to the animal quarters. The silastic tubing and perfusion cap are cleaned with 90% ethanol and forced air. A wire is inserted through the pull tube in the cap while it is not in use.

In most experiments artificial CSF is pumped into the ventricle through the push tube at a rate of 20 μl/min and sequential samples of perfusate (approximately 300 μl are collected every 15 min into the polyethylene microtubes, containing 400 μl of the high-performance liquid chromatography (HPLC) mobile phase (see later). Samples are weighed to estimate the exact volume of perfusate collected and then frozen at −20°C until analyzed.

C. Analytical Detection

Perfusate samples are centrifuged in a Beckman microfuge and the 500 μl are injected directly onto a chromatographic column (μ Bondapak C_{18} column, 30 cm × 3.9 mm i.d.; Waters Associates, Milford, Massachusetts). In some of the initial experiments the samples were filtered (Millipore, 0.22 μm filter membrane) prior to injecting them onto the columns, but this was found to be unnecessary and occasionally resulted in unknown compounds (one of which cochromatographed with DA) being eluted off of the filters.

A model LC-304 liquid amperometric detector was equipped with a TL-5 glassy carbon electrode set at a potential of +0.75 V relative to an Ag^+/AgCl reference electrode. In early experiments a carbon-paste electrode was employed, but it has been replaced by a glassy carbon electrode which is easier to resurface. All chromatographic experiments are performed at ambient temperature (20°–22°C) in an electrically shielded room.

Over the past few years several HPLC mobile phases have been used. These have consisted of either 0.1 *M* phosphate or citrate–phosphate buffers (pH 2–4.9) containing 0.1 m*M* EDTA, 1–8% methanol, and 0.012–0.036% sodium octyl sulfate. The constituents in the mobile phase were altered in order to maintain separation of peaks as the column aged. The buffers were filtered through 0.22 μm Millipore filter membranes and methanol through 0.5 μm Teflon filter membranes (Schleicher and Schnell, Keene, New Hampshire) prior to use.

Peak heights of standards and of compounds in the cerebroventricular perfusates have been recorded on strip chart recorders and recently by a Model 3390A Reporting Integrator (Hewlett Packard, Avondale, Pennsylvania). An example of recording from standards and from two samples of cerebroventricular perfusates is depicted in Fig. 3. There were no peaks in

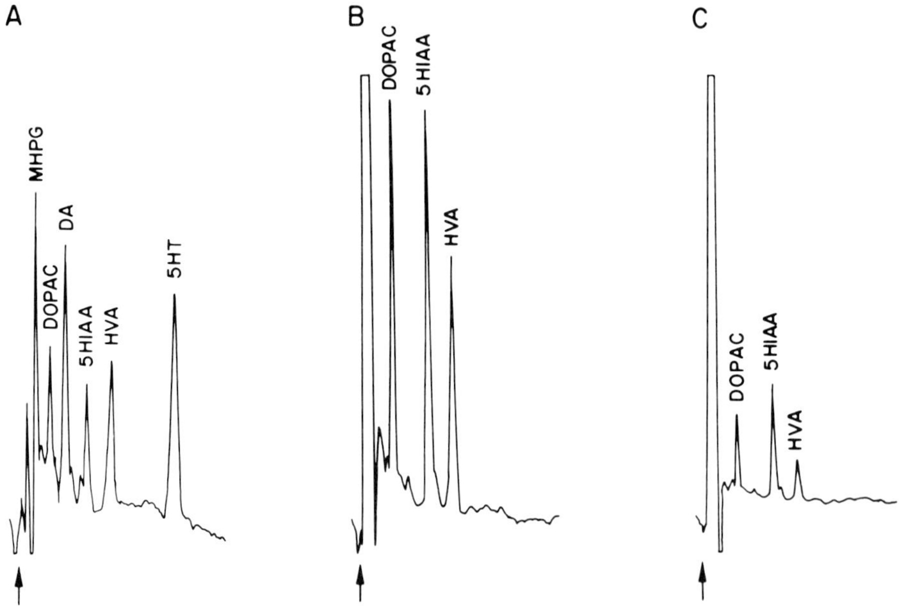

Fig. 3. Chromatograms of standards (A) and of cerebroventricular perfusate samples from a high (B) and a low (C) excretor of amine metabolites. Arrows indicate time of sample injection. Abbreviations: DA, dopamine; DOPAC, dihydroxyphenylacetic acid; 5HIAA, 5-hydroxyindoleacetic acid; 5HT, 5-hydroxytryptamine; HVA, homovanillic acid; MHPG, 3-methoxyl-4-hydroxyphenylglycol.

the perfusate samples with retention times corresponding to DA or 5HT. There were, however, substantial peaks with retention times the same as those for DOPAC, HVA, and 5HIAA. The amount of these metabolites in each sample was determined directly from peak heights of chromatographic standards. The sensitivity of the assays varied depending on the state of the electrode and the age of the μ Bondapak column, but there was no difficulty in detecting 0.6 ng DOPAC, 1.5 ng HVA, and 0.4 ng 5HIAA/ml of perfusate.

II. FINDINGS

Figure 4 is a schematic representation of the biochemical events believed to occur at terminals of central DA and 5HT neurons. In the DA neuron, pictured at the top, DA is synthesized in a two-step process involving the oxidation of tyrosine to form dihydroxyphenylalanine (DOPA) and the subsequent decarboxylation of this precursor to form DA; these reactions are catalyzed by tyrosine hydroxylase and aromatic L-amino acid decarboxylase, respectively. The synthesized DA can be stored or released in response to the arrival at the terminal of nerve action potentials or to the actions of

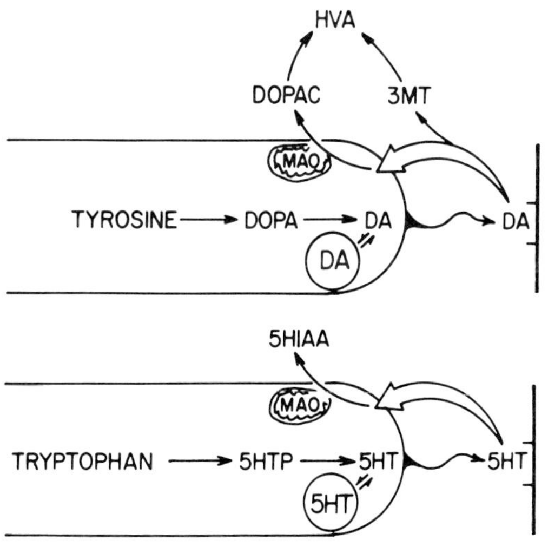

Fig. 4. Schematic diagram of the biochemical events occurring at terminals of a dopaminergic (top) and of a 5-hydroxytryptaminergic neuron (bottom). Abbreviations: DA, dopamine; DOPA, dihydroxyphenylalanine; DOPAC, dihydroxyphenylacetic acid; 5HIAA, 5-hydroxyindoleacetic acid; 5HT, 5-hydroxytryptamine; 5HTP, 5-hydroxytryptophan; HVA, homovanillic acid, MAO, monoamine oxidase; 3MT, 3-methoxytyramine.

drugs. The DA which is released into the synaptic cleft is briefly free to activate DA receptors located on the post- or presynaptic membranes, but it is quickly retrieved by a high-affinity amine transport system located in the presynaptic neuronal terminal. The recaptured DA can be released again, but most appears to be oxidatively deaminated by monoamine oxidase which is located on the surface membranes of mitochondria. The deaminated product of DA, DOPAC, then leaves the neuron and may be further metabolized to the O-methylated deaminated metabolite, HVA. This latter reaction is catalyzed by catechol *O*-methyltransferase, an enzyme that appears to be located primarily in glial cells. At least in the rat brain a small percentage of released DA can be O-methylated to 3-methoxytyramine (3MT) which, in turn, can be deaminated by extraneuronal monoamine oxidase to HVA. The acid metabolites of DA are then transported from the brain and CSF into the blood by an acid transport system.

A similar series of events occurs at the terminals of 5HT neurons. 5HT is synthesized from tryptophan, which is first oxidized to 5-hydroxytryptophan, and then decarboxylated to 5HT. These reactions are catalyzed by tryptophan hydroxylase and aromatic L-amino acid decarboxylase. The synthesized 5HT is then either stored or released into the synaptic cleft. It is quickly recaptured by the presynaptic nerve terminal by means of a high-affinity transport system and is subsequently oxidatively deaminated by mitochondrial monoamine oxidase to 5HIAA. 5HIAA is then removed from the brain by the same acid carrier system that transports DOPAC and HVA.

Our initial efforts were directed toward determining if it was possible to monitor the activity of 5HT and DA neurons in the brains of freely moving rats by measuring the concentrations of these amine neurotransmitters in cerebroventricular perfusates. Despite utilizing a number of different HPLC mobile phases it was not possible to unequivocally identify endogenous DA or 5HT in the perfusates, presumably because the concentrations of these amines were below the sensitivity of the analytical techniques (26). The very low concentration of amines in cerebroventricular perfusates probably results from the fact that the released amines are quickly recaptured by neuronal uptake systems and/or metabolized before they reach the cerebral ventricles.

Although the cerebroventricular perfusates lack significant quantities of DA and 5HT they do contain readily identifiable quantities of acid metabolites of these two amine neurotransmitters. This is depicted in sample chromatograms in Fig. 3. Chromatograms of cerebroventricular samples from two different rats reveal peaks with retention times that correspond with-DOPAC, 5HIAA, and HVA and possibly with 3-methyoxy, 4-hydroxyphenylglycol (MHPG), an O-methylated deaminated metabolite of NE.

The artificial CSF which is pumped into the lateral ventricle mixes with

TABLE I

Basal Efflux of DOPAC and 5HIAA over a 4-Week Period[a]

Time of collection (week)	DOPAC	5HIAA
1	11.3 ± 4.1	15.1 ± 5.7
2	13.8 ± 6.8	19.0 ± 4.7
3	10.3 ± 3.0	16.0 ± 1.7
4	9.7 ± 2.2	17.1 ± 3.6

[a] Values represent the metabolite concentrations (ng/ml; mean ± 1 SE) in perfusate samples collected from 4 rats.

endogenous CSF and this mixture is collected from the pull tube. It is not known what percentage of the collected perfusate is represented by actual CSF, but there is a remarkable constancy in the metabolite concentration in perfusate samples from each animal over time. This is exemplified by the data presented in Table I. The mean concentration of DOPAC and 5HIAA in perfusate samples from 4 rats collected once a week for 4 weeks was relatively constant over this period of time. Note, however, the standard errors are relatively large because of interanimal variation. The perfusate from some animals consistently contains high concentrations of DOPAC, HVA, and 5HIAA, while samples from other animals will almost always contain much lower concentrations of these metabolites (e.g., Fig. 3). The interanimal variation may be related to subtle differences in the placement site of the push–pull cannula in the ventricle. Whatever the reason for the interanimal variation, it can be obviated by having each animal serve as its own control. For example, in studies involving pharmacological manipulations the concentration of the metabolites in perfusate samples collected from each animal before drug administration is subtracted from corresponding values after drug administration. Thus, results are reported as "drug-induced changes."

Examples of drug-induced changes in the efflux of amine metabolites are depicted in Fig. 5. As noted, acid metabolites of DA and 5HT are transported out of the brain and into the blood by an acid transport system. Probenecid blocks this transport system and thereby increases the concentration of these metabolites in the brain and CSF. As expected, probenecid also increased the concentration of DOPAC, HVA, and 5HIAA in the cerebroventricular perfusates. On the other hand, pargyline, a monoamine oxidase inhibitor, prevents the oxidative deamination of DA and 5HT and thereby decreases brain and CSF concentrations of the deaminated metabolites; it also reduces the concentrations of these metabolites in cerebroventricular perfusates. The administration of tryptophan increases the sub-

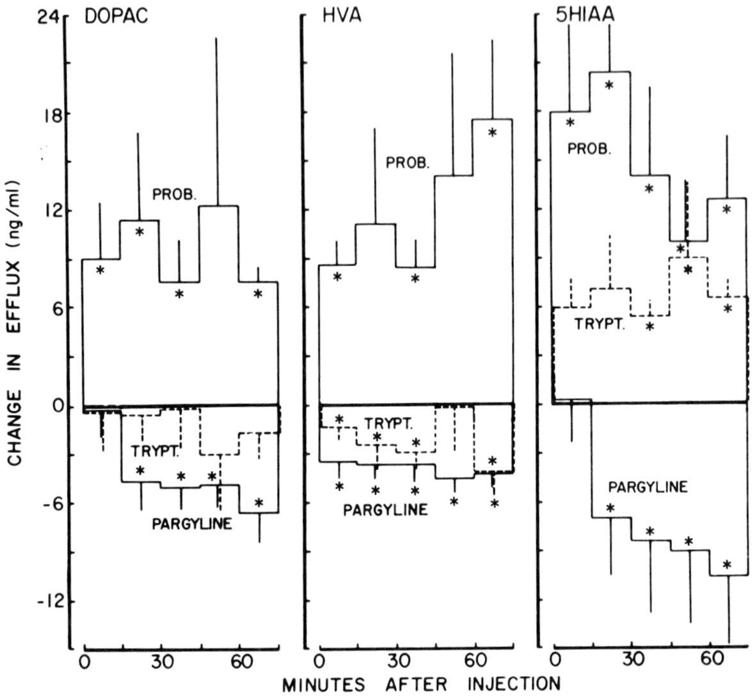

Fig. 5. Effects of systemic injections of probenecid, pargyline or L-tryptophan on the efflux of DOPAC, HVA, and 5HIAA from brain into cerebroventricular perfusates. The lateral cerebral ventricles of 5 rats were perfused for 90 min at weekly intervals with sequential samples collected at 15-min intervals. After collecting the first sample, rats were injected intraperitoneally with probenecid (PROB., 250 mg/kg), L-tryptophan (TRYPT., 100 mg/kg), or pargyline (75 mg/kg). Values represent means and vertical lines 1 SE. (*), Values in drug-treated animals that are significantly different ($p < .05$) from saline-injected animals (changes in efflux of amine metabolites in saline-injected rats were not significantly different from zero, and not reported). [Reprinted from ref. (*23*).]

strate concentration for tryptophan hydroxylase and thereby increases the synthesis of 5HT and consequently the brain concentrations of both 5HT and 5HIAA. Systemic administration of tryptophan increased the perfusate concentration of 5HIAA but was without effect on DOPAC. In this particular experiment tryptophan also caused a slight decrease in the efflux of HVA, but this effect is not observed consistently.

A. Effects of Anesthetics

One of the objectives of the present studies was to carry out cerebroventricular perfusions in unanesthetized rats. Various anesthetics have been reported to alter the concentrations of neurotransmitter metabolites in CSF (*3, 20*) and in cerebroventricular perfusates (*38*). Chloral hydrate has been reported to increase the firing rate of nigrostriatal DA neurons (*8*) and to increase the rate of synthesis of DA in the striatum (*33*). It was not surprising, therefore, that the systemic administration of chloral hydrate increased the efflux of DOPAC and HVA (Fig. 6). This anesthetic tended to reduce the efflux of 5HIAA, but the difference in the concentration of this metabolite in each sample from chloral hydrate-treated animals was not significantly different from corresponding samples from saline-treated animals. On the

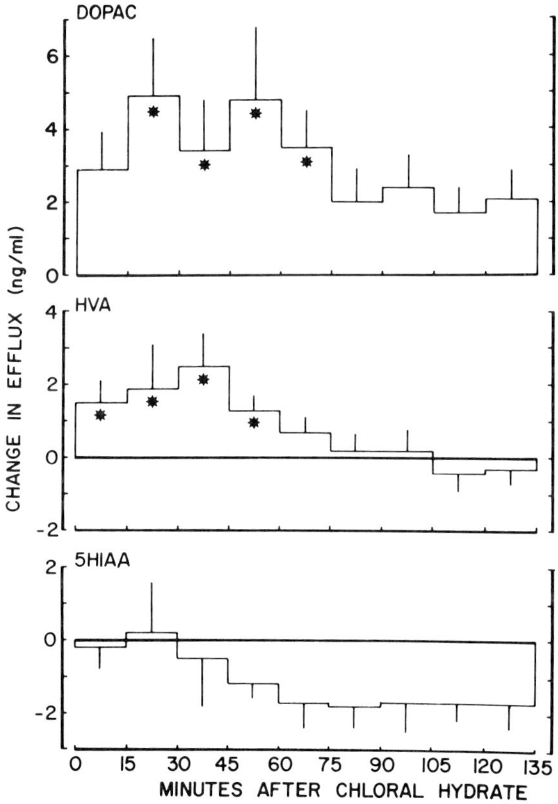

Fig. 6. Efflux of DOPAC, HVA, and 5HIAA into cerebroventricular perfusates of rats treated with chloral hydrate. Columns represent the mean change (vertical lines represent 1 SE, $N=6$) in the concentration of metabolites in 15-min samples collected after injecting chloral hydrate (400 mg/kg, ip) less the mean concentration of metabolites in two samples collected immediately before injecting the anesthetic. (*), Values that are significantly different ($p < .05$) from corresponding values in animals injected with saline. [Reprinted from ref. (*24*). See ref. (*24*) for additional details.]

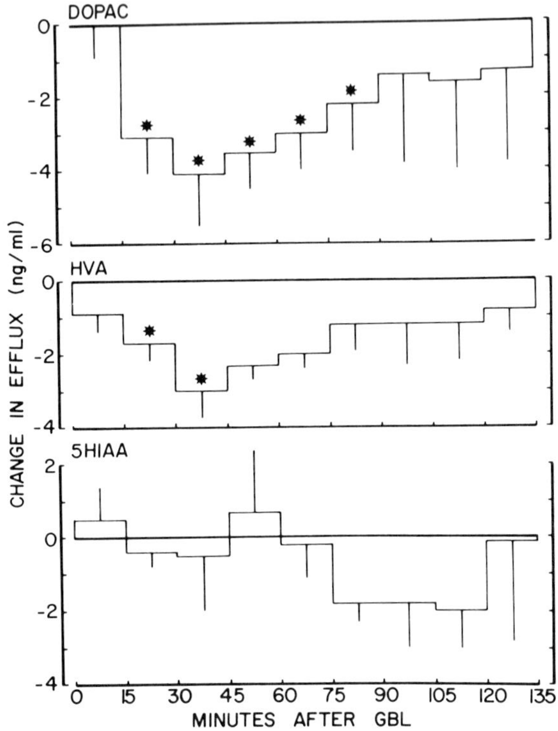

Fig. 7. Efflux of DOPAC, HVA, and 5HIAA into cerebroventricular perfusates of rats treated with γ-butyrolactone (GBL). Columns represent the mean change (vertical lines represent 1 SE, $N=6$) in the concentration of metabolites in 15-min samples collected after injecting GBL (750 mg/kg, ip) less the mean concentration of metabolites in two samples collected immediately before injecting the anesthetic. (*), Values that are significantly different ($p < .05$) from corresponding values in animals injected with saline. [Reprinted from ref. (*24*). See ref. (*24*) for additional details.]

other hand, the systemic administration of γ-butyrolactone (GBL), which is reported to reduce impulse activity in ascending DA neurons (*32*), reduced the efflux of DOPAC and HVA, but was without effect on the efflux of 5HIAA (Fig. 7). These results reveal that anesthetic agents can alter the efflux of DA metabolites into the CSF and suggest that neurochemical studies carried out in anesthetized animals should be interpreted with this in mind.

B. Effects of DA Agonists and Antagonists

The activities of the major ascending DA neurons are regulated, in part, by DA receptor-mediated mechanisms. Activation of postsynaptic DA receptors controlling neuronal feedback loops or of autoreceptors on terminals or cell-body dendrites of the DA neurons decrease the activity and/or release of DA from the terminals of the neurons, while blockade of these receptors results in a compensatory activation of these neurons (see review, *41*). By these mechanisms DA receptor agonists decrease and DA receptor antagonists increase brain and CSF concentrations of DOPAC and HVA (*1, 30–32*). As would be anticipated from these results, it was found that systemic administration of a DA antagonist (haloperidol) increased while a DA agonist (apomorphine) decreased the efflux of DOPAC and HVA into cerebroventricular perfusates (Fig. 8). Haloperidol did not alter the efflux of

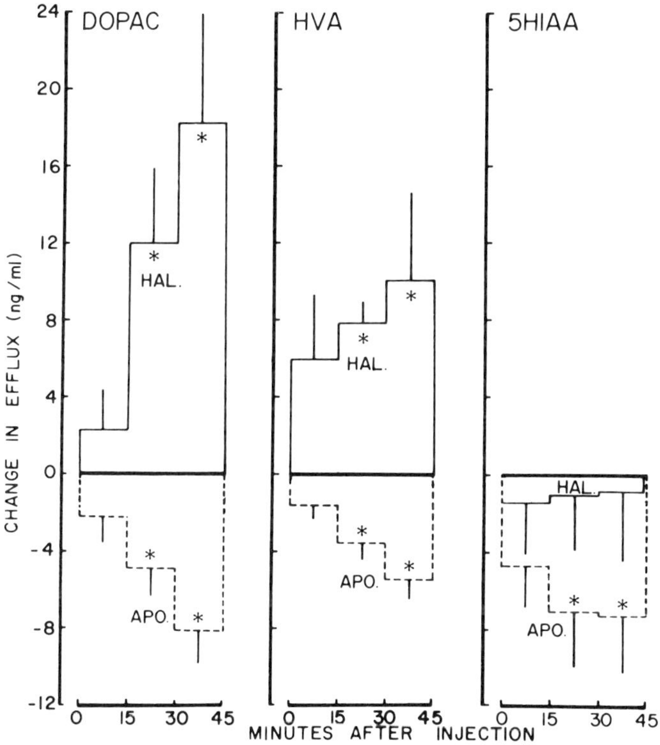

Fig. 8. Effects of systemic injections of haloperidol or apomorphine on the efflux of DOPAC, HVA, and 5HIAA from brain and into cerebroventricular perfusates. At weekly intervals the lateral ventricles of 6 rats were perfused for 90 min. After collecting three 15-min samples the rats were injected subcutaneously with either 0.9% saline, haloperidol (0.1 mg/kg), or apomorphine (0.5 mg/kg). Columns represent the mean change (vertical lines represent 1 SE, $N=6$) in the concentration of metabolites in 15-min samples collected after the systemic injections less the mean concentration of metabolites in two samples collected immediately before injecting the drugs. (*), Values that are significantly different ($p < .05$) from corresponding values in animals injected with saline. [Reprinted from ref. (*23*). See ref. (*23*) for additional details.]

5HIAA while apomorphine caused a slight decrease in the efflux of this metabolite; this latter effect has not been observed in subsequent experiments.

One of the advantages of the present technique is that it permits repeated

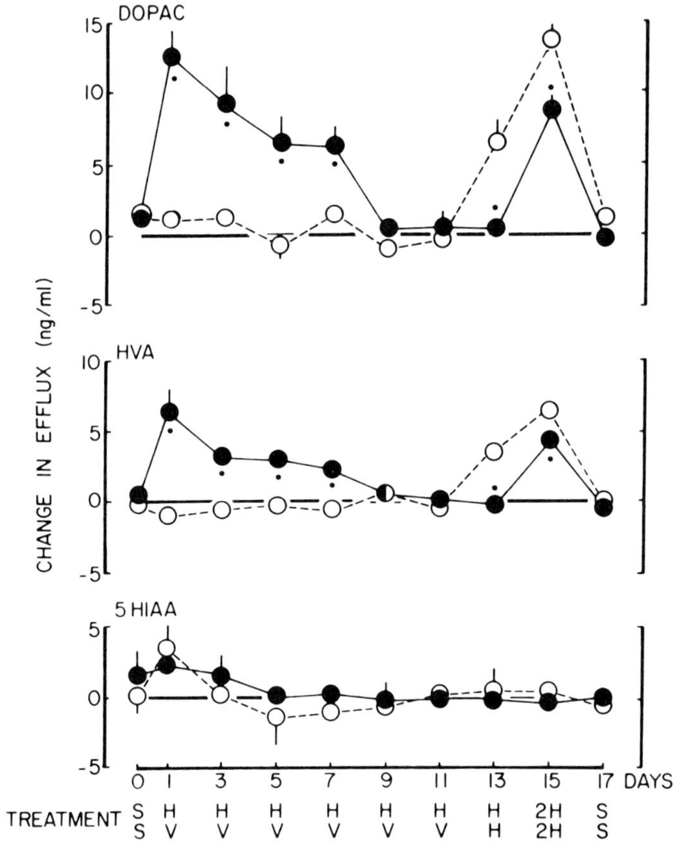

Fig. 9. Effects of repeated injections of haloperidol on the efflux of DOPAC, HVA, and 5HIAA from brain and into cerebroventricular perfusates. The lateral ventricles of two groups of rats were perfused every other day for 75 min with sequential samples collected at 15-min intervals. After collecting two samples the rats were injected subcutaneously as indicated along the abscissa (H and 2H, haloperidol 1 and 2 mg/kg, respectively; S, saline; V, 0.3% tartaric acid vehicle). Symbols (○, chronic vehicle; ●, chronic haloperidol) represent the mean concentrations of metabolites in the sample collected 30–45 min after the injections less the concentration in the sample collected immediately before the injection. Vertical lines projecting upon each symbol represent 1 SE ($N = 3–6$). (*), Significantly different ($p < .05$) from the corresponding value in the chronic vehicle group. [See ref. (*25*) for additional details. Reprinted with permission from *Life Sci.* **31,** J. A. Nielsen, N. J. Duda, and K. E. Moore, Tolerance develops to the haloperidol-induced increase in the efflux of dopamine metabolites from the brains of unanesthetized freely-moving rats. Copyright 1982, Pergamon Press, Ltd.]

cerebroventricular perfusions and thereby allows determination of the neurochemical effects of chronic drug administration in the same animal. The effect of chronic administration of haloperidol is depicted in Fig. 9. In this experiment rats were injected daily with either haloperidol (1 mg/kg) or its 0.3% tartaric acid vehicle. Every second day the cerebral ventricles of these animals were perfused for two 15-min periods, the animals were injected with either haloperidol or vehicle, and the perfusion then continued for another three 15-min periods. The results represent the metabolite concentration in the sample collected 30–45 min after injection less the concentrations in the sample collected immediately before the injection. After the first inection of haloperidol there was a marked increase in the efflux of DOPAC and HVA (see also Fig. 8). This effect declined progressively during each subsequent perfusion session so that by days 9, 11, and 13 haloperidol no longer altered the efflux of the DA metabolites. When the dose of haloperidol was doubled on day 15 the animals did exhibit an increased efflux of DOPAC and HVA. At no time was there a significant change in the efflux of 5HIAA. Thus, tolerance develops to the haloperidol-induced efflux of DA metabolites. This is consistent with previous reports on the development of tolerance to DA antagonist-induced changes in unit activity (*7*) and in the neurochemical dynamics of DA neurons (*34*).

C. Long-Term Perfusions of Cerebral Ventricles

In experiments already described the cerebral ventricles of individual animals were perfused for up to 4 weeks. It was deemed of interest to determine if the ventricles of individual rats could be perfused for longer periods of time. The "basal" concentrations of DOPAC and 5HIAA in cerebroventricular perfusates collected at 2, 9, and 16 months of age from two individual rats are summarized in Table II. The absolute concentration of metabolites differed substantially in the ventricular perfusates of the two

TABLE II

Basal Efflux of DOPAC and 5HIAA over a 14-Month Period[a]

Rat	Metabolite	2 months	9 months	16 months
No. 76	DOPAC	10.6 ± 1.1	10.5 ± 2.0	8.3 ± 4.2
	5HIAA	6.1 ± 0.7	4.5 ± 0.5	4.1 ± 1.1
No. 80	DOPAC	15.2 ± 1.8	17.5 ± 3.6	19.3 ± 2.5
	5HIAA	15.1 ± 2.4	26.2 ± 1.4	21.5 ± 5.8

[a] Values represent the metabolite concentrations (ng/ml; mean ± 1 SE) in 3 perfusate samples collected at approximately 7-day intervals from 2 individual rats at 2, 9, and 16 months of age.

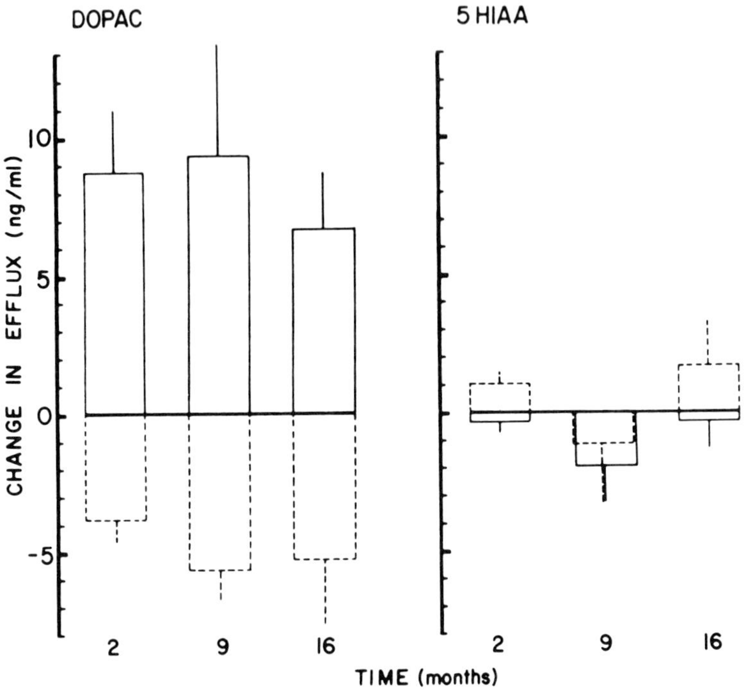

Fig. 10. Effects of systemically administered haloperidol or apomorphine on concentrations of DOPAC and 5HIAA in cerebroventricular perfusates from rats at 2, 9, and 16 months of age. Columns represent the mean change (vertical lines represent 1 SE, $N=6$ at 2 and 9 months and $N=3$ at 16 months) in the concentrations of DOPAC and 5HIAA collected during the 45-min period after the injection of the drug less the mean concentration in two samples collected before the drugs were administered (——, haloperidol 1 mg/kg, sc; ---, apomorphine, 0.5 mg/kg sc). The mean predrug concentrations of metabolites did not change significantly over the 14-month period (see Table II).

animals (No. 76 being a low excretor and No. 80 a high excretor), but the efflux of both DOPAC and 5HIAA was remarkably constant over the 14-month period. Furthermore, the responses to drugs were also maintained over this period. As shown in Fig. 10, the haloperidol-induced increase and the apomorphine-induced decrease in the ventricular perfusate concentrations of DOPAC were essentially the same at 2, 9, and 16 months of age. These results suggest that it is possible to monitor neurochemical indices of DA and 5HT neuronal activity in unanesthetized rats for prolonged periods of time.

One of the problems encountered in this study was that between 9 and 16 months of age one of the six animals in the study died of unknown causes and two forcibly removed their cannulas. In addition, histological examination of the brains of the 16-month animals revealed that the ventricles were enlarged and the ventricular lining of two animals showed signs of inflammatory responses. When brains were perfused over shorter periods of time (4 weeks) there was often some evidence of ventricular enlargement and occasionally some gliosis and infiltration of macrophages near the ventricular lining. For the most part, however, the ventricular lining appeared to be anatomically normal.

D. Consequences of Destroying DA and 5HT Neurons

It is generally assumed that DA and 5HT metabolites in the CSF (and consequently cerebroventricular perfusates) orginate from DA and 5HT neu-

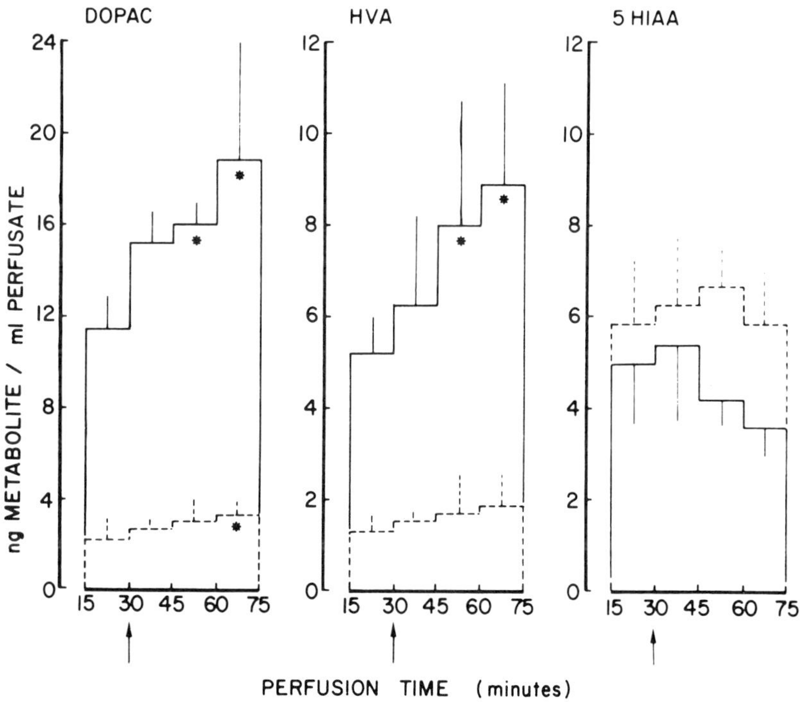

Fig. 11. Effects of haloperidol on DOPAC, HVA, and 5HIAA concentrations in cerebroventricular perfusates of unanesthetized rats before and after treatment with 6-hydroxydopamine. The lateral cerebroventricles of 6 rats were perfused with artificial cerebrospinal fluid for 75 min with sequential samples collected at 15-min intervals. Each animal was injected with haloperidol (1 mg/kg, sc) at 30 min as indicated by the arrows. Approximately 2 hr after the end of the perfusion, 6-OHDA (200 μg/rat) was injected i.vent, and this was repeated 7 days later. Seven days after the second 6-OHDA injection the animals were again perfused and injected with haloperidol. Values represent the mean perfusate concentrations of DOPAC, HVA, and 5HIAA before (——) and after (---) treatments with 6-OHDA. Vertical lines represent 1 SE; (*), Haloperidol-induced changes in metabolite concentrations ($p < .05$).

rons terminating in regions bordering the cerebral ventricles. To test this directly, rats were treated with neurotoxins that selectively destroy DA or 5HT neurons.

In animals treated 14 days previously with an intracerebroventricular injection of 6-hydroxydopamine (6-OHDA) the basal efflux of DOPAC and HVA, but not of 5HIAA, was markedly reduced (Fig. 11). Prior to 6-OHDA treatment haloperidol increased the efflux of DA metabolites (see also Figs. 8 and 9), whereas after 6-OHDA this action of haloperidol was greatly attenuated.

In animals treated 10 days previously with 5,7-dihydroxytryptamine (5,7DHT) the basal efflux of 5HIAA was drastically reduced while the efflux of DOPAC and HVA was not altered (Fig. 12). Prior to the administration of

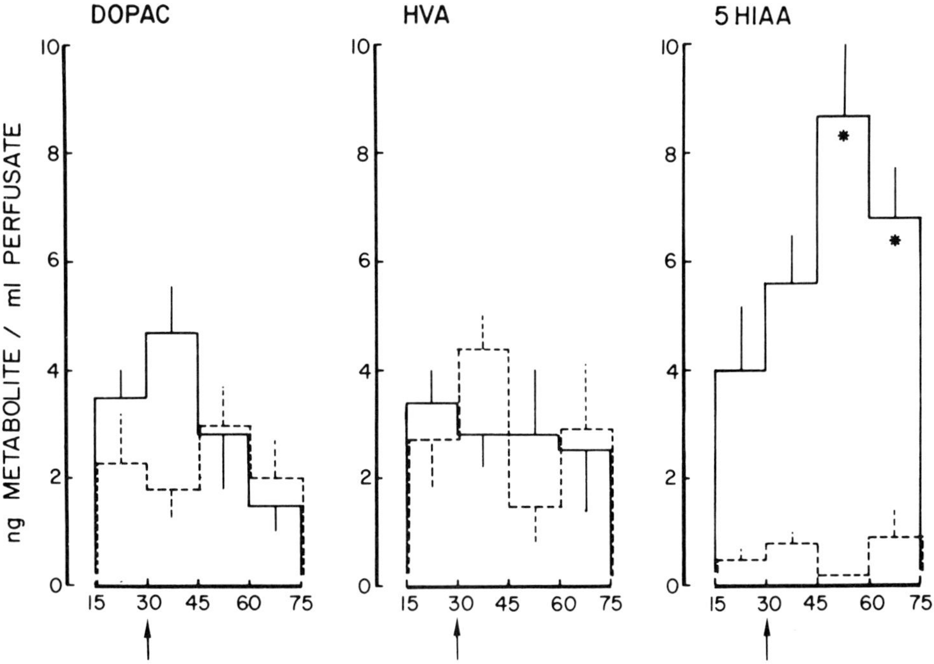

Fig. 12. Effects of L-tryptophan on DOPAC, HVA, and 5HIAA concentrations in cerebroventricular perfusates of unanesthetized rats before and after treatment with 5,7-DHT. The lateral cerebroventricles of 4 rats were perfused with artificial cerebrospinal fluid for 75 min with sequential samples collected at 15-min intervals. Each animal was injected with L-tryptophan (100 mg/kg, ip) at 30 min as indicated by the arrows. Approximately 2 hr after the end of the perfusion, 5,7-DHT (200 μg/rat) was injected i.vent. Ten days later the animals were again perfused and injected with L-tryptophan. Values represent the mean perfusate concentrations of DOPAC, HVA, and 5HIAA before (——) and after (---) treatment with 5,7-DHT. Vertical lines represent 1 SE; (*), L-tryptophan-induced changes in metabolite concentrations ($p < .05$). [Reprinted from ref. (*42*).]

5,7DHT an injection of L-tryptophan increased the efflux of 5HIAA; this effect was not observed following treatment with 5,7DHT.

Since intracerebroventricular injections of 6-OHDA destroy catecholaminergic neurons and injections of 5,7DHT destroy 5HT neurons, it is not surprising that these two neurotoxins selectively reduced the cerebroventricular perfusate concentrations of DA and 5HT metabolites, respectively. The results of these two experiments indicate, however, that the DOPAC and HVA and the 5HIAA which appear in cerebroventricular perfusates do originate from DA and 5HT neurons in the brain, presumably from terminals in brain regions lying adjacent to the lateral cerebral ventricles.

III. PERSPECTIVES

A technique is described which permits repeated noninvasive sampling of CSF from unanesthetized and unrestrained rats. The technique involves permanent implantation of a cannula such that the tip is located within a lateral cerebral ventricle. Perfusion of the ventricle is effected by inserting a push cannula into the chronically implanted pull cannula and pumping artificial CSF into the lateral cerebral ventricle. The artificial CSF apparently mixes with the endogenous CSF and serial samples of the mixture are then collected over time and analyzed for putative neurotransmitters and their metabolites using HPLC coupled to an electrochemical detector. This analytical procedure is relatively simple and inexpensive (when compared to radioactive tracer techniques) and since endogenous compounds are analyzed, some of the problems which occasionally confound results of studies using radioactive tracers (alterations in pool size, radioactive impurities, etc.) are avoided. The deaminated metabolites of DA and 5HT are easily identified in the cerebroventricular perfusates although, unfortunately, the method is not sensitive enough to quantify the small amounts of the parent amines present in the CSF. Nevertheless, pharmacological manipulations which alter DA and 5HT neuronal activity or which alter the metabolism and/or transport of the amines or their metabolites, and thereby cause characteristic changes in the concentrations of the amine metabolites in brain tissue, cause comparative changes in the cerebroventricular perfusate concentrations of these metabolites. These pharmacological studies support the proposal that the concentrations of metabolites in cerebroventricular perfusate samples reflect, to a large extent, the activity of central DA and 5HT neurons.

One advantage of the technique is that it can be carried out in unanesthetized animals so that the effects of physiological and pharmacological manipulations on the efflux of DA and 5HT metabolites are not confounded by the presence of anesthetics, which are shown to alter the efflux of these metabolites. Furthermore, since the animals do not need to be restrained, perfusions can be carried out in the animals' home cages thereby eliminating possible influences of novel environments on the results.

Another advantage of the technique is that since the tip of the push–pull cannula is within the cerebral ventricle there is less likelihood of collecting perfusate from damaged tissue as may be the case when the tip of the cannula is in brain tissue per se. On the other hand, the precise source of the amine metabolites in the cerebroventricular perfusates is unknown, although presumably the metabolites originate from nerve terminals in tissues bordering the lateral cerebral ventricles. Although the presence of the push–pull cannula within the cerebral ventricles appears to cause little tissue damage, the results should be tempered by the fact that the pressure or turbulence produced during the perfusions may cause some structural alteration in the ventricular lining or brain. Nevertheless, the metabolite concentrations in perfusates collected over several months from individual animals are remarkably constant, and are consistently altered in response to repeated drug administration. Thus, it is possible with this technique to follow the effects of repeated pharmacological or other manipulations in the same animal over periods of weeks or even months.

ACKNOWLEDGMENTS

The authors gratefully acknowledge the assistance of Diane Hummel in preparing the manuscript. The authors' studies have been supported by USPHS grant NS15911.

REFERENCES

1. Andén, N.-E., Roos, B.-E., and Werdinius, B. Effects of chlorpromazine, haloperidol and reserpine on the levels of phenol acids in rabbit corpus striatum. *Life Sci.* **3** (1974) 140–159.
2. Ashkenazi, R., Holman, R. B., and Vogt, M. Release of transmitters on stimulation of the nucleus linearis raphé in the cat. *J. Physiol.* (*London*) **223** (1972) 255–259.
3. Barkai, A. I. Dopamine turnover in the intact rabbit brain: effect of pentobarbital or haloperidol. *J. Pharmacol. Exp. Ther.* **205** (1978) 133–140.
4. Besson, M. J., Cheramy, A., Feltz, P. and Glowinski, J. Dopamine: spontaneous and drug-induced release from the caudate nucleus in the cat. *Brain Res.* **32** (1971) 407–424.
5. Bhattacharya, B. K., and Feldberg, W. Perfusion of cerebral ventricles: effects of drugs on outflow from the cisterna and the aqueduct. *Br. J. Pharmacol.* **13** (1958) 156–162.
6. Bhattacharya, B. K., and Feldberg, W. Perfusion of cerebral ventricles: assay of pharmacologically active substances in the effluent from the cisterna and the aqueduct. *Br. J. Pharmacol.* **13** (1958) 163–174.
7. Bunney, B. S., and Grace, A. A. Acute and chronic haloperidol treatment, comparison of effects of nigral dopaminergic cell activity. *Life Sci.* **23** (1978) 1715–1728.
8. Bunney, B. S., Walters, J. R., Roth, R. H., and Aghajanian, G. K. Dopaminergic neurons:

effect of antipsychotic drugs and amphetamine on single cell activity. *J. Pharmacol. Exp. Ther.* **185** (1973) 560–571.
9. Carmichael, E. A., Feldberg, W., and Fleischauer, K. Methods for perfusing different parts of the cat's cerebral ventricles with drugs. *J. Physiol. (London)* **173** (1964) 354–367.
10. Carr, L. A., and Moore, K. E. Effects of amphetamine on the contents of norepinephrine and its metabolites in the effluent of perfused cerebral ventricles of the cat. *Biochem. Pharmacol.* **19** (1970) 2361–2374.
11. Chiueh, C. C., and Moore, K. E. Effects of dopaminergic agonists and electrical stimulation of the midbrain raphe on the release of 5-hydroxytryptamine from the cat brain *in vivo*. *J. Neurochem.* **26** (1976) 319–324.
12. Chiueh, C. C., and Kopin, I. J. Radioenzymatic paper-chromatographic assay for dopamine and norepinephrine in cerebroventricular cisternal perfusate of cat following administration of cocaine or *d*-amphetamine. *J. Neurochem.* **31** (1978) 561–564.
13. Feldberg, W., and Meyers, R. D. Appearance of 5-hydroxytryptamine and an unidentified pharmacologically active lipid acid in effluent from perfused cerebral ventricles. *J. Physiol. (London)* **184** (1966) 837–855.
14. Gallager, D. W., and Aghajanian, G. K. Effects of chlorimipramine and lysergic acid diethylamide on efflux of precursor-formed ^{3}H-serotonin: correlations with serotonergic impulse flow. *J. Pharmacol. Exp. Ther.* **193** (1975) 785–795.
15. Gallager, D. W., Sanders-Bush, E., Aghajanian, G. K., and Sulser, F. An evaluation of the use of intraventricularly administered ^{3}H-5-hydroxytryptamine as a marker for endogenous brain 5-hydroxytryptamine. *Brain Res.* **93** (1975) 111–122.
16. Goodrich, C. A. Effect of monoamineoxidase inhibitors on 5-hydroxytryptamine output from perfused cerebral ventricles of anaesthetized cats. *Br. J. Pharmacol.* **37** (1969) 87–93.
17. Guldberg, H. C., and Yates, C. M. Some studies of the effects of chlorpromazine reserpine and dihydroxyphenylalanine on the concentrations of homovanillic acid, 3,4-dihydroxyphenylacetic acid and 5-hydroxyindole-3-acetic acid in ventricular cerebrospinal fluid of the dog using the technique of serial sampling of the cerebrospinal fluid. *Br. J. Pharmacol.* **33** (1968) 457–471.
18. Guldberg, H. C., Ashcroft, G. W., and Crawford, T. B. B. Concentrations of 5-hydroxyindoleacetic acid and homovanillic acid in the cerebrospinal fluid of the dog before and during treatment with probenecid. *Life Sci.* **5** (1966) 1571–1575.
19. Homan, R. B., and Vogt, M. Release of 5-hydroxytryptamine from caudate nucleus and septum. *J. Physiol. (London)* **223** (1972) 243–254.
20. Isaac, L. Temperature alteration of monoamine metabolites in cerebrospinal fluid. *Nature (London)* **243** (1973) 269–271.
21. Loullis, C. C., Hingtgen, J. N., Shea, P. A., and Aprison, M. H. *In vivo* determination of endogenous biogenic amines in rat brain using HPLC and push–pull cannula. *Pharmacol. Biochem. Behav.* **12** (1980) 959–964.
22. Moore, K. E. The actions of amphetamine on neurotransmitters: a brief review. *Biol. Psychiat.* **12** (1977) 451–462.
23. Nielsen, J. A., and Moore, K. E. Measurement of metabolites of dopamine and 5-hydroxytryptamine in cerebroventricular perfusates of unanesthetized, freely moving rats. *Pharmacol. Biochem. Behav.* **16** (1982) 131–137.
24. Nielsen, J. A., and Moore, K. E. Effects of chloral hydrate, γ-butyrolactone, and equithesin on the efflux of dopamine and 5-hydroxytryptamine metabolites into cerebroventricular perfusates of rats. *J. Neurochem.* **39** (1982) 235–238.
25. Nielsen, J. A., Duda, N. J., and Moore, K. E. Tolerance develops to the haloperidol-induced increase in the efflux of dopamine metabolites from the brains of unanesthetized freely moving rats. *Life Sci.* **31** (1982) 1495–1500.

26. Palfreyman, M. G., Huot, S., and Wagner, J. Value of monoamine metabolite determinations in CSF as an index of their concentrations in rat brain following various pharmacological manipulations. *J. Pharmacol. Meth.* **8** (1982) 174–183.
27. Pellegrino, L., J., and Cushman, A. J. "A Stereotaxic Atlas of the Rat Brain," 1967. Appleton, New York.
28. Portig, P. J., and Vogt, M. Release into the cerebral ventricles of substances with possible transmitter function in the caudate nucleus. *J. Physiol. (London)* **204** (1969) 687–715.
29. Portig, P. J., Sharman, D. F., and Vogt, M. Release by tubocurarine of dopamine and homovanillic acid from the superfused caudate nucleus. *J. Physiol. (London)* **194** (1968) 565–572.
30. Post, R. M., and Goodwin, F. K. Approaches to brain amines in psychiatric patients: a reevaluation of cerebrospinal fluid studies. *In* "Handbook of Psychopharmacology," Vol. 13, (L. L. Iversen and S. H. Snyder, eds.), 1978, pp. 147–185. Plenum, New York.
31. Roos, B.-E. Decrease in homovanillic acid as evidence for dopamine receptor stimulation by apomorphine in the neostriatum of the rat. *J. Pharm. Pharmacol.* **21** (1969) 263–264.
32. Roth, R. H., Walters, J. R., and Aghajanian, G. K. Effect of impulse flow on the release and synthesis of dopamine in the rat striatum. *In* "Frontiers in Catecholamine Research," (E. Usdin and S. H. Snyder, eds.), 1973, pp. 567–574. Pergamon, New York.
33. Roth, R. H., Walters, J. R., Murrin, L. C., and Morgenroth, V. H. Dopaminergic neurons: role of impulse flow and presynaptic receptors in the regulation of tyrosine hydroxylase. *In* "Pre- and Postsynaptic Receptors," (E. Usdin and W. E. Bunney, es.), 1975, pp. 5–46. Dekker, New York.
34. Scatton, B. Differential regional development of tolerance to increase in dopamine turnover upon repeated neuroleptic administration. *Eur. J. Pharmacol.* **46** (1977) 363–369.
35. Sparber, S. B. Perfusion techniques. *Carrier* **2** (1975) 1–5.
36. Ternaux, J. P., Birreau, A., Bourgoin, S., Hamon, M., Hery, F., and Glowinski, J. *In vivo* release of 5-HT in the lateral ventricle of the rat: effects of 5-hydroxytryptophan and tryptophan. *Brain Res.* **101** (1976) 533–548.
37. Tilson, H. A., and Sparber, S. B. On the use of the push–pull cannula as a means of measuring biochemical changes during on-going behavior. *Behav. Res. Meth. Instrum.* **2** (1970) 131–134.
38. Vogt, M. Release from brain tissue of compounds with possible transmitter function: interaction of drugs with these substances. *Br. J. Pharmacol.* **37** (1969) 325–337.
39. Von Voigtlander, P. F., and Moore, K. E. Involvement of nigro-striatal neurons in the *in vivo* release of dopamine by amphetamine, amantadine and tyramine. *J. Pharmacol. Exp. Ther.* **184** (1973) 542–552.
40. Wagner, J., Vitali, P., Palfreyman, M. G., Zraika, M., and Huot, S. Simultaneous determination of 3,4-dihydroxyphenylalanine, 5-hydroxytryptophan, dopamine, 4-hydroxy-3-methoxyphenylalanine, norepinephrine, 3,4-dihydroxyphenylacetic acid, homovanillic acid, serotonin, and 5-hydroxyindoleacetic acid in the rat cerebrospinal fluid and brain by HPLC with electrochemical detection. *J. Neurochem.* **38** (1982) 1241–1254.
41. Wuerthele, S. M., and Moore, K. E. Regulation of nigrostriatal and tuberoinfundibular-hypophyseal dopaminergic neurons. *In* "Progress in Neurobiology," Vol. 13, (G. A. Kerkut and J. W. Phillis, eds.), 1979, pp. 325–359. Pergamon, New York.
42. Nielson, J. A., and Moore, K. E. 6-Hydroxydopamine and 5,7 dihydroxytryptamine selectively reduce dopamine and 5-hydroxytryptamine metabolites in cerebroventricular perfusates of rats. *Pharmacol. Biochem. Behav.* **19** (1983) 905–907.

12

Hippocampal Involvement in the Effects of Ethyl Alcohol: *In Vivo* and *In Vitro* Levels of Analysis

H. S. SWARTZWELDER

Department of Medicine
Division of Neurology
Duke University Medical Center
Durham, North Carolina

I. INTRODUCTION

The limbic system consists of a group of interconnected structures of the forebrain and diencephalon. Although diverse in morphology, this limbic circuit has been hypothesized to participate in the modulation of learning and memory (*28*), behavioral reactivity (*6*), motivation (*36*), and emotionality (*45*). The structures of the limbic system include the hippocampus, amygdala, cingulate gyrus, and septum. With the exception of the hippocampus, these structures are clearly of a non-cortical nature; however, certain cortical and diencephalic structures are crucial components of the integrated limbic system. Entorhinal, pyriform, and frontal cortical areas are reciprocally interconnected with the primary limbic components mentioned

IN VIVO PERFUSION AND RELEASE
OF NEUROACTIVE SUBSTANCES

ISBN 0-12-083350-6

above, as are the dorsomedial thalamic nucleus and mammillary bodies of the hypothalamus.

The limbic system is, therefore, in an ideal position anatomically to act as an interface between the diencephalon and the neocortex, and its interconnections with these areas would suggest a modulatory role for its core structures. In fact, this position is supported at the functional level by the observation that many of the effects of lesions or stimulation of extrahypothalamic limbic structures may be replicated by stimulation or lesion of hypothalamic nuclei [see ref. (*28*)]. Of particular interest in this regard are the extensive connections of the entorhinal cortex with the hippocampus. Polysensory information from this association area is relayed directly to the hippocampal formation over an excitatory pathway (discussed later). Thus, the limbic system and in particular the hippocampus seem to be positioned strategically for the integration of both internal and external stimuli. The possibility then arises that a rudimentary level of stimulus evaluation may occur in this system prior to or simultaneously with cortical processing.

The evolutionary or adaptive import of such an integrative and modulatory mechanism is obvious, and the limbic system has continued to evolve along with the hominid neocortex. Despite the fact that the limbic structures themselves have remained rudimentary and small in volume relative to the expanding primate neocortex, the amount of limbic-cortical connection has increased through evolution; that is, the number of axons in the fiber tracts leading to and from the limbic system and cortex have increased both in absolute volume and relative to the fiber systems supporting other central nervous system (CNS) interconnections. In fact, Isaacson (*28*) points out that in man there are five times as many fibers in the fornix as in the optic tracts. The adaptive importance of the hypothalamic–limbic–cortical interface is suggested by this evolutionary development.

In the context of psychopharmacology and drug addiction, it seems likely that the limbic system and in particular the hippocampus may play a crucial role in both integrating the sensory and visceral effects of psychoactive compounds as well as in modulating the behavioral reactivity (including addictive behaviors) of the animal to a drug effect. That the hippocampus is particularly sensitive to the effects of various drugs, toxicants, and disease states will be a consistent theme throughout the remainder of this chapter, and provides the primary rationale for my suggestion that this may be a fertile structure in which to study drug effects via chemical stimulation techniques. However, prior to outlining the interactions of alcohol effects with hippocampal function, a brief outline of hippocampal anatomy and vulnerability is in order.

Both the morphology and physiological integrity of the hippocampus are altered following chronic electrical stimulation via the perforant path (*49*).

Seizure activity will produce similar changes whether induced by bicuculline (*37*), allylglycine (*37*), kainic acid (*42*), or dipiperidinoethane (*44*). Hippocampal tissue is similarly compromised under conditions of idiopathic epilepsy (*13, 18*). In addition, anoxia, produced by occlusion of the carotid artery, results in selective damage to the hippocampus (*8, 29*) while carbon monoxide hypoxia alters the responsiveness of this structure to a stimulating electrical current (*15*). Finally, the alkyl tin derivative, trimethyltin, produces a rather selective pattern of damage to the hippocampal formation (*8, 16, 40, 54, 63*). Thus, the hippocampus is a structure that is particularly susceptible to pharmacological and toxicological insult, while possibly serving the function of integrating the information from these stimuli and modulating the reactivity of the organism to the particular drug or toxic state.

II. OVERVIEW OF HIPPOCAMPAL ANATOMY

As already implied, the hippocampus may be considered a cortical structure by virtue of its laminar morphology. Although Ramon y Cajal (*46*) suggested a seven-layered concept of the hippocampal formation, his subdivisions included white matter and epithelial zones as distinct layers. Similar zones in neocortex are not traditionally considered discrete layers, and therefore Isaacson (*28*) portrays the hippocampus as having three layers.

Briefly, these layers are arranged as follows: A molecular layer includes the outermost zone of the hippocampus and dentate gyrus (unless otherwise specified I will consider the dentate gyrus as an integral part of the hippocampal formation). This region contains many fibers, some of which project to the subiculum or pyramidal cell layer below. In addition, some of the cells in this layer form intranuncial connections. The pyramidal cell layer includes three to four rows of large, densely packed cells. Some of the processes from these neurons descend to the alveus and course through the fornix to other diencephalic and telencephalic structures., while others project to the stratum oriens and terminate there. In addition, collaterals of the pyramidal cell fibers provide primary intralaminar connections. The dendritic arborizations of these cells extend both toward the molecular layer and the stratum oriens. This distinguishes them from the pyramidal cells found in mammalian neocortex since neocortical pyramids have only a single apical dendritic projection. Herrick (*27*) observed that this double dendritic projection is characteristic of the cells of reptilian cortex, and suggested that hippocampal pyramidal cells may represent a reptilian component of the mammalian brain. The stratum oriens is the third hippocampal layer and the cells which comprise this zone resemble those found in the deep layers of the neocortex. Axons from these neurons project to the molecular layer to terminate there or arch back into diverse terminations in the pyramidal cell layer.

Despite the clear laminar divisions of the hippocampus, the subdivisions suggested by the great anatomist Lorente de No actually provide a more convenient and perhaps physiologically relevant visualization of this structure. Basically, the focus is upon the pyramidal cell layer and the cells of the dentate gyrus. He has divided the pyramidal cell layer into four divisions: Cornu Ammunis (CA) 1–4. CA1 consists of densely packed pyramids; CA2 is a loosely defined transitional zone where the dense packing begins to dissipate; the cells in CA3 are rather loosely packed as the cell band curves into the intrahilar region of the dentate gyrus; and CA4 consists of fully dispersed pyramidal cells in this region. The dentate gyrus proper consists of three zones: a molecular zone which contains few neurons and short processes, a granule cell layer which projects to the hippocampal pyramidal cells, and a layer of polymorphic cells.

The main input to the hippocampus is from two sources: neocortex and other limbic and diencephalic structures. Polysensory areas of the entorhinal cortex project via the perforant path both directly to CA3 and to the granule cells of the dentate gyrus which innervate CA3 over mossy fibers. Both of these inputs to CA3 are highly excitatory. The other main input system to the hippocampus is via the fornix. This tract contains commissural fibers from the contralateral hippocampus as well as connections with the hypothalamus and septum. Thus, the hippocampus is primarily connected with structures providing information about sensory, visceral, and regulatory events. For a more detailed review of limbic neuroanatomy, the chapters on this topic by Isaacson (*28*) are highly recommended.

III. FINDINGS

A. Alcohol and the Hippocampus

Ethyl alcohol is a known neurotoxin which is addictive, ubiquitous, and produces a variety of affective, mnemonic, and motor effects after both acute and chronic administration. A considerable amount of evidence has accumulated which may suggest an involvement of the hippocampus in alcohol toxicity and/or the etiology of addiction to this drug.

B. Clinical and Behavioral Evidence

It is well known that chronic alcohol drinking in man is accompanied by disruption of mnemonic function (*55*). Although this deficit has been attributed to thiamine deficiency in the alcoholic (*57*), brain damage and mental deterioration have been increasingly reported among alcoholics with no history or clinical evidence of malnutrition or trauma (*7, 26, 30, 51*). A strikingly similar set of behavioral and mnemonic symptoms has been reported in humans suffering hippocampal damage (*38, 39*). Although evidence from the clinic is clearly suggestive of a hippocampal lesion in the chronic alcoholic, limitations on behavioral and histological assessment render conclusions problematic.

A number of behavioral studies with animals have provided an interesting corollary with the clinical literature. For example, Walker and Hunter (*62*) demonstrated that rats that were chronically exposed to alcohol through a liquid diet were impaired on problems involving the consolidation of short-term memory. Under normal conditions, the rat will learn an alternation task rapidly and tolerate rather long intertrial intervals (ITIs) before a performance deficit is observed. In such a task the rat is trained to press a lever for food reinforcers. After initial training, a bar is presented on each of several discrete trials and removed during the ITI. Bar presses are only reinforced on odd-numbered trials. Presumably the rat must remember its response on the previous trial in order to respond correctly on the following trial. Although the alcohol-treated rats performed well when the ITIs were relatively short, a profound deficit in response efficiency was observed in these animals when the ITI was lengthened. This suggests that chronic exposure to alcohol results in an inability to consolidate a new memory over long retention intervals. A very similar deficit is commonly observed in chronic alcoholics (*9*) and patients with hippocampal damage (*39*). Moreover, when rats are given direct lesions to the hippocampus their performance on an alternation task is virtually identical to that of the chronically alcoholized rat (*60, 61*).

The chronically alcoholized animal also performs poorly on behavioral tasks that require the animal to respond to time cues. Differential reinforcement of low rates of responding (DRL) techniques allow for the assessment of timing efficacy in the rat, and performance on this schedule is markedly impaired both in animals with direct hippocampal lesions and those that have been exposed to alcohol for long periods (*56, 58*). These findings suggest that following both direct lesions and chronic alcohol drinking, a deficit in the ability to withhold responding may emerge.

A more general type of behavioral deficit which accompanies both hippocampal lesions and prolonged exposure to alcohol is an increase in locomotor and exploratory behavior (*14, 31, 34*). Again, this increase in the basal rate of behavior may be interpreted as either a deficit in response inhibition or as a reflection of a diminished fear or neophobic response. Both of these interpretations have been suggested in the context of the assessment of limbic function (*50, 52*).

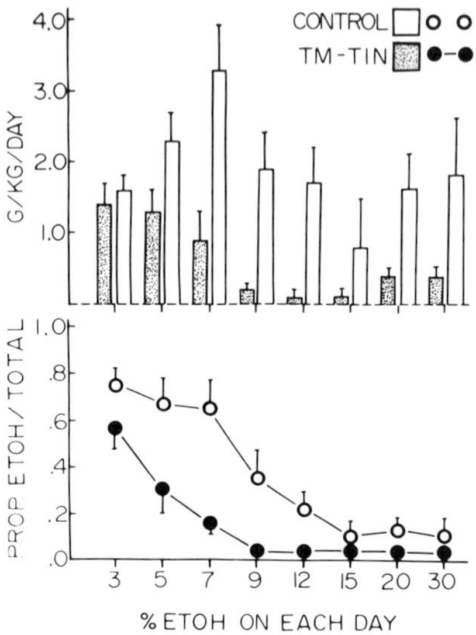

Fig. 1. Number of grams/kg/day (top) of alcohol consumed and proportion of alcohol to total fluid (bottom) consumed by rats treated with either trimethyltin (7.0 mg/kg) or the saline vehicle. The rats were tested on consecutive days with a 3-bottle/2-choice preference using an ascending series of ethanol concentrations and tap water. [From ref. (40).]

Finally, experimental manipulation of the hippocampus has resulted in an altered pattern of alcohol self-selection by the rat. For example, the hippocampus is one of the few areas where an injection of a tetrahydroisoquinoline alkaloid will result in an increase in alcohol drinking (*41*). In addition, exposure to the neurotoxin trimethyltin produces a decrease in alcohol drinking in the rat (Fig. 1) (*40*). Trimethyltin is known to produce a rather specific lesion to hippocampal tissue when administered systemically. Specifically, after a single oral dose of 7.0 mg/kg a clear loss of cells may be visualized in area CA3 of the hippocampus (Fig. 2) (*8, 16, 54*). This TMT-induced decrease in alcohol consumption is not an artifact of either a learned taste aversion or disrupted gustatory sensitivity (*40*). Moreover, the decrease is observed even in rats that typically self-select only between 1 and 2 g/kg/day of alcohol as a baseline. Taken together, these results may suggest that the hippocampus plays a role in the modulation of behavioral reactivity (i.e., drinking behavior) to the sensory or pharmacological effects of alcohol.

C. Electrophysiological Evidence

Both macroelectrical and microelectrical recording techniques have demonstrated that alcohol has specific effects upon the hippocampal formation.

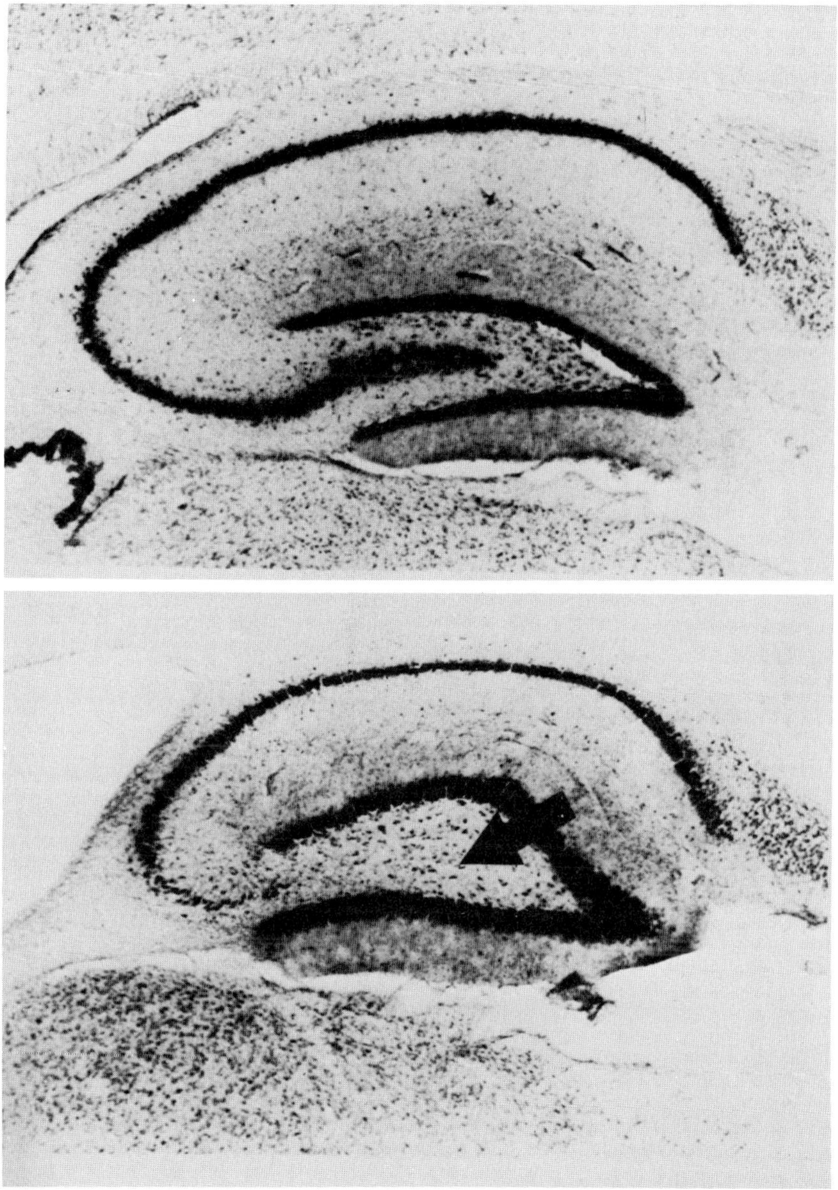

Fig. 2. Sagittal sections through hippocampus of control (top) and trimethyltin-treated (bottom) (7.0 mg/kg) rats. Arrow highlights damage in the CA3–4 cell fields. [From ref. (40).]

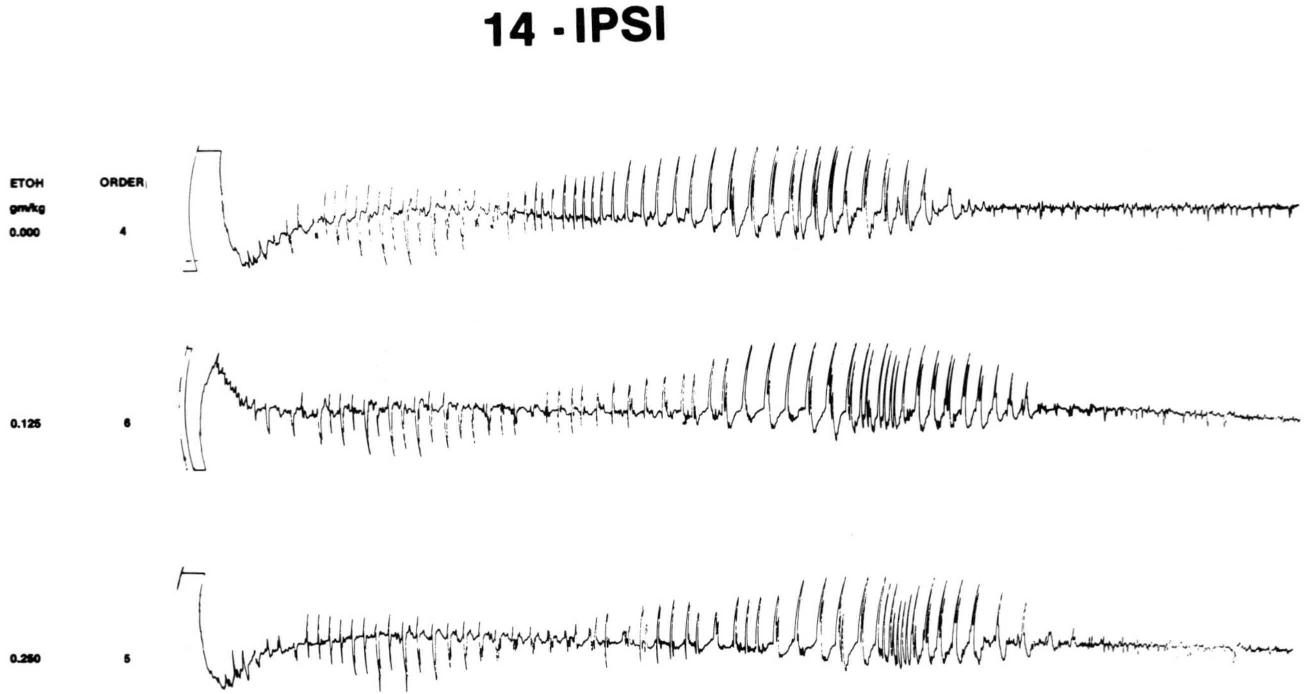

Fig. 3. Representative EEGs from a rat that received repeated testing with a range of concentrations of alcohol. After-discharges were recorded from dorsal hippocampus. [From ref. (53).]

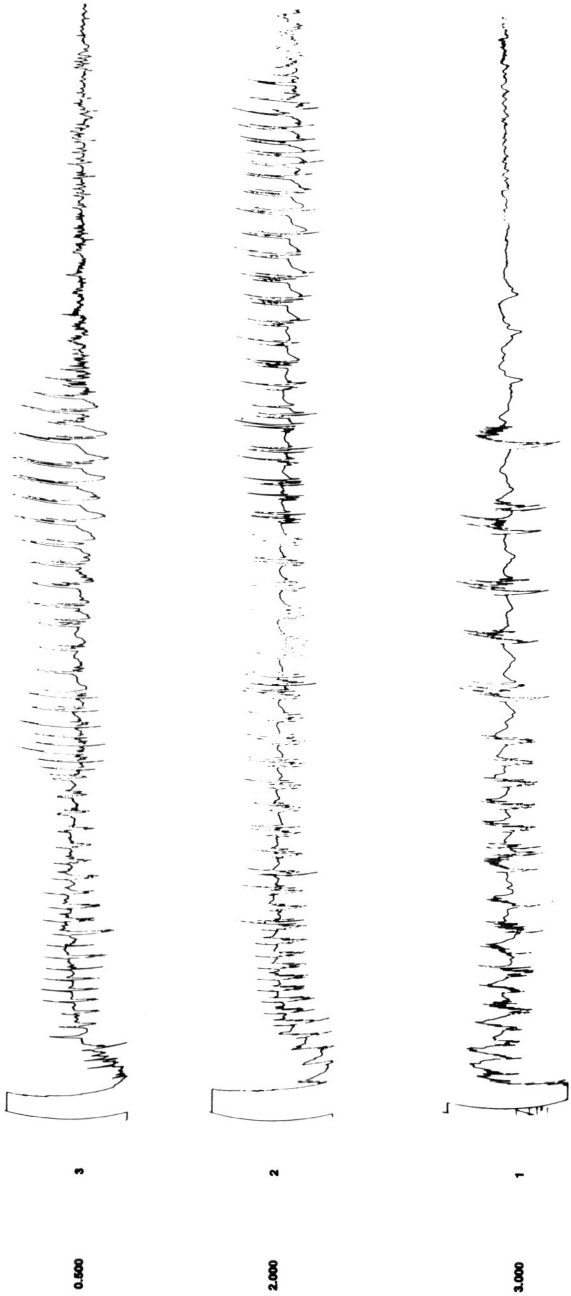

Fig. 3B.

Freeman (*20*) showed that rats kindled from a hippocampal focus had higher thresholds for the production of both epileptiform after-discharges and motor seizures following a challenge dose of alcohol than did animals kindled from other limbic regions. In addition, a dissociation of after-discharge and motor seizures after a dose of alcohol (1.6 g/kg ip) was noted more often when seizures were generated through the hippocampus. These findings are in agreement with those of Swartzwelder *et al.* (*53*), who found that hippocampal after-discharges and after-discharge thresholds were affected biphasically across a range of doses of alcohol (Figs. 3 and 4). Moreover, an elevation in the threshold for production of seizures from a chemically induced hippocampal focus has been reported following acute treatment with alcohol, although an increase in epileptiform activity was observed after direct injection of alcohol into the hippocampus (*4*).

The hippocampus appears to be particularly sensitive to the effects of alcohol when the activity of single and multiple units is measured. For example, Klemm and his colleagues (*32, 33*) have shown that both single-

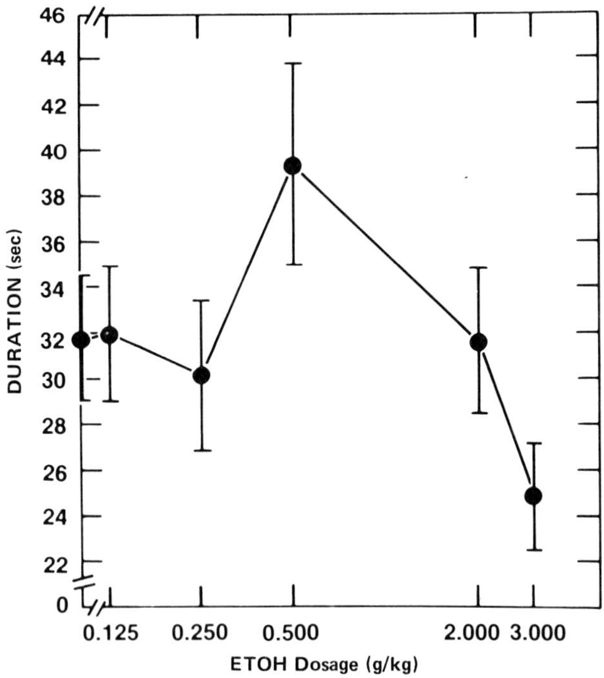

Fig. 4. Effect of ethanol upon the duration of hippocampal after-discharges across a range of dosages. [From ref. (53).]

unit and multiple-unit activity in the hippocampus are altered markedly by low doses of alcohol. In addition, Grupp (*24*) measured biphasic responses of cells in the dorsal hippocampus after a low dose of alcohol. As the dose was increased, the unit responses became more uniformly depressed, corroborating the depressive effect of alcohol upon macroelectrical recordings from this region.

The relationship between hippocampal and cortical activity following an alcohol challenge has been initially investigated by Grupp and Perlanski (*23*). In these studies a decrease in hippocampal unit firing was accompanied by high-amplitude slow wave activity in the frontal cortex. The doses used in this study were similar to those used by Swartzwelder *et al.* (*53*) to induce a decrease in the responsiveness of the hippocampus to electrical stimulation. Thus, the effect of alcohol upon hippocampal activity may alter cortical responsiveness.

As previously discussed, the hippocampus receives input to CA3 via two pathways: the mossy fibers from dentate granule cells and commissural fibers. Both of these pathways are highly excitatory, and a brief period of inhibition may be observed following a burst of input to CA3. Recently, a single exposure to alcohol was shown to increase both the excitation elicited in CA3 following stimulation of these pathways, and the period of poststimulus inhibition (*43*). Since these investigators failed to see any change in the spontaneous firing of CA3 cells after similar treatment, they suggested that alcohol may have specific effects upon synaptic rather than membrane mechanisms in CA3.

Chronic alcohol treatment also produces changes in hippocampal function measured electrophysiologically. Although acute treatment with alcohol decreases the amplitude of the population spike evoked from CA1 after stimulation of the stratum radiatum, this effect diminishes with chronic treatment (*11*). This change in responsiveness over time may be an indication that functional tolerance is manifested in the activity of hippocampal cells. That this effect may be specific to the hippocampus is suggested by the fact that no such effect is observed at the neuromuscular junction. Clearly, more work is necessary in order to determine whether such an effect may be observed in other central structures.

During chronic treatment with alcohol, the threshold for producing epileptiform signs via electrical stimulation of the hippocampus is increased (*22*). The threshold was decreased during the first 72 hr of withdrawal, but not at 1 week after the termination of exposure. Although these data would suggest no long-term effect of chronic alcohol treatment upon hippocampal excitatory mechanisms, the period of chronic exposure in this study was only 19–22 days, a period considerably shorter than is used in many chronic alcohol studies.

The population spikes elicited from CA1 during paired pulse stimulation over Schaffer collaterals and commissural fibers are increased in the chronically alcoholized rat (*3*). In addition, the alcohol-treated animals showed a trend toward greater facilitation of the population spike during 5 and 10 Hz tetani, though no effects upon long-term potentiation were observed. It is possible, then, that chronic treatment with alcohol may disrupt intrinsic inhibitory transmission in the hippocampus.

That alcohol disrupts the normal function of hippocampal cells and cell fields after both acute and chronic exposure suggests the possibility that the well-known deficits in memory formation after a single high dose of alcohol may be in part attributable to this disruption. Moreover, chronic alteration of the processes which modulate hippocampal function may underlie the memory deficits observed in chronic alcoholics and patients suffering Korsakoff's syndrome.

D. Morphological Evidence

Initial demonstrations of the effect of chronic alcohol exposure upon CNS morphology were provided by Walker and his colleagues (*47, 59*). These studies show very clearly that the pyramidal cells of CA1 and the granule cells of the dentate gyrus suffer a loss of dendritic spines and arborization after long-term alcohol drinking in the mouse. Moreover, this effect was replicated in the rat, and an actual loss of cells in these regions could be visualized. This loss of cells is accompanied by distinct damage to the commissural fiber pathway to CA3 (*2*) and by a loss of entorhinal afferents to the molecular layer of the dentate gyrus (*1*). This damage would clearly diminish the amount of polysensory input to the hippocampus over this pathway.

In this connection, a lesion of the entorhinal cortex will typically result in compensatory sprouting of the remaining afferents in the dentate gyrus. Chronic exposure to alcohol results in a diminution of this compensatory plasticity (*65*). Therefore, not only is input to the hippocampus disrupted following alcohol exposure, but the compensatory mechanisms unique to this region appear to be compromised as well.

Finally, prenatal exposure to alcohol results in a decrease in the number of hippocampal pyramidal cells in the adult rat (*5*) and in abnormally distributed mossy fibers connecting cells of the dentate gyrus to those of CA3 (*64*).

Thus, it seems clear that the normal integrative function of the hippocampus is markedly compromised after alcohol exposure, since the cells of this structure and the fiber systems connecting it to the cortex are damaged as a result of this treatment.

E. Evidence from the Membrane

Several recent studies have suggested that calcium may play a role in mediating the effects of alcohol upon the CNS. The divalent cation, calcium, is known to initiate the release of neurotransmitter from the bouton via exocytosis. When the depolarization associated with action potential production reaches the presynaptic terminal, calcium channels are opened and the cation flows down a concentration gradient to cross the cell membrane. Although the precise mechanisms whereby exocytosis is initiated remain unclear, calcium is crucial for this process to occur. Since the synapse is perhaps the most vulnerable point in CNS circuitry to chemical intervention, and since calcium–membrane interaction is central to the process of synaptic transmission, it seems likely that the calcium channel is altered by exposure to psychoactive drugs in general and alcohol in particular.

Although the uptake of calcium into brain synaptosomes has been shown to decrease under certain conditions of *in vitro* alcohol exposure (*25*), other investigators have shown increases in synaptosomal calcium accumulation after alcohol exposure *in vitro* (*21*). The latter investigators also studied calcium uptake in the brains of alcohol-treated mice. Synaptosomal preparations from mice given one acute injection of alcohol accumulated a high amount of calcium after an *in vitro* ethanol challenge. In contrast, if the mouse was treated chronically with alcohol prior to sacrifice, the synaptosomal preparation accumulated considerably less calcium following an *in vitro* challenge. These findings strongly suggest that physiological tolerance to alcohol may be related to an alteration of CNS calcium dynamics.

At the behavioral level, an intracerebroventricular (ICV) injection of calcium has been shown to increase the period of time that an animal will sleep following a hypnotic dose of alcohol (*17*). In addition, the calcium ionophores X537A and A23187 accentuated the effect of the calcium treatment, whereas the calcium chelators EDTA and EGTA decreased sleeping time. It seems, therefore, that CNS calcium may exist in an extracellular pool, the membrane dynamics of which mediate the intoxicating effect of alcohol. The question remains, however, as to a specific neural structure that may be particularly sensitive to these effects of alcohol or may modulate the behavioral changes associated with these effects.

Ross and his colleagues (*48*) showed a naloxone-reversible decrease in the concentration of calcium in a number of central structures including the hippocampus after acute treatment with alcohol. A similar effect was observed in the hypothalamus, midbrain, and pons medulla region after a single high dose (*19*).

In the hippocampal slice preparation Carlen *et al.* (*12*) demonstrated that alcohol increased both EPSPs and IPSPs when perfused in the bathing medium. When applied to apical dendrites in the stratum radiatum, where there are many excitatory synapses, alcohol caused an increase in EPSPs but not in orthodromically stimulated IPSPs. Conversely, when alcohol was microinfused onto the cell bodies in this region, an area rich in inhibitory synapses, it increased only the IPSPs. These results indicate that alcohol increases the amount of neurotransmitter release in the hippocampus regardless of the type of synapse (excitatory or inhibitory). Therefore the suggestion that alcohol increases the uptake of calcium at the synaptic terminal is supported by these electrophysiological data.

Using *in vivo* perfusion of the hippocampus, we have recently shown that calcium membrane kinetics may mediate the *in vivo* actions of alcohol and acetaldehyde. Push–pull guide tubes were implanted into the dorsal hippocampus of male rats (Fig. 5). After recovery from surgery, the hippocampus was labeled with 45 Ca^{2+} which was allowed to equilibrate for 12–18 hr. A 10–15 sample series of 5-min push–pull perfusions was then initiated. Although the results are preliminary at this writing, a high dose of alcohol in the perfusion medium generally resulted in a decrease in the number of labeled calcium ions released at the region of the cannula tip (Fig. 6). This initial decrease was often followed by a rebound of calcium release. A lower

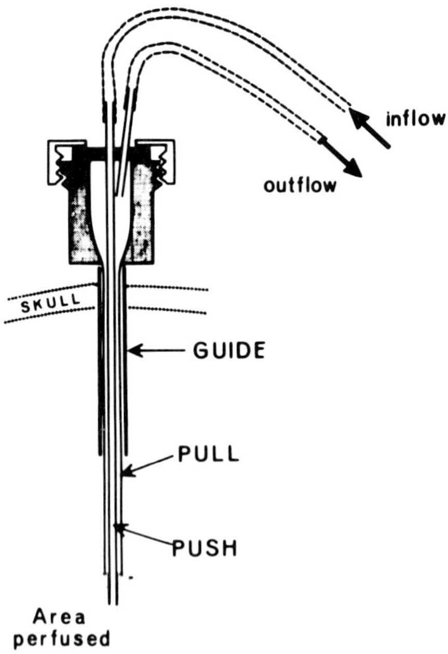

Fig. 5. Collosin-type cannula used for *in-vivo* push–pull perfusion of brain tissue. [From ref. (66).]

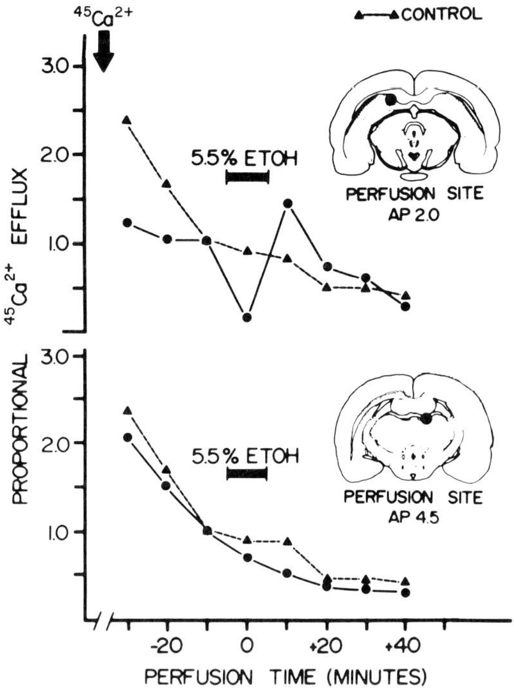

Fig. 6. Ethanol-induced efflux of labeled calcium from dorsal hippocampus (top) and lack of effect in nonhippocampal tissue (bottom).

dose of alcohol ordinarily evoked only an efflux of calcium ions (Fig. 7). In addition, acetaldehyde evoked an immediate release of calcium but *tert*-butanol produced no consistent effect upon calcium dynamics.

Taken together, these studies suggest that calcium ions play an important role in the responsiveness of the CNS and in particular the hippocampus to alcohol. Moreover, since the hippocampus is particularly susceptible to neurotoxic insult in general, and the effects of alcohol specifically, future research should focus upon hippocampal calcium dynamics using the methods of *in vitro* and *in vivo* chemical stimulation.

IV. SUMMARY AND CONCLUSIONS

Several lines of evidence have been outlined in support of the possibility that the hippocampal formation may (1) be particularly sensitive to the effects of acute or chronic exposure to physiological doses of ethyl alcohol and/or (2) mediate the behavioral sequelae (including addictive behaviors

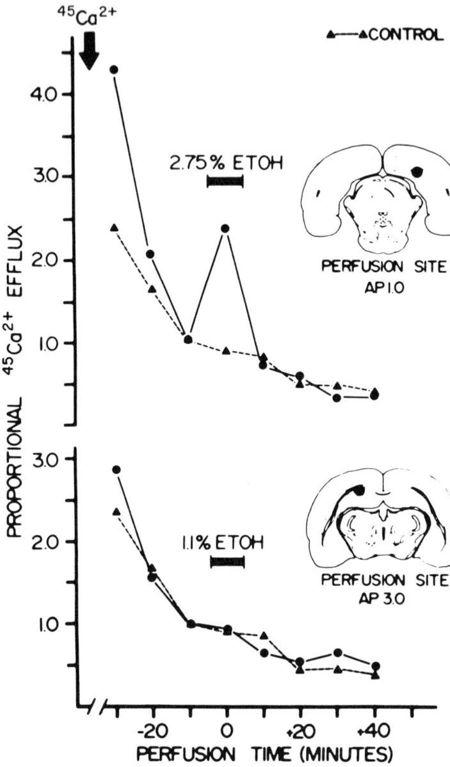

Fig. 7. Effect of low concentrations of ethanol upon calcium efflux using the push–pull perfusion technique in hippocampus.

and learning deficits) associated with the use of this drug. Behaviorally, both chronic alcohol drinking and direct lesions to the hippocampal formation produce similar deficits in learning and memory. This, in concert with the fact that chronic alcohol consumption produces clear morphological damage to the hippocampus, would suggest an etiological connection between the hippocampal damage and learning deficits associated with chronic alcoholism. Moreover, electrophysiological evidence strongly supports the notion that the hippocampus is a structure which is particularly susceptible to the pharmacological and toxicological properties of ethanol. Finally, the membrane dynamics of Ca^{2+} appear to be markedly altered following both *in vivo* and *in vitro* exposure to alcohol, thus suggesting that a chronic membrane alteration may underlie some of the electrophysiological and morphological changes observed after chronic exposure to alcohol.

Although these data strongly indicate hippocampal involvement in the actions and consequences of alcohol drinking, we have not yet come to a level of analysis that will allow clear mechanistic or etiological interpretations. Perhaps the effects of ethanol upon the membrane dynamics of calcium come closest to this level, although interpretations of the results of such studies is often problematic and more research into these relationships is necessary. If, as our preliminary findings suggest, there are dose–response relationships between alcohol and calcium release at the membrane, it will be important to assess the time course of such changes and their responsiveness to pharmacological manipulation. Such experiments are currently possible using push–pull perfusion techniques, and should provide important insights into the mechanisms whereby alcohol produces alterations in neuronal function.

REFERENCES

1. Abraham, W., and Hunter, B. An electrophysiological analysis of chronic ethanol neurotoxicity in the dentate gyrus: distribution of entorhinal afferents. *Exp. Brain Res.* **47** (1982) 61–68.
2. Abraham, W., Manis, P., Hunter, B., Zornester, S., and Walker, D. Electrophysiological analysis of synaptic distribution in CA1 of the rat hippocampus after chronic ethanol exposure. *Brain Res.* **237** (1982) 91–105.
3. Abraham, W., Hunter, B., Zornester, F., and Walker, D. Augmentation of short term plasticity in CA1 of rat hippocampus after chronic ethanol treatment. *Brain Res.* **221** (1981) 271–287.
4. Baker, W., and Benedict, F. Effects of alcohol on chemically induced hippocampal foci. *Arch. Int. Pharmacodyn.* **162** (1966) 170–179.
5. Barnes, D., and Walker, D. Prenatal ethanol exposure permanently reduces the number of pyramidal neurons in rat hippocampus. *Brain Res.* **227** (1981) 333–340.
6. Blanchard, R., and Blanchard, D. Effects of hippocampal lesions on the rat's reaction to a cat. *J. Comp. Physiol. Psychol.* **78** (1972) 77–82.
7. Brewer, C., and Perrett, L. Brain damage due to alcohol consumption: an air-encephalographic, psychometric and electroencephalographic study. *Br. J. Addict.* **66** (1971) 170–182.
8. Brown, A., Aldridge, W., Street, B., and Verschoyle, R. The behavioral and neuropathologic sequelae of intoxication by trimethyltin compounds in the rat. *Am. J. Pathol.* **97** (1979) 59–82.
9. Butters, N., Cermack, L., Montgomery, K., and Adinolfi, A. Some comparisons of the memory and visuoperceptive deficits of chronic alcoholics and patients with Korsakoff's disease. *Alcoholism Clin. Exp. Res.* **1** (1977) 73–80.
10. Butters, N., and Cermack, L. Some analyses of amnesic syndromes in brain damaged patients. *In* "The Hippocampus: Neurophysiology and Behavior" (R. L. Isaacson and K. H. Pribram, eds.), Vol 2, 1975, pp. 377–407. Plenum, New York.
11. Carlen, P., and Corrigall, W. Ethanol tolerance measured electrophysiologically in hippocampal slices and not in neuromuscular junctions from chronically ethanol-fed rats. *Neurosci. Lett.* **17** (1980) 95–100.
12. Carlen, P. R., Gurevich, N., and Durand, D. Ethanol in low doses augments calcium-mediated mechanisms measured intracellularly in hippocampal neurons. *Science* **215** (1982) 306–308.

13. Dam, A. M. Epilepsy and neuron loss in the hippocampus. *Epilepsia* **21** (1980) 617–629.
14. Douglas, R. The hippocampus and behavior. *Psychol. Bull.* **67** (1967) 416–422.
15. Dyer, R. S., Burden, E., Hulebak, K., Schultz, N., Swartzwelder, H., and Annau, Z. Hippocampal afterdischarges and their post-ictal sequelae in rats: effects of carbon monoxide hypoxia. *Neurobehav. Toxicol.* **1** (1979) 21–25.
16. Dyer, R., Dashields, T., and Wonderlin, W. Trimethyltin-induced changes in gross morphology of the hippocampus. *Neurobehav. Toxicol. Teratol.* **4** (1982) 141–147.
17. Erickson, C. K., Tyler, T. D., and Harris, R. A. Ethanol: modification of acute intoxication by divalent cations. *Science* **199** (1978) 1219–1221.
18. Falconer, M., Serefetinides, E., and Corsellis, J. Etiology and pathogenesis of temporal lobe epilepsy. *Arch. Neurol.* **10** (1964) 233–248.
19. Ferko, A., and Bobyock, E. A study on regional brain calcium concentrations following acute and prolonged administration of ethanol in rats. *Toxicol. Appl. Pharmacol.* **55** (1980) 179–187.
20. Freeman, F. Effects of alcohol on kindled seizure thresholds in rats. *Pharmacol. Biochem. Behav.* **8** (1978) 641–644.
21. Friedman, M. B., Erickson, C. K., and Leslie, S. W. Effects of acute and chronic ethanol administration on whole mouse brain synaptosomal calcium influx. *Biochem. Pharmacol.* **29** (1980) 1903–1908.
22. Greisler, R., Hunter, B., and Walker, D. Ethanol dependence in the rat: temporal changes in neuroexcitability following withdrawal. *Psychopharmacology* **56** (1978) 287–292.
23. Grupp, L. A., and Perlanski, E. Ethanol-induced changes in the spontaneous activity of single units in the hippocampus of the awake rat: a dose–response study. *Neuropharmacology 18* (1979) 63–70.
24. Grupp, L. A. Biphasic action of ethanol on single units of the dorsal hippocampus and the relationship to the cortical EEG. *Psychopharmacology* **70** (1980) 95–103.
25. Harris, R. A., and Hood, W. F. Inhibition of synaptosomal calcium uptake by ethanol. *J. Pharmacol. Exp. Ther.* **213** (1980) 562–568.
26. Haug, J. Pneumoencephalographic evidence of brain damage in chronic alcoholics. *Acta Psychiat. Scand.* (Suppl.) **203** (1968) 135–143.
27. Herrick, C. J. "Brains of Rats and Men." 1926. Univ. of Chicago Press, Chicago, Illinois.
28. Isaacson, R. L. "The Limbic System." 1978. Plenum, New York.
29. Ito, U., Spatz, M., Walker, J., and Klatzo, I. Experimental cerebral ischemia in mongolian gerbils. *Acta Neuropathol.* **32** (1975) 209–223.
30. Jones, B., and Parsons, O. Impaired ability in chronic alcoholics. *Arch. Gen. Psychiat.* **24** (1971) 71–75.
31. Kimble, D. Hippocampus and internal inhibition. *Psychol. Bull.* **70** (1968) 285–295.
32. Klemm, W. R., Dreyfus, L., Forney, E., and Mayfield, M. Differential effects of low doses of ethanol on the impulse activity in various regions of the limbic system. *Psychopharmacology* **50** (1976b) 131–138.
33. Klemm, W. R., Mallari, C., Dreyfus, L., Fiske, J., Forney, E., and Mikeska, J. Ethanol-induced regional and dose–response differences in multiple unit activity in rabbits. *Psychopharmacology* **49** (1976a) 235–244.
34. Liljequist, S., Ahlenius, S., and Engel, J. The effect of chronic ethanol treatment on behavior and central monoamines in the rat. *Arch. Pharmacol.* **300** (1977) 205–216.
35. Llinas, R., and Walton, K. Voltage-dependent calcium conductances in neurons. *In* "The Cell Surface and Neuronal Function," (C. Cotman, G. Poste, and G. Nicolson, eds.), 1980, pp. 88–110. Elsevier, Amsterdam.
36. MacLean, P. The triune brain, emotion and scientific bias. *In* "The Neurosciences Second Study Program," (F. O. Schmidt, ed.), 1970, pp. 336–349. Rockefeller University Press, New York.

37. Meldrum, B., and Brierley, J. Prolonged epileptic seizures in primates: ischemic cell changes and its relation to ictal physiological events. *Arch. Neurol.* **28** (1973) 10–17.
38. Milner, B. The memory deficit in bilateral hippocampal lesions. *Psychiat. Res. Rep.* **11** (1959) 43–52.
39. Milner, B., Corkin, S., and Teuber, H. Further analysis of the hippocampal amnesic syndrome. *Neuropsychology* **6** (1968) 267–282.
40. Myers, R. D., Swartzwelder, H. S., and Dyer, R. S. Acute treatment with trimethyltin alters alcohol self-selection. *Psychopharmacology* **78** (1982) 19–22.
41. Myers, R. D., and Hoch, D. Localization of sites in the brain mediating alcohol drinking induced by THP. *Curr. Alcohol.* **5** (1979) 29–44.
42. Nadler, J., Perry, B., and Cotman, C. Intraventricular kainic acid preferentially destroys hippocampal pyramidal cells. *Nature (London)* **271** (1978) 676–677.
43. Newlin, S., Mancillas-Trevino, J., and Bloom, F. Ethanol Causes increases in excitation and inhibition in area CA3 of the dorsal hippocampus. *Brain Res.* **209** (1981) 113–128.
44. Olney, J., Fuller, T., Collins, R., and de Gubareff, T. Systemic dipiperidinoethane mimics the convulsant and neurotoxic actions of kainic acid. *Brain Res.* **200** (1980) 231–235.
45. Papez, J. A proposed mechanism of emotion. *Arch. Neurol. Psychiat.* **38** (1937) 725–744.
46. Ramon y Cajal, S. "The Structure of Ammon's Horn." 1968. Thomas, Springfield, Illinois.
47. Riley, J., and Walker, D. Morphological alterations in hippocampus after long-term alcohol consumption in mice. *Science* **201** (1978) 646–648.
48. Ross, D. H., Medina, I. A., and Cardenas, H. L. Morphine and ethanol: selective depletion of regional brain calcium. *Science* **185** (1974) 63–65.
49. Sloviter, R. S., and Damino, B. Sustained electrical stimulation of the perforant path duplicates kainic acid-induced electrophysiological effects and hippocampal damage in rats. *Neurosci. Lett.* **24** (1981) 279–284.
50. Slotnick, B. Fear behavior and passive avoidance deficits in mice with amygdala lesions. *Physiol. Behav.* **11** (1973) 717–720.
51. Smith, J., Burt, D., and Chapman, R. Intelligence and brain damage in alcoholics: a study of patients of middle and upper social class. *Quart. J. Stud. Alc.* **34** (1973) 414–422.
52. Swartzwelder, H. S. Deficits in passive avoidance and fear behavior following bilateral and unilateral amygdala lesions in mice. *Physiol. Behav.* **26** (1981) 323–326.
53. Swartzwelder, H. S., Johnson, C., Cooley, B., Howell, W., and Dyer, R. S. Alcohol-induced alterations in hippocampal afterdischarges and afterdischarge thresholds: dose–response studies. *Neurobehav. Toxicol.*, 1 (1979) 253–258.
54. Swartzwelder, H. S., Hepler, J., Holahan, W., King, S., Leverenz, H., Miller, P., and Myers, R. D. Impaired maze performance in the rat caused by trimethyltin treatment: problem solving deficits and perseveration. *Neurobehav. Toxicol. Teratol.* **4** (1982) 169–176.
55. Talland, G. "Deranged Memory." 1965. Academic Press, New York.
56. Van Hartesveldt, C. Size of reinforcement and operant responding in hippocampectomized rats. *Behav. Biol.* **8** (1973) 347–356.
57. Victor, M., and Adams, R. On the etiology of the alcoholic neurologic diseases with special reference to the role of nutrition. *Am. J. Nutr.* **9** (1961) 379–397.
58. Walker, D., and Freund, G. Impairment of timing behavior after prolonged alcohol consumption in rats. *Science* **182** (1973) 597–599.
59. Walker, D., Barnes, D., Zornester, S., Hunter, B., and Kubanis, P. Neuronal loss in hippocampus induced by prolonged ethanol consumption in rats. *Science* **209** (1980) 711–713.
60. Walker, D., Messer, L., Freund, G., and Means, L. Effect of hippocampal lesions and intertrial interval on single alternation performance in the rat. *J. Comp. Physiol. Psychol.* **80** (1972) 469–477.

61. Walker, D., and Means, L. Single alternation performance in rats with hippocampal lesions: disruption by an irrelevant task interposed during the intertrial interval. *Behav. Biol.* **9** (1973) 93–104.
62. Walker, D., and Hunter, B. Short-term memory impairment following chronic alcohol consumption in rats. *Neuropsychology* **16** (1978) 545–553.
63. Walsh, T., and Tilson, H. Neurobehavioral toxicology of the organoleads. *Neurotoxicology* (in press) (1985).
64. West, J., Hodges, C., and Black, A. Prenatal exposure to ethanol alters the organization of hippocampal mossy fibers in rats. *Science* **211** (1981) 957–959.
65. West, J., Lind, M., Demuth, R., Parker, E., Alkana, R., Cassell, M., and Black, A. Lesion-induced sprouting in the rat dentate gyrus is inhibited by repeated ethanol administration *Science* **218** (1982) 809–810.
66. Myers, R. D. Methods for perfusing different structures of the brain. *In* "Methods in Psychobiology," Vol. 2 (R. D. Myers, ed.). 1972, pp. 169–212. Academic Press, New York.

13

The Use of Push–Pull Cannulae for Superfusing Various Hypothalamic Areas in Anesthetized and Conscious, Freely Moving Animals

ATHINEOS PHILIPPU

Department of Pharmacodynamics and Toxicology
University of Innsbruck
Innsbruck, Austria

I. INTRODUCTION

A possible approach to the functional significance of neurotransmitters of the brain is the superfusion of distinct brain areas and the determination of endogenous neurotransmitters in the superfusate. Superfusion of various hypothalamic areas through push–pull cannulae has been used in our laboratory to investigate the patterns of release of endogenous catecholamines, GABA, and histamine, and to elucidate the involvement of central neurotransmitters in the regulation of the arterial blood pressure. In the following results are presented that were obtained in anesthetized and conscious, freely moving animals.

IN VIVO PERFUSION AND RELEASE
OF NEUROACTIVE SUBSTANCES

ISBN 0-12-083350-6

II. METHODS

A. Cannulae

Push–pull cannulae with the following diameters have been used.

1. CAT

Outer cannula: 1.8 mm o.d., 1.5 mm i.d.; inner cannula: 0.5 mm o.d., 0.3 mm i.d. (Fig. 1A). The outer surface of the outer cannula was electrically insulated (*14*). Thus, the cannula might be used as a monopolar electrode to stimulate the area that is superfused. Before insertion the outer surface of the outer cannula was coated with paraffin oil to reduce tissue damage. It is

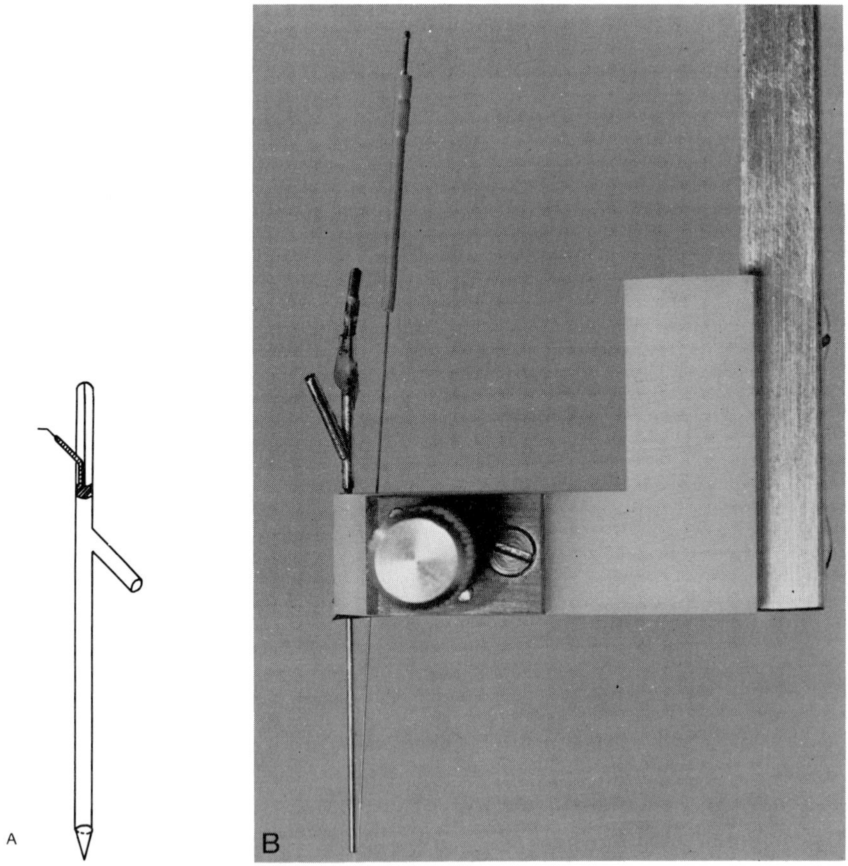

Fig. 1. (A) The push–pull cannula used for superfusion of the cat hypothalamus. (B) Combination of the push–pull cannula with a microelectrode. (Reproduced by courtesy of H. Wilson and K. C. F. Fone.) For details see Section IV.

possible to fix more than one cannula into an appropriate frame and to superfuse simultaneously various hypothalamic regions.

In order to investigate effects of drugs on the activity of brain neurons the push–pull cannula may be combined with a microelectrode in juxtaposition (diameter of the tip: 1 μm). The push–pull cannula illustrated in Fig. 1B has the following diameters: outer cannula: 0.6 mm o.d., 0.3 mm i.d.; inner cannula: 0.2 mm o.d., 0.1 mm i.d. Because of the small diameters of the outer cannula, a second pump may be used to pull cerebrospinal fluid (CSF).

2. RABBIT

Guide cannula: 1.3 mm o.d., 0.85 mm i.d.; push–pull cannula: outer cannula: 0.8 mm o.d., 0.5 mm i.d.; inner cannula: 0.3 mm o.d., 0.15 mm i.d. Two push–pull cannulae were fixed into an appropriate frame, thus making possible the simultaneous superfusion of left and right hypothalamic areas (*11*).

3. RAT

Guide cannula: 1.25 mm o.d., 0.9 mm i.d.; push–pull cannula: outer cannula: 0.7 mm o.d., 0.5 mm i.d.; inner cannula: 0.2 mm o.d., 0.1 mm i.d. (*18*).

B. Surgical and Superfusion Procedures

In the anesthetized cat (sodium pentobarbitone, 36 mg/kg ip), the hypothalamus was superfused as previously described (*14*). The push–pull cannula with its stylet was stereotaxically inserted (*17*) and the hypothalamus was superfused with artificial CSF, pH 7.2. When the release of endogenous catecholamines was determined in the superfusate, CSF contained 10^{-4} *M* pargyline (*12*). The superfusion rate was usually 150 μl/min; it was kept constant by a peristaltic pump. Because of the relatively large space between outer surface of the inner cannula and inner surface of the outer cannula only one peristaltic pump was necessary to push the superfusing fluid through the push–pull cannula (see later). When this technique is used, the superfusate may be continuously collected in from 1- to 15-min periods. Determination of neurotransmitters was carried out in 100–200 μl of the superfusate. To collect the superfusate in 10-sec periods it was necessary to appropriately increase the rate of superfusion (*16*).

At the end of the experiment an overdose of sodium pentobarbitone was injected intravenously. The brain was removed and immersed in formaldehyde solution. The localization of the cannula was verified microscopically in histological slides stained with Cresyl Violet.

In the anesthetized rabbit (sodium pentobarbitone, 40 mg/kg ip), the guide cannula with its stylet was stereotaxically (6) inserted into the brain. To avoid damage of the tissue, the cannula was inserted until its tip was 2 or 4 mm above the hypothalamic area to be superfused. In some experiments catheters were inserted into the jugular vein and the carotid artery for intravenous injections of drugs and for recording of the arterial blood pressure, respectively (*11, 15*).

Some days after operation the stylet of the guide cannula was removed and replaced by a push–pull cannula which was longer than the guide cannula in order to reach the hypothalamic area. The animal was placed in a cage (0.13 m^2) and the push–pull cannula was connected with tubing with two peristaltic pumps, one to push and another to pull the fluid (*10, 11*). The hypothalamus was superfused with CSF at a rate of 150 μl/min and the superfusate was collected in from 1- to 10-min periods.

At the end of the experiment an overdose of sodium pentobarbitone was injected. A minute amount of Cresyl Violet was injected into the hypothalamus through the inner cannula to facilitate visualization of the tip of the cannula. The localization of the push–pull cannula was carried out in histological slides.

In rats anesthetized with sodium pentobarbitone (44 mg/kg ip) or chloral hydrate (300 mg/kg ip) the guide cannula with its stylets was stereotaxically (*8*) inserted and fixed on the skull with resin cement and screws. The guide cannula did not reach the area to be superfused, but it ended 2 mm above its dorsal surface. Some days after operation a push–pull cannula was inserted and the hypothalamus was superfused with CSF at a rate of 150 μl/min. The push–pull cannula was 2 mm longer than the guide cannula, thus reaching the region to be superfused. As for the superfusion of the rabbit hypothalamus, the push–pull cannula was connected with tubing to two peristaltic pumps and the superfusate was collected at from 1- to 10-min time periods (*18*).

C. Determination of Neurotransmitters in the Superfusate

Catecholamines and histamine were determined in the superfusate by radioenzymatic assays (*9, 13*). GABA was determined by a radioreceptor assay (*4*).

III. FINDINGS

A. Optimization of the Experimental Procedure

When push–pull cannulae with relatively large diameters are used to superfuse the cat hypothalamus, coating of the cannulae with paraffin oil before inserting reduces tissue damage. Very recently, thin push–pull cannulae (outer cannula: 1.25 mm o.d., 0.9 mm i.d.; inner cannula: 0.2 mm o.d., 0.1 mm i.d.) have been used successfully (in preparation).

The success of the experiments mainly depends on the localization of the cannulae. In 60–70% of the experiments positioning was good. Bleedings were negligible and rates of superfusion and volume of superfusate remained constant throughout the experiment.

B. Neurobiological Applications

1. PATTERNS OF RESTING RELEASE OF NEUROTRANSMITTERS IN THE HYPOTHALAMUS

To investigate the patterns of release of neurotransmitters, the posterior hypothalamus of anesthetized cats as well as the anterior and posterior hypothalamus of freely moving rabbits were superfused for 6 hr and the superfusates continuously collected in 15-min (cat) or 10-min (rabbit) periods. The rates of release of dopamine, noradrenaline, adrenaline, GABA, and histamine in the two hypothalamic areas seemed to vary rhythmically with time. Synchronization of the rates of release in the various experiments (see Fig. 2) revealed a phasic release of the neurotransmitters. Phases of high rate of release were separated from each other by phases of low rates of release, the time period between two adjacent phases of high rates of release being 60–70 min (Fig. 2). In the posterior hypothalamus of the anesthetized cat, the peaks of the three catecholamines coincided fairly well with each other.

In the conscious, freely moving rabbit, the posterior and anterior hypothalamic areas were superfused simultaneously. The last three or four peaks of high rate of release of the catecholamines in the anterior hypothalamus coincided reasonably well with those in the posterior hypothalamus. In both areas the phases of high rates of release of dopamine corresponded to those of adrenaline rather than to noradrenaline. On the other hand, the phases of high rates of release of histamine in the anterior hypothalamus of the freely moving rabbit coincided with those in the posterior hypothalamus.

2. ARTERIAL BLOOD PRESSURE AND RELEASE OF CATECHOLAMINES IN THE HYPOTHALAMUS

Experiments in anesthetized cats have shown that experimentally induced changes in the arterial blood pressure alter the release of catecholamines in the anterior and posterior hypothalamus. A rise in blood pressure enhances the rates of release of dopamine, noradrenaline, and adrenaline in the anterior hypothalamus, while the release in the posterior hypothalamus is reduced. However, a fall of blood pressure increases the rates of release of the catecholamines in the posterior hypothalamus, whereas the rates of release in the anterior hypothalamus are decreased (*5, 11, 16*). The changes in the

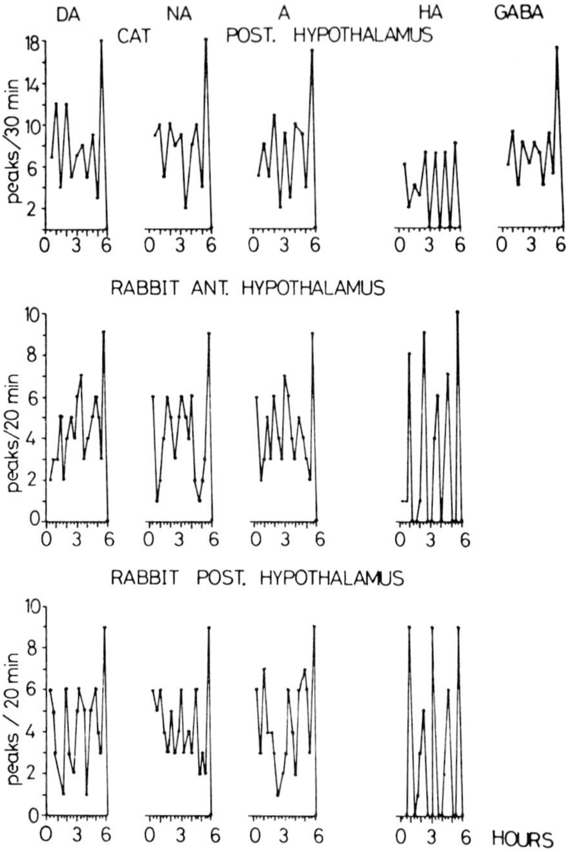

Fig. 2. Resting release of dopamine (DA), noradrenaline (NA), adrenaline (A), histamine (HA), and GABA in the posterior hypothalamus of anesthetized cats and conscious, freely moving rabbits. To synchronize the phases in the various experiments the last peak of high rate of release of each experiment was taken as the antepenultimate (cat) or penultimate (rabbit) sample and the preceding and following samples were rearranged accordingly. Subsequently, frequency polygons were drawn by plotting number of peaks per 30 min (cat) or number of peaks per 20 min (rabbit) against time. Mean values of 9–17 experiments [Reproduced from refs. (*4, 12, 13, 15*).]

rates of release in the opposite direction in the two hypothalamic areas may indicate the involvement of catecholaminergic systems of the hypothalamus in the homeostasis of the arterial blood pressure.

Since these experiments were carried out in anesthetized animals it cannot be excluded that anesthesia interfered with or even falsified the alterations in the rates of release of catecholamines elicited by changing the arterial blood pressure. For this reason a series of experiments was carried

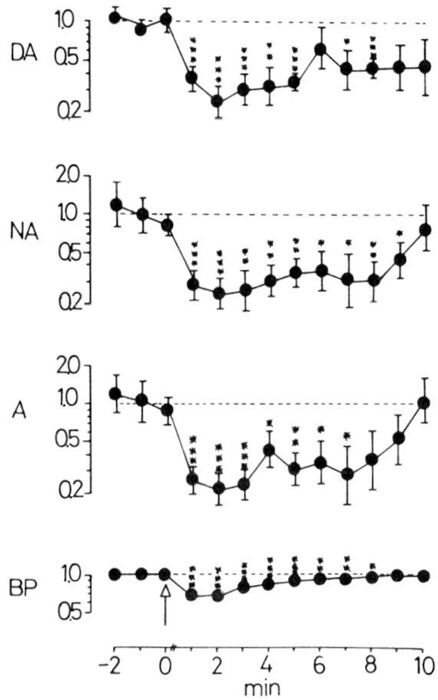

Fig. 3. Effects of sodium nitroprusside on the release of catecholamines in the anterior hypothalamus and on arterial blood pressure of conscious, freely moving rabbits. Arrow indicates intravenous injection of nitroprusside (200 μg/kg). Mean values ± SE of 10 injections in 5 animals. **p* < .05, ***p* < .01, ****p* < .001. [Reproduced from ref. (*15*).]

out in conscious, freely moving rabbits, in which push–pull cannulae were implanted under anesthesia some days prior to hypothalamic superfusion.

Figures 3 and 4 show the effects of intravenous injection of nitroprusside on the arterial blood pressure and on the release of catecholamines in the anterior and posterior hypothalamus of the freely moving rabbit. In the anterior hypothalamus, the fall of blood pressure elicited by nitroprusside was associated with a marked decrease in the rates of release of dopamine, noradrenaline, and adrenaline. The changes in the rates of release of the catecholamines lasted approximately as long as the depressor response to nitroprusside. On the other hand, the rates of release of the three catecholamines were increased in the posterior hypothalamus of the rabbit. Again, commencement and duration of the enhanced release of the catecholamines coincided with commencement and duration of the fall of blood pressure.

These results show that anesthesia does not modify the pattern of response of the hypothalamus when the arterial blood pressure is changed. Pentobarbitone seems to reduce the responsiveness of the two hypothalamic areas in counteracting blood pressure changes because the alterations in the rates of

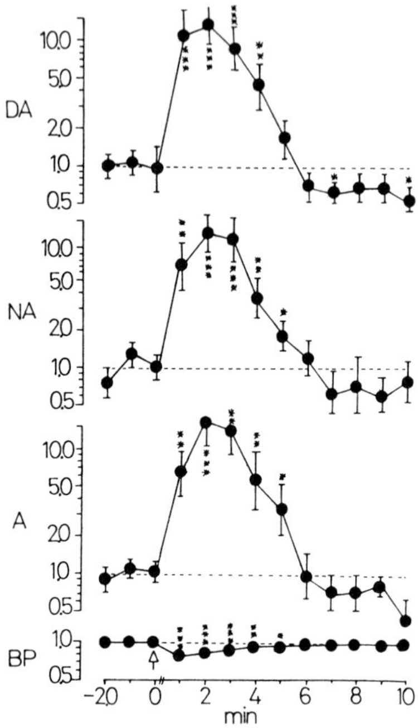

Fig. 4. Effects of sodium nitroprusside on the release of catecholamines in the posterior hypothalamus and on arterial blood pressure of conscious, freely moving rabbits. Arrow indicates intravenous injection of nitroprusside (100 μg/kg). Mean values of 9 injections in 5 animals. *$p < .05$, **$p < .01$, ***$p < .001$. [Reproduced from ref. (*11*).]

release of the catecholamines in the conscious rabbit were much more pronounced than those found in the anesthetized cat. However, species differences might also be responsible for various degrees of responsiveness of the hypothalamic catecholamines to blood pressure changes.

3. RELEASE OF CATECHOLAMINES, HISTAMINE, AND GABA IN THE HYPOTHALAMUS OF NORMOTENSIVE AND SPONTANEOUSLY HYPERTENSIVE RATS

Catecholaminergic systems of the hypothalamus have been implicated in the development and/or maintenance of the elevated blood pressure of spontaneously hypertensive (SH) rats (*9*). Histamine levels have been found to be either unaltered (*2*) or increased in the hypothalamus of SH rats (*3*). Recently, we investigated the rates of resting release of catecholamines and histamine in the posterior hypothalamus of conscious, freely moving nor-

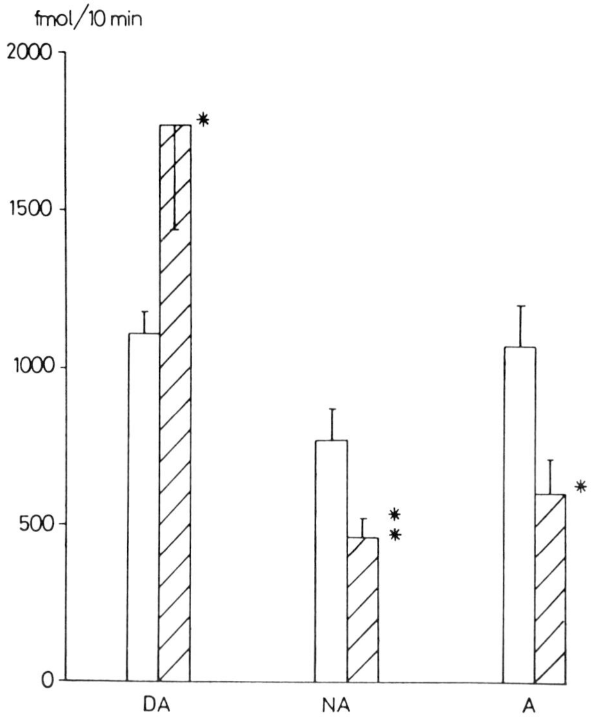

Fig. 5. Resting release of dopamine, noradrenaline, and adrenaline in the posterior hypothalamus of normotensive and spontaneously hypertensive rats. Open columns: WKy rats (N = 8); striped columns: SH rats (N = 9). Mean values ± SE. *$p < .05$, **$p < .01$. [Reproduced from ref. (*18*).]

motensive Wistar Kyoto (WKy) and SH rats. We also studied the rate of release of GABA in normotensive and hypertensive rats because central application of GABA affects the arterial blood pressure (*1, 7, 14*).

The release of neurotransmitters was studied in 60-day-old WKy and SH rats. The rates of release of dopamine and histamine were higher in SH than in normotensive WKy rats. However, the rates of noradrenaline and adrenaline were lower in SH than in WKy rats, while hypertension did not affect the rate of release of GABA (Figs. 5 and 6). These findings show that hypertension is associated with profound changes in the release of catecholamines and histamine in the posterior hypothalamus. Additional experiments are necessary to prove whether these changes are due to or whether they are evoked by the elevated blood pressure.

Since the rate of release of GABA was found to be similar in the hypo-

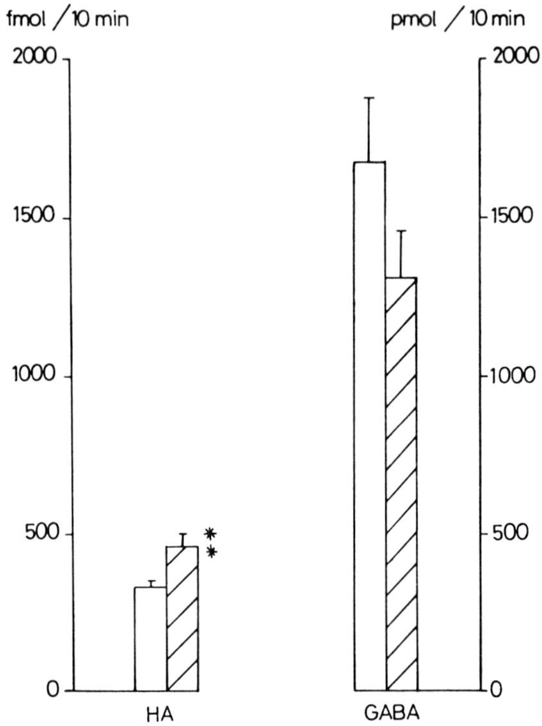

Fig. 6. Resting release of histamine and GABA in the posterior hypothalamus of normotensive and spontaneously hypertensive rats. Open columns: WKy rats ($N = 8$–9); striped columns: SH rats ($N = 9$). Mean values ± SE. $^{**}p < .01$. [Reproduced from ref. (*18*).]

thalamus of WKy and SH rats, GABA neurons of the posterior hypothalamus do not seem to be involved in hypertension.

IV. PERSPECTIVES

The previously described technique makes possible the superfusion of distinct brain areas through push–pull cannulae and the continuous determination of the release of endogenous neurotransmitters in the superfusate. It is possible to determine the rates of release of neurotransmitters in 10-sec time periods. Thus, this technique may be used to closely correlate experimentally induced changes in functions of peripheral organs with alterations in the rates of release of endogenous neurotransmitters. In this way conclusions may be drawn concerning functions of neurotransmitters in the central nervous system. The main advantage of the superfusion technique combined with the subsequent determination of transmitters in the superfusate is versatility and high specificity of the detection assays. Probably the main disadvantage of the technique is the time-consuming detection of the endogenous compounds.

The push–pull cannula has been recently combined with a microelectrode for recording activity of brain stem neurons. Figure 7 shows that a long-lasting superfusion of the respiratory center with CSF through the push–pull cannula does not affect the firing of a superfused inspiratory neuron. Hence, it is possible to investigate the effects of locally applied drugs on the activity of single neurons (H. Wilson, personal communication). A combination of this technique with the determination of neurotransmitters in the superfusate may further extend the usefulness of the superfusion technique in elucidating the functional importance of brain neurons and in identifying their neurotransmitters as well. The development of more sensitive assays for the direct determination of transmitters in the superfusate will greatly facilitate the procedure.

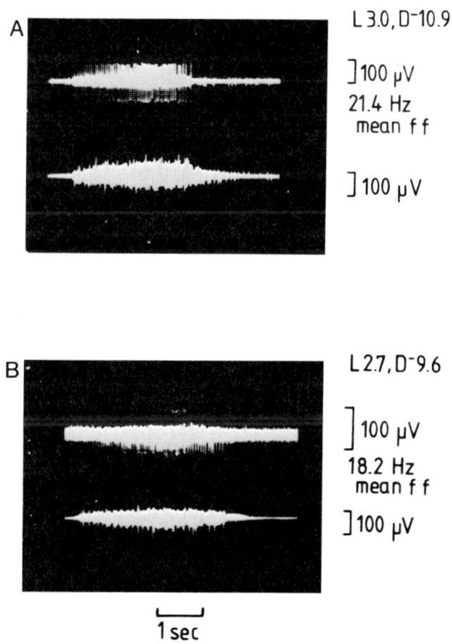

Fig. 7. Extracellular recordings from a phasically active inspiratory neuron (A) and the correlation of this discharge to the electromyogram of the diaphragm (B) in two spontaneously breathing cats. (A) Neuronal activity was recorded with the microelectrode. (B) The microelectrode was fixed in juxtaposition to the push–pull cannula. Superfusion rate: 92 µl/min. L, lateral; D, vertical; P, posterior to the zero point [stereotaxic atlas of Snider and Niemer (*17*)]; ff, firing frequency. (Reproduced by courtesy of H. Wilson and K. C. F. Fone.)

REFERENCES

1. Antonaccio, M. J., and Taylor, D. G. Involvement of central GABA receptors in the regulation of blood pressure and heart rate of anesthetized cats. *Eur. J. Pharmacol.* **46** (1977) 283–287.
2. Chalmers, J. P., Howe, P. R. C., Provis, J. C., and West, M. J. Cardiac and central histamine in spontaneously hypertensive and stroke-prone rats. *In* "Nervous System and Hypertension," (P. Meyer and H. Schmitt, eds.), 1979. pp. 244–251. Wiley, New York.
3. Correa, F. M., and Saavedra, J. M. Increase in histamine concentration in discrete hypothalamic nuclei of spontaneously hypertensive rats. *Brain Res.* **205** (1981) 445–451.
4. Dietl, H., and Philippu, A. *In vivo* release of endogenous GABA in the cat hypothalamus. *Naunyn-Schmiedeberg's Arch. Pharmacol.* **308** (1979) 143–147.
5. Dietl, H., Eisert, A., Kraus, A., and Philippu, A. The release of endogenous catecholamines in the cat hypothalamus is affected by spinal transection and drugs which change the arterial blood pressure. *J. Auton. Pharmacol.* **1** (1981) 279–286.
6. Fifkova, E., and Marsala, J. Stereotaxic atlases for the cat, rabbit and rat. *In* "Electrophysiological Methods in Biological Research" (3rd edition) (J. Bures, M. Petran, and J. Jachar, eds.), 1967, pp. 653–711. Academic Press, New York.
7. Guertzenstein, P. G. Blood pressure effects obtained by drugs applied to the ventral surface of the brainstem. *J. Physiol.* **229** (1973) 395–408.
8. König, J., and Klippel, R. "The Rat Brain. A Stereotaxic Atlas," 1963. Krieger, Huntington.
9. Philippu, A. Regulation of the arterial blood pressure. *In* "Adrenergic Activators and Inhibitors," (L. Szekeres ed.), 1979, pp. 521–548. Springer-Verlag, Berlin.
10. Philippu, A. Use of push–pull cannulae to investigate the release of endogenous neurotransmitters in distinct brain areas of anaesthetized or freely moving animals. *In* "Measurement of Neurotransmitter Release *in Vivo*," (C. A. Marsden, ed.), 1984, pp. 3–37. Wiley, New York.
11. Philippu, A., Dietl, H., and Eisert, A. Hypotension alters the release of catecholamines in the hypothalamus of the conscious rabbit. *Eur. J. Pharmacol.* **69** (1981) 519–523.
12. Philippu, A., Dietl, H., and Sinha, J. N. *In vivo* release of endogenous catecholamines in the hypothalamus. *Naunyn-Schmiedeberg's Arch. Pharmacol.* **308** (1979) 137–142.
13. Philippu, A., Hanesch, U., Hagen, R., and Robinson, R. Release of endogenous histamine in the hypothalamus of anaesthetized cats and conscious, freely moving rabbits. *Naunyn-Schmiedeberg's Arch. Pharmacol.* **321** (1982) 282–286.
14. Philippu, A., Przuntek, H., and Roensberg, W. Superfusion of the hypothalamus with gamma-aminobutyric acid: effect on release of noradrenaline and blood pressure. *Naunyn-Schmiedeberg's Arch. Pharmacol.* **276** (1973) 103–118.
15. Robinson, R., Dietl, H., Bald, M., Kraus, A., and Philippu, A. Effects of short-lasting and long-lasting blood pressure changes on the release of endogenous catecholamines in the hypothalamus of the conscious, freely moving rabbit. *Naunyn-Schmiedeberg's Arch. Pharmacol.* **322** (1983) 203–209.
16. Sinha, J. N., Dietl, H., and Philippu, A. Effect of a fall of blood pressure on the release of catecholamines in the hypothalamus. *Life Sci.* **26** (1980) 1751–1760.
17. Snider, R. S., and Niemer, W. T. "A Stereotaxic Atlas of the Cat Brain," 1961. Univ. of Chicago Press, Chicago, Illinois.
18. Tuomisto, L., Yamatodani, A., Dietl, H., Waldmann, U., and Philippu, A. *In vivo* release of endogenous catecholamines, histamine and GABA in the hypothalamus of Wistar Kyoto and spontaneously hypertensive rats. *Naunyn-Schmiedeberg's Arch. Pharmacol.* **323** (1983) 183–187.

14

Release of Arginine Vasopressin from the Brain: Correlation with Physiological Events

WILLIAM D. RUWE, WARREN L. VEALE, QUENTIN J. PITTMAN, NORMAN W. KASTING,* AND K. LEDERIS

Department of Medical Physiology
Faculty of Medicine
University of Calgary
Calgary, Alberta, Canada

**Department of Physiology*
University of British Columbia
Vancouver, British Columbia, Canada

I. INTRODUCTION

Arginine vasopressin (AVP) long has been known primarily for its functional roles as a pressor hormone affecting peripheral vasomotor tone and as an antidiuretic hormone affecting water retention in the kidneys. Recently, the neuroparacrine function of this peptide has been recognized. AVP, now implicated as a potential neurotransmitter, may participate in the control

IN VIVO PERFUSION AND RELEASE
OF NEUROACTIVE SUBSTANCES

ISBN 0-12-083350-6

mechanisms which subserve (1) modulatory influence on the electrical activity of certain neuronal populations (*3*), (2) the stimulation of ACTH release from the adenohypophysis (*37, 64*), (3) the regulation of brain water permeability (*54*), (4) the functional regulation of cerebrospinal fluid (CSF) formation and its chemical composition (*58, 59*), (5) the control of central and peripheral fluid electrolyte balance (*53*), (6) well-identified deficiency syndrome, diabetes insipidus (DI) (*52*), (7) the cortical appreciation of thirst (*45, 46*), (8) the pathophysiology of affective disorders (*19, 55, 70*), (9) the mediation of certain cognitive processes of learning and memory in man (*20*) and in animals, and (10) the development of tolerance to ethanol and/or drugs (*24, 51*).

The presence of this putative neurotransmitter in the brain has been adequately demonstrated. Immunocytochemistry (*4, 5, 11, 16, 62, 69, 75*) revealed the presence of this nonapeptide in the hypothalamus within the magnocellular and parvocellular neurons of the paraventricular nucleus (PVN), supraoptic nucleus (SON), and suprachiasmatic nucleus (SCN) and arcuate nucleus (*17*). Electrophysiological (*14, 36, 56*) and retrograde transport studies (*2, 15, 60, 66*) indicate that these nuclei send projections to a number of extrahypothalamic areas. In keeping with these observations are the neuroanatomical investigations indicating the presence of AVP and oxytocin and their related neurophysins in neuronal fibers in many limbic system structures including the septum, habenula, and amygdala (*5, 61, 63, 65*). Other structures involved in the control of vital autonomic functions which may be innervated by AVP-containing fibers include the nucleus of the tractus solitarius (NTS), the dorsal motor nucleus of the vagus (DMN), midbrain periaqueductal gray (*5, 47, 61, 63, 65*), the fiber systems of the choroid plexi, and the spinal cord.

An important criterion for the establishment of a biochemical substance as a neurotransmitter is that of release from appropriate biological tissue (*38*). Currently, both indirect and direct evidence has been obtained to demonstrate that AVP is released within the central nervous system (CNS). First, it is well known that hemorrhage is a potent stimulus for the neurohypophyseal release of AVP (*18*). This reduction in total blood volume may mimic the effect of an intracerebroventricular (ICV) injection of AVP in sensitizing the rat to the convulsant action of this neuropeptide. The direct infusion of AVP into the lateral cerebral ventricle of the rodent evokes a generalized seizure with myoclonic/myotonic convulsions (*30*). This seizure-like activity is observed but only after an initial comparable injection of the peptide which, it is believed, sensitizes the brain to the seizure-inducing effects of AVP (*30, 50*). Similarly, gross motor disturbances including barrel rotations and/or convulsions are evoked by an ICV injection of AVP when, instead of the initial microinjection of AVP, the animal is subjected to sequential hemorrhages (6). It is thought that during the hemorrhage, the central release of AVP or a related substance occurs, thus sensitizing the brain to the convulsive actions of the subsequent ICV injection of neuropeptide.

Additional more direct evidence that AVP is released centrally has been obtained by measuring the circulating levels of immunoassayable AVP or antidiuretic activity in the CSF in any of a number of species (*13, 23, 26, 57, 72, 73*). Certain physiological events such as vagal stimulation, the administration of pentobarbital, and hemorrhage are known to cause the release of neurohypophyseal AVP (*50*). Stimuli such as these have been shown to elicit an increase in the antidiuretic activity of the CSF of rabbits (*23, 72*).

The present experiments were undertaken to obtain further direct evidence that AVP has a functional role as a neurotransmitter within the brain; that is, since stimuli are known to cause an evoked release of AVP into the circulation or into CSF, can we in turn identify physiological events that are effective in causing the release of this neuropeptide from specific brain structures?

II. METHODS

A. Series 1

Male New Zealand white rabbits were housed individually in a colony room that was maintained at an ambient temperature of 20°–22°C and illuminated on a 12-hr light–dark cycle. Each animal was anesthetized with sodium pentobarbital injected intravenously into the marginal ear vein. A stereotaxic headplate was affixed to the calvarium of each animal and a chronic jugular catheter was implanted according to surgical procedures described previously (*71*). During a 5-day recovery period, the animals were habituated to the experimental surrounds.

To determine the activity of the endogenous stores of AVP, sites within the lateral septum or the amygdala were perfused using the push–pull technique (*42*). As described previously, the inner or push cannula cut from 29-ga thin-walled stainless-steel tubing was inserted into an outer or pull cannula consisting of 23-ga thin-walled stainless-steel tubing. The beveled tip of the push cannula was extended 0.5–1.0 mm beyond the tip of the pull cannula. With this separation of the cannulae, it was possible to bathe a sphere of tissue approximately 1.0 mm in diameter (*44*). The depth of penetration was predetermined by a set-screw spacer affixed to the outer pull cannula.

The push and pull cannulae were connected by PE-20 and PE-50 tubing, respectively, to calibrated 2.0-ml gas-tight glass syringes which were mounted on a Harvard infusion–withdrawal pump. Glassware and related equipment used for injections and perfusions were kept sterile and pyrogen free by baking at 180°C for 3 hr or placing them in benzalkonium chloride for 24 hr. All solutions were passed through a 13-mm Swinnex Millipore filter with a 0.22-μm pore size. The cannula assembly, tubing, and syringes were stored in 70% ethanol between experiments and flushed repeatedly with ethanol and a sterile physiological solution prior to an experiment.

A sterile physiological solution was perfused through the cannula at a rate of 35–40 μl/min for three successive 30-min periods. The perfusate was collected on ice and then frozen immediately at −70°C. If the pull side of the system gave signs of occlusion or if the perfusate became discolored, the perfusion experiment was terminated immediately.

Upon completion of the first 30-min perfusion period and concurrent with the beginning of the second perfusion period, either 8.0 ml of sterile 3 *M* NaCl was infused over 10 min into the jugular catheter or 0.1 μg/10.0 μl of *Salmonella abortus equi* (SAE; Difco Laboratories) was injected into the marginal ear vein. Following infusion of the NaCl, blood osmolarity was increased to approximately 345 mOsm. The increase in blood osmolarity represents a potent stimulus for the release of AVP from the pituitary (*48*). Within 20–30 min after the ICV infusion of the pyrogen, a marked fever was elicited. The third and final 30-min push–pull perfusion was conducted 30 min after completion of the second perfusion.

Perfusates were assayed using a high-specificity radioimmunoassay with sensitivity to less than 1.0 pg/ml and very little cross-reactivity to other related peptides (*41*).

B. Series 2

Mature female Suffolk, Dorset, and crossbred sheep were housed in a colony room that was maintained at an ambient temperature of 18°–20°C and illuminated on a 12-hr light–dark cycle. Each animal was shorn and allowed to acclimate to laboratory conditions. An array of 17-ga stainless-steel guide tubes was implanted above several regions of the hypothalamus and septum. Each guide tube was fitted with an indwelling stylet to occlude the cannnulae when they were not in use and to maintain sterility. The cannulae were securely affixed to the calvarium with cranioplastic cement. A polyethylene pedestral with a protective cap was placed over the guide tubes and secured to the skull with steel screws. The cap both protected and assured the patency of the array of cannulae, and maintained an aseptic preparation for the duration of the experiments.

A YSI thermistor probe was inserted approximately 10 cm into the vagina. The sheep's vaginal temperature was monitored and recorded continuously on a Bedman pen recorder. The baseline temperature of each sheep was obtained for at least 30 min before injection of endotoxin and for 200 min thereafter. At regular intervals throughout the course of an experiment, respiratory rate, postural adjustments, and shivering were assessed by observation and recorded.

The push–pull perfusion procedures utilized in this series of experiments were identical to those used in Series 1. Injection of the exogenous pyrogen and commencement of the push–pull perfusion occurred simultaneously. The sequence of perfusions with the different substances was carried out in a random order at weekly intervals. The solution used for the push–pull perfusion was either 260 m*M* sucrose or 260 m*M* sucrose with AVP at a concentration of 0.8, 2.0, or 4.0 μg/ml. AVP was stored as a stock solution of 1.0 mg/ml in 0.25% acetic acid at 4.0°C. AVP exhibited an activity of 360 rat pressor units/mg and 360 rat antidiuretic units/mg. The exogenous pyrogen used in this series was derived from *Salmonella abortus equi* (Difco Laboratories). A standard dose of SAE, 30.0 μg/3.0 ml sterile physiological saline, evoked a biphasic fever with a maximum rise of 1.36 ± 0.06°C at 200 min when injected intravenously in mature, unoperated ewes.

As in Series 1, the interval of perfusion was 30 min. A successive series of perfusions was conducted during the development of the pyrogen-induced fever. The perfusions were undertaken primarily in sites of the brain in which AVP perfusions had been determined previously to be effective in reducing the febrile response.

Upon completion of both series of experiments, each animal was given an overdose of sodium pentobarbital. After the heart was clamped, saline followed by 10% neutral Formalin was perfused through the common carotid arteries. The brain was blocked in the coronal plane and then sectioned on a freezing stage microtome and stained for cells and fibers. The stained site of each perfusion was localized under light microscopy and mapped anatomically using histological reconstructions.

III. FINDINGS

A. Series 1

Increasing the blood osmolarity in the rabbit is associated with increased levels of AVP from sites located in the limbic system. Levels of AVP in the control perfusates ranged from less than 1.5 pg/ml (i.e., undetectable) to 135 pg/ml. As illustrated in Fig. 1, after intravenous injection of the hypertonic saline, the levels of immunoassayable AVP were increased above these resting values. In perfusion sites located in the lateral septum, AVP

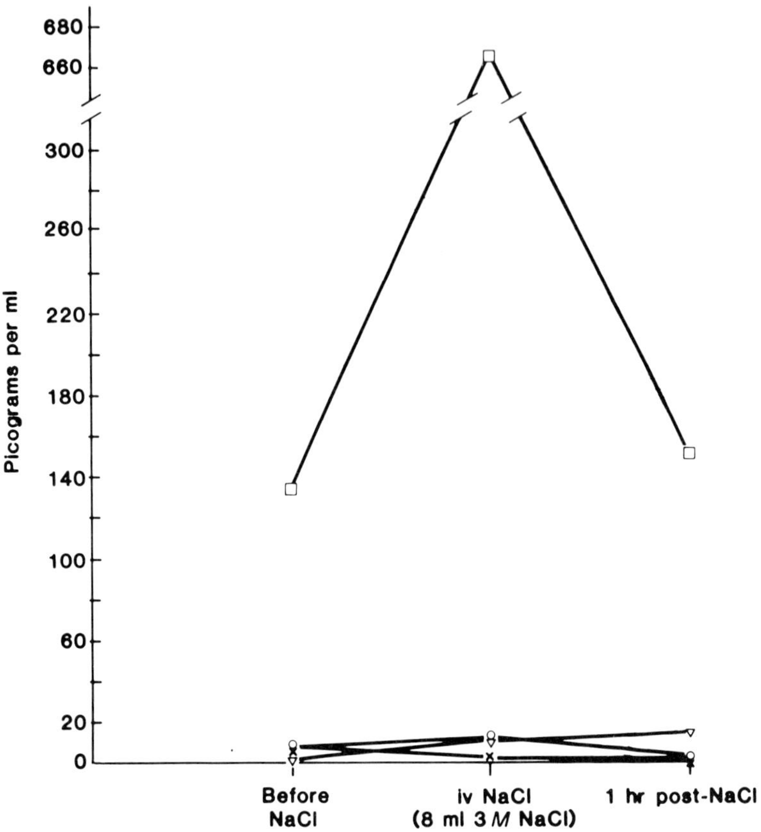

Fig. 1. Levels of arginine vasopressin (AVP), in picograms per milliliter, detected by radioimmunoassay in perfusates collected from limbic system sites of an unanesthetized rabbit. Push–pull perfusions were carried out over a 30-min period before, during, and 1 hr after an intravenous injection of 3 *M* NaCl/8.0 ml (open squares). Site specificity is indicated by the minimal response to the hypertonic saline in three other sites in the limbic system.

levels rose by 316%. Perfusates collected from sites in the amygdala increased by 299%. In other central sites, the perfusates collected after plasma osmolarity was increased showed no appreciable difference in the amounts of AVP (see Fig. 1). Perfusates collected during the third and final perfusion contained levels of AVP that were still elevated above the resting levels observed prior to injection of the sterile saline. Similar perfusions carried out sequentially from sites displaying elevated AVP levels after increased osmolarity did not show such elevations after intravenous infusion of 0.9% NaCl.

B. Series 2

Within certain limbic system sites in the sheep and the rabbit, the release of AVP is altered during the pathogenesis of fever; that is, push–pull perfusates collected as the core temperature increases contained lesser amounts of AVP than those collected during a decline in temperature. Figure 2 depicts the decreasing amounts of AVP that were released into the extracellular fluid as the core temperature rose during the initial stages of the pyrogen-

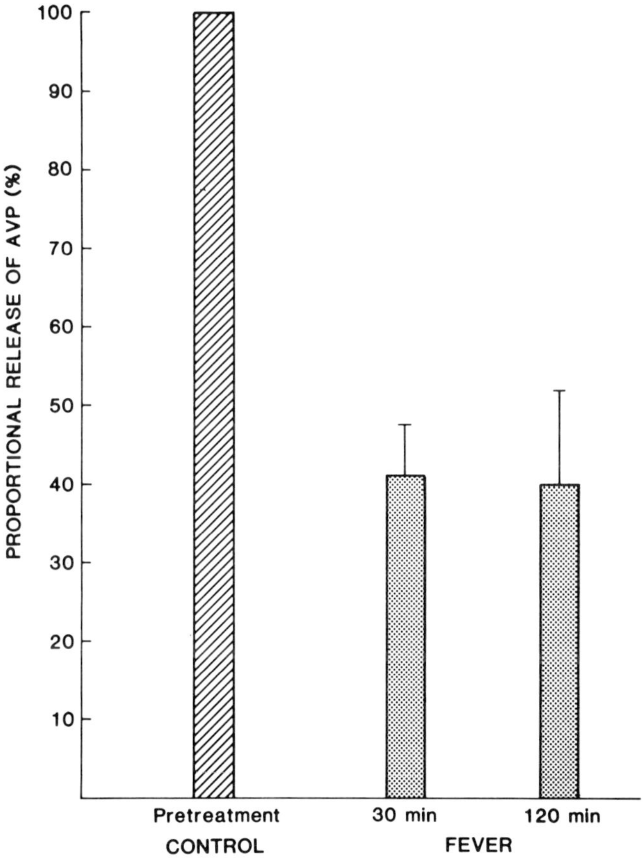

Fig. 2. Changes in the levels of arginine vasopressin (AVP) detected by radioimmunoassay in perfusates of a site in the lateral septum of the unanesthetized rabbit plotted as proportional release or percentage change. Push–pull perfusions were carried out over a 30-min period before (pretreatment control; resting level = 100%) and during two stages of a pyrogen-induced fever (30 and 120 min). Absolute values of AVP contained in the perfusate ranged from 17.5 to 193 pg/ml.

induced fever. Even at 2 hr following injection of the pyrogen, the amount of AVP released was reduced below that observed during the pretreatment or control perfusion. The sites in which the push–pull perfusions were carried out were located primarily within the septal area, 2–3 mm rostral to the anterior commissure.

When AVP was perfused into punctate regions in the brain of the sheep or rabbit, the pyrogen-induced fever was suppressed. The infusion of comparable quantities of AVP was without effect on the core temperature of an afebrile animal. During a perfusion interval of 200 min in which approximately 32 ng of AVP were delivered in 1 min, there was a marked reduction of nearly 1.0°C in the febrile response. The absolute magnitude of the fever was reduced in a dose-dependent manner when 0.8 μg AVP/ml to 4.0 μg AVP/ml was perfused proximal to or directly within the septal area. The febrile response obtained following perfusion of the sites with AVP was significantly lower than that obtained with perfusion of sucrose only or without a perfusion ($p < .0005$). Moreover, physiological changes normally associated with the activation of heat conservation/heat production mechanisms characteristic of fever, such as shivering, decreased respiratory rate, and a huddled posture, were not observed in animals receiving AVP.

Although effective in the septal area and perhaps the diagonal band of Broca or closely related sites, AVP had no effect on the core temperature of either a febrile or an afebrile animal following perfusion within the anterior hypothalamus, the preoptic area, the fornix, or the rostrum of the corpus callosum.

Comparable infusions of other peptide neurohormones were without effect on the fever. Perfusions of oxytocin, somatostatin, angiotensin II, and substance P did not alter the febrile response. A structurally similar neuropeptide, arginine vasotocin, caused a partial antagonism of the fever when infused into the AVP-sensitive sites within the septal area. Bombesin also reduced core temperature of the febrile animal as it was perfused into these sites in the limbic system. However, since this neuropeptide also decreased the core temperature of an afebrile animal, it is likely that bombesin has a nonspecific effect on the thermoregulatory mechanisms of the animal. Following perfusion of these septal sites with a specific antiserum to AVP, the fever developed more quickly and body temperature increased much more rapidly. The febrile response during perfusion of the anti-AVP antiserum was significantly greater than the control febrile response for nearly 3 hr after injection of the pyrogen. Similarly, when an AVP analog, desamino-dicarba-AVP, was perfused into these sites, the febrile response again was enhanced. The latency to onset was shorter and the rate of increase in core temperature was more pronounced than the control febrile response.

IV. DISCUSSION

The results of this series of experiments indicate that it is possible to identify certain physiological events that are highly correlated with the release of AVP from the brain. The evoked release of this neurohypophyseal peptide in the brain suggests that, in addition to its typical neuroendocrine role, AVP may function in the CNS as a neurotransmitter or neuromodulator. Indeed, previous investigators (*67*) have suggested that neurohypophyseal peptides could provide the means by which the vital autonomic and neuroendocrine mechanisms can be integrated centrally. It may be that these neuropeptides are released centrally within the animal as it responds to a perturbation in its homeostatic processes (*32*). Observations such as these raise the interesting possibility that neuropeptides in the brain and neurohypophyseal peptide systems could function in a highly coordinated manner to maintain the important balances within the system which insure homeostasis.

Results from the first series of experiments indicate that, in accordance with electrophysiological studies (*50*), physiological events that are known to trigger the release of neurohypophyseal hormones into the periphery are also capable of causing the release of the same peptide centrally. Moreover, this evoked release is specific to very circumscribed sites in the limbic system, suggesting that such a release is not the result of a generalized activation of a variety of neural networks. These results are consistent with reports that other stimuli that are known to cause the neurohypophyseal release of AVP also elicit the central release of this peptide into the lateral cerebral ventricles (*72*). Thus, another physiological event that alters the hemodynamics of the organism in such a manner as to activate the neurohypophysis also may simultaneously activate certain brain structures, thus releasing the peptide both peripherally and centrally. It is currently believed that the blood CSF barrier is impervious to penetration by this neurohypophyseal hormone (*72, 74*). Thus, it is quite probable that the levels of immunoassayable AVP detected in the push–pull perfusate reflect primarily an alteration in the central release of this peptide rather than changes in peripheral levels of the neurohormone.

The second series of experiments provides additional compelling evidence for the central release of AVP from brain tissue in response to a specific physiological event. In this case, the pathogenesis of a fever may serve as a potent stimulus for the eventual release of this neuropeptide as the infected organism attempts to achieve thermal homeostasis. That AVP is not released during the initial phase of the febrile response, nor even during the asymptotic phase, may indicate that so long as the postulated set-point shift (*43*) has occurred, the release of this endogenous antipyretic is not necessary. It may be that during the initiation of defervescence, as the set point returns to normal, the vasopressinergic system is activated to restore the organism's thermal balance.

It is clear from this series of experiments that AVP, when administered directly into brain tissue, has a definite physiological action. The effective dosage of this neuropeptide, 6.4 μg over a 200-min period, is well within the range for an effective dose of a central injection of an antipyretic (9) or an anti-inflammatory steroid (7), both of which effectively antagonize the febrile response. Moreover, the thermolytic property of AVP appears to be specific to the febrile condition since the peptide does not lower the normal body temperature of an afebrile animal.

How might the central release of AVP function to maintain the homeostasis of an organism? There is now a considerable body of evidence that suggests that AVP may function as a natural or endogenous antipyretic. As summarized in Table I, there are four sets of evidence for the involvement of central stores of AVP in the postulated mechanism for endogenous antipyresis. This evidence has been derived from both indirect and direct neuroanatomical, physiological, and pharmacological investigations in a variety of species, including man. In the light of such evidence, it becomes increasingly apparent that not only is AVP released from tissues of various brain structures, but that this neurohypophyseal peptide acts centrally as a neuromodulator or neurotransmitter in the maintenance of thermal homeostasis. Indeed, the febrile response appears to be one physiological event in which the important neuroparacrine function that AVP plays is brought to the forefront.

Although it is now clear that this neurohypophyseal peptide can be released from structures within the brain in response to certain identifiable physiological stimuli, such as increased blood osmolarity or fever, much more research will be required before the precise role of AVP can be determined. For example, the mode of action of AVP, the neuroanatomical areas and pathways in and through which AVP is active, and the complex interactions in which AVP is involved have yet to be defined with certainty. Initially, it must be demonstrated more fully that the release of AVP within these brain structures is definitely a specific response to a given physiological event. Other areas of the brain will require thorough exploration to identify all the neuroanatomical loci at which AVP may be released. Concurrently, the release of other neurohormones should be examined. In addition to correlating the release of AVP with the release of other neuroactive agents, other stimuli should be utilized to ascertain whether they, too, might evoke the release of such neurohypophyseal peptides. It is obvious that the innovative nature of the push–pull technique will be supplanted by the nature of necessity as it is employed in these efforts to delineate the complex function of AVP in the brain.

TABLE I

Summary of Evidence for Arginine Vasopressin as a Centrally Acting Endogenous Antipyretic

A. Indirect evidence
1. Central warming of the basal forebrain area of an animal elicits an increase in plasma concentrations of AVP (*68*), whereas cooling this area causes a reduction in plasma concentrations of AVP (*22*).
2. Exposure to heat evokes a marked increase in the release of AVP from the neurohypophysis of an animal (*25*).
3. Electrical stimulation of sites in the limbic system elicits an increase in plasma concentrations of AVP and a concomitant decrease in body temperature (*21*).
4. Concurrent with the hemorrhage-induced release of AVP into plasma (*18*) and CSF (*72*) is a reduction in the magnitude of the febrile response (*31*).
5. AVP, known to evoke seizures or seizure-like activity (*30*), may be involved in the etiology of febrile convulsions (*34*).

B. Neuroanatomical evidence
1. AVP-containing neuronal elements and axonal projections are present in known thermoregulatory areas of the brain (*39*).
2. Coincident with the period of the diminished febrile response, an increase in the amount of vasopressin-reactive material occurs in the nuclear regions of the mediobasal hypothalamus (*40*).
3. Effective antipyresis can be achieved only when AVP is perfused within a very circumscribed region of the brain, the septal area only 2–3 mm rostral to the anterior commissure (*8*).
4. Owing to the neuroanatomical location and the nature of these affected structures, it is unlikely that AVP leaks into the peripheral circulation to exert its antipyretic action there (*27*).

C. Pharmacological evidence
1. Direct intracerebroventricular injections of small quantities of neurohypophyseal extracts or AVP produce a profound hypothermia in the animal (*3,10,30*).
2. Push–pull perfusion of small quantities of AVP into punctate regions of the mammalian brain evokes a dose-dependent reduction in the febrile response (*8*).
3. Push–pull perfusion of the control or vehicle solution, oxytocin, somatostatin, angiotensin, and substance P does not affect the febrile response (*35*).
4. Infusion of a specific antiserum to AVP disrupting AVP's neurochemical function interrupts the antipyretic action of AVP (*27*).
5. Infusion of desamino-dicarba-AVP, an AVP analog which alters the receptor population, interrupts the antipyretic action of AVP (*27*).

D. Physiological evidence
1. Coincident with the periparturient period when circulating levels of AVP are markedly enhanced (*1*) the febrile response is greatly diminished (*28*).
2. Fetal and maternal leukocytes are capable of being stimulated to produce endogenous pyrogen (*29*).
3. During the pathogenesis of fever, the release of central AVP is negatively correlated with fever: as body temperature increases, there is a decrease in the amount of AVP released into the extracellular fluid (*3*).
4. Intravenous administration of even very high concentrations of AVP is ineffective in antagonizing the febrile response (*8*).

ACKNOWLEDGMENTS

This research was supported by the Medical Research Council (MRC) of Canada and the Alberta Heritage Foundation for Medical Research (AHFMR). The authors wish to thank E. Annand, J. Disturnal, D. Ko, T. Malkinson, C. Nagata, and J. Simpson for their technical assistance and help in collection of the data. Thanks to G. Olmstead for typing the manuscript. WDR is an AHFMR Fellow, QJP and NWK are MRC Scholars, and KL is a Career Investigator of the MRC.

REFERENCES

1. Alexander, D. P., Bashore, R. A., Britton, H. G., and Forsling, M. A. Maternal and fetal arginine vasopressin in the chronically catheterized sheep. *Biol. Neonate* **25** (1974) 242–248.
2. Alexander, W. E., Warach, S., Hatton, G. J., and McNeill, T. H. Subnuclei in the rat hypothalamic paraventricular nucleus: a cytoarchitectural, horseradish peroxidase and immunocytochemical analysis. *Neuroscience* **5** (1980) 1931–1958.
3. Barker, J. L., Ifshin, M. S., and Gainer, H. Studies on bursting pacemaker potential activity in molluscan neurons. III. Effects of hormones. *Brain Res.* **84** (1975) 501–513.
4. Buijs, R. M. Intra- and extrahypothalamic vasopressin and oxytocin pathways in the rat. *Cell Tiss. Res.* **192** (1978) 423–435.
5. Buijs, R. M., Swaab, D. F., Dogterom, J., and van Leeuwen, F. W. Intra- and extra-hypothalamic vasopressin and oxytocin pathways in the rat. *Cell Tiss. Res.* **186** (1978) 423–433.
6. Burnard, D. M., Pittman, Q. J., and Veale, W. L. Vasopressin-induced convulsions: sensitization by hemorrhage. *Proc. Can. Fed. Biol. Soc.* **24** (1981) 171.
7. Chowers, I., Confarti, N., and Feldman, S. Local effect of cortisol in the preoptic area on temperature regulation. *Am. J. Physiol.* **214** (1968) 538–542.
8. Cooper, K. E., Kasting, N. W., Lederis, K., and Veale, W. L. Evidence supporting a role for endogenous vasopressin in natural suppression of fever in the sheep. *J. Physiol. (London)* **295** (1979) 33–45.
9. Cranston, W. I., and Rawlins, M. D. Effects of intracerebral microinjection of sodium salicylate on temperature regulation in the rabbit. *J. Physiol. (London)* **222** (1972) 257–266.
10. Cushing, H. "*Papers Relating to the Pituitary Body, Hypothalamus and Parasympathetic Nervous System*," 1932, pp. 59–110. Thomas, Springfield, Illinois.
11. Defendini, R., and Zimmerman, E. A. The magnocellular neurosecretory system of the mammalian hypothalamus. *In* "The Hypothalamus," (S. Reichlin, R. J. Baldessarini, and J. B. Martin eds.), 1978, pp. 137–152. Raven, New York.
12. deWied, D. Behavioral effects of intraventricularly administered vasopressin and vasopressin fragments. *Life Sci.* **19** (1976) 685–690.
13. Dogterom, J., van Wimersma Greidanus, T. B., and Swaab, D. F. Evidence for the release of vasopressin and oxytocin into cerebrospinal fluid: measurements in plasma and CSF of intact and hypophysectomized rats. *Neuroendocrinology* **24** (1977) 108–118.
14. Dreifuss, J. J., Harris, M. C., and Tribollet, E. Excitation of phasically firing hypothalamic supraoptic neurones by carotid occlusion in rats. *J. Physiol. (London)* **257** (1976) 337–354.
15. Fisher, A. W. F., Price, P. G., Burford, G. D., and Lederis, K. A reappraisal of the topography of the rat's hypothalamoneurohypophysial system. *In* "Current Studies of Hy-

pothalamic Function 1978," Vol. 1, (W. L. Veale and K. Lederis eds.), 1978, pp. 1–14. S. Karger, Basel.
16. Fisher, A. W. F., Price, P. G., Burford, G. D., and Lederis, K. A 3-dimensional reconstruction of the hypothalamoneurohypophysial system of the rat. *Cell Tiss. Res.* **204** (1979) 343–354.
17. George, J. M., and Jacobowitz, D. M. Localization of vasopressin in discrete areas of the rat hypothalamus. *Brain Res.* **93** (1975) 363–366.
18. Ginsburg, M., and Brown, L. M. Effect of anaesthetics and haemorrhage on the release of neurohypophysial and antidiuretic hormone. *Br. J. Pharmacol.* **11** (1956) 236–244.
19. Gold, P. W., and Goodwin, F. K. Vasopressin in affective illness. *Lancet* **1** (1978) 1233–1236.
20. Gold, P. W., Weingartner, H. L., Ballenger, J. C., Goodwin, F. K., and Post, R. M. Effects of 1-desamo-8-D-arginine vasopressin on behaviour and cognition in primary affective disorders. *Lancet* **2** (1979) 992–994.
21. Hayward, J. N. Amygdala and thermoregulation: implications for temporal lobe seizures. *In* "Brain Dysfunction in Infantile Febrile Convulsions," (Brazier, M. H. B. and Coceani, F., eds.) 1976, pp. 179–185. Raven, New York.
22. Hayward, J. N., and Baker, M. A. Diuretic and thermoregulatory responses to preoptic cooling in the monkey. *Am. J. Physiol.* **214** (1968) 843–850.
23. Heller, H., Hansan, S. H., and Saifi, A. W. Antidiuretic activity in the cerebrospinal fluid. *J. Endocr.* **41** (1968) 273–280.
24. Hoffman, P. L., Ritzmann, R. F., Walter, R., and Tabakoff, B. Arginine vasopressin maintains ethanol tolerance. *Nature (London)* **276** (1978) 614–616.
25. Itoh, S. The release of antidiuretic hormone from the posterior pituitary body on exposure to heat. *Jpn. J. Physiol.* **4** (1954) 185–190.
26. Jenkins, J. S., Mather, H. M., and Ang, V. Vasopressin in human cerebrospinal fluid. *J. Clin. Endocr. and Metab.* **50** (1980) 364–367.
27. Kasting, N. W. *An Antipyretic System in the Brain and the Role of Vasopressin.* Ph.D. Thesis, University of Calgary, Calgary, Canada (1980).
28. Kasting, N. W., Veale, W. L., and Cooper, K. E. Evidence for a centrally active, endogenous antipyretic near parturition. *In* "Current Studies of Hypothalamic Function" (Veale, W. L. and Lederis, K., eds.), 1978, pp. 63–71. S. Karger, Basel.
29. Kasting, N. W., Veale, W. L., and Cooper, K. E. Endogenous pyrogen release by fetal sheep and pregnant sheep blood leukocytes. *Can. J. Physiol. Pharmacol.* **57** (1979) 1453–1456.
30. Kasting, N. W., Veale, W. L., and Cooper, K. E. Convulsive and hypothermic effects of vasopressin in the brain of the rat. *Can. J. Physiol. Pharmacol.* **58** (1980) 316–319.
31. Kasting, N. W., Veale, W. L., Cooper, K. E., and Lederis, K. Effects of hemorrhage on fever: the role of vasopressin. *Can. J. Physiol. Pharmacol.* **59** (1981) 324–328.
32. Kasting, N. W., Veale, W. L., and Cooper, K. E. Vasopressin: a homeostatic effector in the febrile response. *Neurosci. Biobehav. Rev.* **6** (1982) 215–222.
33. Kruk, Z. L., and Brittain, R. T. Changes in body core and skin temperature following intracerebroventricular injection of substances in the conscious rat: interpretation of data. *J. Pharm. Pharmac.* **24** (1972) 835–837.
34. Lederis, K., Veale, W. L., Kasting, N. W., Cooper, K. E., and Haslam, R. H. A. Febrile convulsions in animals and children: the role of vasopressin. *Proc. West. Pharmacol. Soc.* **24** (1981) 97–99.
35. Lederis, K., Pittman, Q. J., Kasting, N. W., Veale, W., and Cooper, K. E. Central neuromodulatory role of vasopressin in antipyresis and in febrile convulsions. *Biomed. Res.* **3** (1982) 1–5.

36. Lincoln, D. W. Investigation of hypothalamic function: anatomical and physiological studies. *In* "The Endocrine Hypothalamus," (S. L. Jeffcoate and J. S. M. Hutchinson eds.), 1978, pp. 35–74. Academic Press, New York.
37. Luerssen, T. G., and Robertson, G. L. Cerebrospinal fluid vasopressin and vasotocin in health and disease. *In* "Neurobiology of Cerebrospinal Fluid," (J. H. Wood, ed.), 1980, pp. 613–623. Plenum, New York.
38. McGeer, P., Eccles, J. C., and McGeer, E. G. "Molecular Neurobiology of the Mammalian Brain," 1978. Plenum, New York.
39. Merker, G., Zeisberger, E., Bergheim-Hackmann, E., and Brück, K. Lower brain stem projections to the thermointegrative area of the hypothalamus, identified by the horse-radish peroxidase (HRP) technique. *Proc. 27th Int. Congr. Physiol. Soc., Paris* **13**(1487) (1977) 502.
40. Merker, G., Blähser, S., and Zeisberger, E. Reactivity of vasopressin-containing neurons and its relation to the antipyretic reaction in the pregnant guinea pig. *Cell Tiss. Res.* **212** (1980) 47–61.
41. Moore, G., Lutterodt, A., Burford, G., and Lederis, K. A highly specific antiserum for arginine vasopressin. *Endocrinology* **101** (1977) 1421–1435.
42. Myers, R. D. Methods for chemical stimulation of the brain. *Meth. Psychobiol.* **1** (1971) 247–280.
43. Myers, R. D. The role of ions in thermoregulation and fever. *In* "Pyretics and Antipyretics: Handbook of Experimental Pharmacology," (A. S. Milton, ed.), Vol. 60, 1982, pp. 151–196. Springer-Verlag, New York.
44. Myers, R. D., and Veale, W. L. Body temperature: possible ionic mechanism in the hypothalamus controlling the set point. *Science* **170** (1970) 95–97.
45. Pasqualini, R. Q. Diabetes insipidus without thirst. *Lancet* **1** (1959) 889–890.
46. Pasqualini, R. Q., and Codevilla, A. Thirst suppressing ("antidipsetic") effect of pitressin in diabetes insipidus. *Acta Endocrinol.* **30** (1959) 37–41.
47. Pittman, Q. J., Blume, H. W., Kearney, R. E., and Renaud, L. P. Influence of midbrain stimulation on the excitability of neurons in the medial hypothalamus of the rat. *Brain Res.* **174** (1979) 39–53.
48. Pittman, Q. J., Malkinson, T. J., Veale, W. L., and Lederis, K. Central release of arginine vasopressin (AVP) in rabbit brain. *Soc. Neurosci. Abstr.* **7** (1981) 506.
49. Pittman, Q. J., Lawrence, D., and McLean, L. Central effects of arginine vasopressin on blood pressure in rats. *Endocrinology* **110** (1982) 1058–1060.
50. Pittman, Q. J., Veale, W. L., and Lederis, K. Central neurohypophyseal peptide pathways—interactions with endocrine and other autonomic functions. *Peptides* **3** (1982) 515–520.
51. Pittman, Q. J., Rogers, J., and Bloom, F. E. Arginine vasopressin deficient Brattleboro rats fail to develop tolerance to the hypothermic effects of ethanol. *Reg. Peptides* **4** (1982) 33–41.
52. Post, R. M., Gold, P., Rubinow, D. R., Ballenger, J. C., Bunney, Jr., W. E., and Goodwin, F. K. Peptides in the cerebrospinal fluid of neuropsychiatric patients: an approach to central nervous system peptide function. *Life Sci.* **31** (1982) 1–15.
53. Raichle, M. E. Hypothesis: a central neuroendocrine system regulates brain ion homeostasis and volume. *In* "Neurosecretion and Brain Peptides: Implications for Brain Function and Neurological Disease," (J. B. Martin, S. Reichlin, and K. L. Birck eds.), 1981, pp. 329–333. Raven, New York.
54. Raichle, M. E., and Grubb, R. L. Regulation of brain water permeability by centrally released vasopressin. *Brain Res.* **143** (1978) 191–194.
55. Raskind, M. A., Weitzman, R. E., Orenstein, H., Fisher, D. A., and Courtney, N. Is

antidiuretic hormone elevated in psychosis? A pilot study. *Biol. Psychiatry* **13** (1978) 385–390.
56. Renaud, L. P., Pittman, Q. J., and Blume, H. W. Neurophysiology of hypothalamic peptidergic neurons. *In* "Central Regulation of the Endocrine System," (K. Fuxe, T. Hokfelt, and R. Luft, eds.), 1979, pp. 119–135. Plenum, New York.
57. Reppert, S. M., Artman, H. G., Swaminathan, S., and Fisher, D. A. Vasopressin exhibits a rhythmic daily pattern in cerebrospinal fluid but not in blood. *Science* **213** (1981) 1256–1257.
58. Rodriguez, E. M. Morphological and functional relationship between the hypothalamo-neurohypophyseal system and cerebrospinal fluid. *In* "Aspects of Neuroendocrinology," (W. Bargmann and E. Scharrer, eds.), 1969, pp. 354–365. Springer-Verlag, New York.
59. Rodriguez, E. M., and Heller, H. Antidiuretic activity and ultrastructure of the toad choroid plexus. *J. Endocrinol.* **46** (1970) 83–91.
60. Sherlock, D. A., Field, P. M., and Rainsman, G. Retrograde transport of horseradish peroxidase in the magnocellular neurosecretory system of the rat. *Brain Res.* **88** (1975) 403–414.
61. Sofroniew, M. V. Projections from vasopressin, oxytocin, and neurophysin neurons to neural targets in the rat and human. *J. Histochem. Cytochem.* **285** (1980) 475–478.
62. Sofroniew, M. V., and Glasman, W. Golgi-like immunoperoxidase staining of hypothalamic magnocellular neurons that contain vasopressin, oxytocin or neurophysin in the rat. *Neuroscience* **5**(4) (1981) 619–643.
63. Sofroniew, M. V., and Weindl, A. Extrahypothalamic neurophysin-containing perikarya, fiber pathways and fiber clusters in the rat brain. *Endocrinology* **102** (1978) 334–337.
64. Stillman, M. A., Recht, L. D., Rosario, S. L., Seif, S. M., Robinson, A. G., and Zimmerman, E. A. The effects of adrenalectomy and glucocorticoid replacement on vasopressin and vasopressin-neurophysin in the zona externa of the median eminence of the rat. *Endocrinology* **101** (1977) 42–49.
65. Swanson, L. W. Immunohistochemical evidence for a neurophysin-containing autonomic pathway arising in the paraventricular nucleus of the hypothalamus. *Brain Res.* **128** (1977) 346–353.
66. Swanson, L. W., and Kuypers, H. G. J. M. The paraventricular nucleus of the hypothalamus: cytoarchitectonic subdivisions and organization of projections to the pituitary, dorsal vagal complex, and spinal cord as demonstrated by retrograde fluorescence double-labeling methods. *J. Comp. Neurol.* **194** (1980) 555–570.
67. Swanson, L. W., and Sawchenko, P. E. Paraventricular nucleus: a site for the integration of neuroendocrine and autonomic mechanisms. *Neuroendocrinology* **31** (1980) 410–417.
68. Szczepanska-Sadowska, E. Plasma ADH increase and thirst suppression elicited by preoptic heating in the dog. *Am. J. Physiol.* **226** (1974) 155–161.
69. Vandesande, F., Dierickx, K., and De Mey, J. The origin of the vasopressinergic and oxytocinergic fibres of the external region of the median eminence of the rat hypophysis. *Cell Tiss. Res.* **180** (1977) 443–452.
70. Van Kammen, D. P., and Sternberg, D. E. Cerebrospinal fluid studies in schizophrenia. *In* "Neurobiology of Cerebrospinal Fluid," (J. H. Wood, ed.), 1980, pp. 719–742. Plenum, New York.
71. Veale, W. L. A stereotaxic method for the push–pull perfusion of discrete regions of brain tissue of the unanesthetized rabbit. *Brain Res.* **42** (1972) 479–481.
72. Vorherr, H., Bradbury, M. W. B., Hoghoughi, M., and Kleeman, C. R. Antidiuretic hormone in cerebrospinal fluid during endogenous and exogenous changes in in its blood level. *Endocrinology* **83** (1968) 246–250.
73. Wang, B. C., Share, L., Crofton, J. T., and Kimura, T. Changes in vasopressin concentra-

tion in plasma and cerebrospinal fluid in response to hemorrhage in anesthetized dogs. *Neuroendocrinology* **33** (1981) 61–66.

74. Zaidi, S. M., and Heller, H. Can neurohypophysial hormones cross the blood-cerebrospinal fluid barrier? *J. Endocrinol.* **60** (1974) 195–196.
75. Zimmerman, E. A., Stillman, M. A., Recht, L. D., Michaels, J., and Nilaver, G. The magnocellular neurosecretory system: pathways containing oxytocin, vasopressin and neurophysins. *In* "Celluar Biology of Hypothalamic Neurosecretory Processes," (C. Kordon and J. D. Vincent, eds.), 1978, pp. 375–389. Collogues Internationaux du CNRS, Paris.

15

The Push–Pull Perfusion Technique in Neuroendocrinology

VICTOR D. RAMÍREZ

Department of Physiology and Biophysics
University of Illinois
Urbana, Illinois

I. INTRODUCTION

Twenty years ago the push–pull cannula (PPC) was first introduced by Gaddum (*31*) to study brain secretory function. Typically, this invasive method (*74*) was used in anesthetized (*3, 8, 25, 47, 55, 70*) or in immobilized (*32, 52*) animal preparations. In 1980 we introduced such a device in the field of neuroendocrinology and successfully estimated the *in vivo* output of LHRH from the median eminence (ME) of conscious, unrestrained rats (*42*). Aside from LHRH the *in vivo* output of neuropeptides like somatostatin (*1, 39*), enkephalin (*4, 5*), vasopressin (*16, 64*), and TRH (*2*) as well as neurotransmitters (*45, 56, 58, 66, 69*) and amino acids (*48*) have also been estimated from brain areas of conscious, unrestrained animals.

It is the intent of this article to (1) discuss some methodological issues as related to push–pull perfusion (PPP) of central nervous structures (CNS), (2) illustrate the applicability of this technique for estimating the *in vivo* output of neuroactive substances from the mediobasal hypothalamus (MBH) and from the caudate nucleus (CN) of conscious, freely behaving rats, and (3)

ISBN 0-12-083350-6

offer some speculations on the future trends of such a device in furthering the neuroendocrinology field, particularly as related to the action of hormones on neurosecretory functions of selective brain structures in conscious, unrestrained animals.

II. METHODS

The estimation with PPP of *in vivo* output of neuroactive substances from the brain of freely behaving rats requires the solution of at least three basic technical problems: (1) construction of a cannula of the smallest size possible to minimize tissue damage and allow chronic brain implantation and yet be compatible with successful perfusion performance, (2) selection of a perfusion medium that mimics brain extracellular fluid and permits measurable output of neuroactive substances during prolonged perfusion sessions, (3) development of highly sensitive and suitable assay methods to reliably measure the extremely low output of the majority of neuroactive substances, and (4) devising an ideal procedure to measure immediately the concentration of neuroactive substances as they are collected. In my laboratory we have partially resolved some of these technical issues and successfully applied a homemade PPC to estimate the output of LHRH and of several brain neurotransmitters in conscious rats.

The PPC assembly consists of an outer 22-ga needle syringe (0.7 mm o.d.) which is permanently implanted into the brain of the animal using stereotaxic techniques; a removable stylette 28 to 29-ga size tubing extending about 1 mm past the tip of the outer cannula; and an inner perfusion assembly cannulae made of a straight push 31-ga tubing (0.25 mm o.d.) extending only 0.5–0.7 mm past the tip of the outer cannula and a short bent pull 28-ga tubing that is adjacent to the push tubing but extending only to the bottom of a base that fits tightly into the hub of a 22-ga needle. The base is prepared by cutting off the bottom of a 1-ml plastic syringe at approximately the 0.05-ml level. Details of the construction of the assembly and stylette are available upon request (see Fig. 1).

The major problem in perfusing brain tissue of conscious, freely moving animals is the clogging of the PPC. The main reason for the clogging appears to be the tissue damage at the tip of small-sized PPC. We have found that at least 4–5 days should pass between implantation and first perfusion to permit complete stabilization of the healing process around the tip of the cannula, thereby reducing incidence of clogging of the cannula by cellular debris.

A modified Krebs–Ringer phosphate (KRP) medium (consisting of NaCl, 123 mM; KCl, 4.8 mM; $MgSO_4$, 1.2 mM; $CaCl_2$, 0.78 mM; Na_2HPO_4, 85

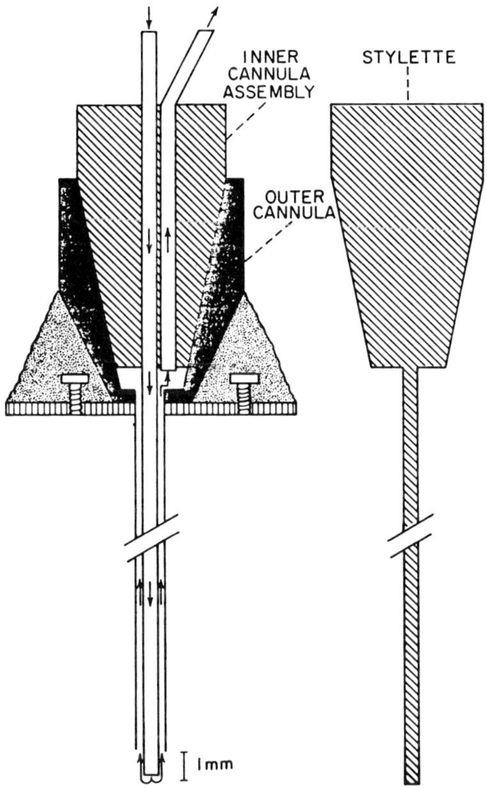

Fig. 1. The push–pull cannula assembly and stylette. The shaft of the permanently implanted outer cannula (left) has an outer diameter of 0.70 mm. The inner cannula and the stylette have outer diameters of 0.35 mm and inner diameters of 0.18 mm. [Reproduced from ref. (*42*). © 1980, The Endocrine Society.]

m*M*; and NaH_2PO_4, 15 m*M*) adjusted to pH 7.4 and delivered at a flow rate of 18–24 μl/min appears to be an adequate and suitable perfusion medium permitting reliable estimates of the output of LHRH and neurotransmitters. This medium appears relatively innocuous to the animal since no gross alterations in behavior were observed; in contrast, when a saline phosphate medium, pH 7.4, was perfused through a PPC placed in the CN, the majority of the animals showed clear signs of hyperactivity and abnormal alertness. The relatively low concentration of $CaCl_2$ in the KRP medium has also helped to reduce the incidence of clogging of the PPC without significant changes in the estimated normal output of ME LHRH and CN neurotransmitters or modifications of typical rat behavior. Of 30 experiments 24 have been successfully accomplished using these PPP conditions irrespective of

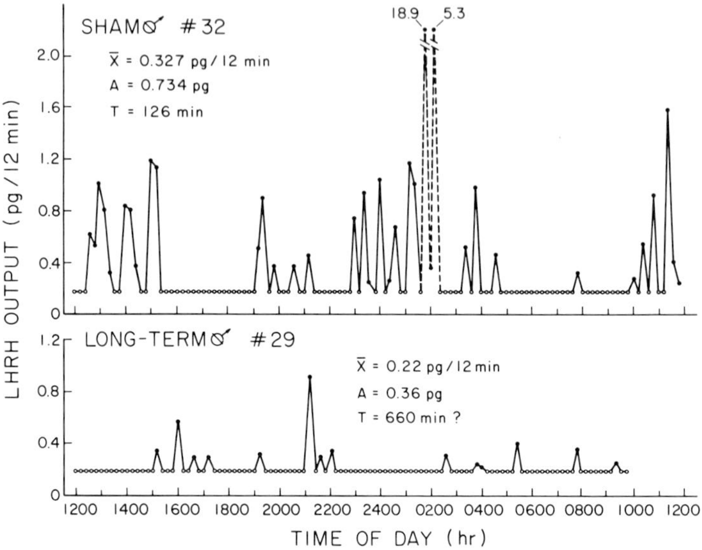

Fig. 2. LHRH secretory profile during a 24-hr PPP of a sham-castrated (upper panel) and a long-term (30 day) castrated rat (lower panel). The animals were brought to the laboratory and push–pull perfusions started approximately at 1200 hr and continued for 24 hr. Notice that in both cases the *in vivo* output of LHRH occurs in a burst of activity followed by silent periods. Interspersed among this type of activity large pulses of LHRH ("surge type") are seen only in the sham-castrated rat. The mean LHRH release, amplitude, and period were calculated using a cycle detector program (*14*). In each animal the tip of the cannula laid in the rostral and lateral portion of the ME.

PPC placement (either in the ME or CN). Moreover, as illustrated in Fig. 2, continuous perfusion for 24 hr was performed in male rats without detecting abnormal behaviors or changes in the profile pattern of LHRH output.

Because the neuroactive substances are released in small quantities and only a fraction of the total is collected (*25, 65*) in the fluid of the pull cannula, highly sensitive assays are required. Presently, these are the limiting factors in expanding the use of this technique to estimate *in vivo* output of an array of known neuroactive substances produced by the brain. For the estimation of LHRH output we have taken advantage of a highly sensitive, accurate, and specific radioimmunoassay (RIA) developed in my laboratory that detects 0.2 pg of LHRH per assay tube at 90% binding (*40*). Figure 3 presents an example of a composite standard curve from pooled data from several assays corresponding to different experiments in which the *in vivo* output of this neuropeptide from the rat ME was measured. It would be also highly desirable to develop analytical procedures permitting immediate measurements of the concentration of several neuroactive substances while

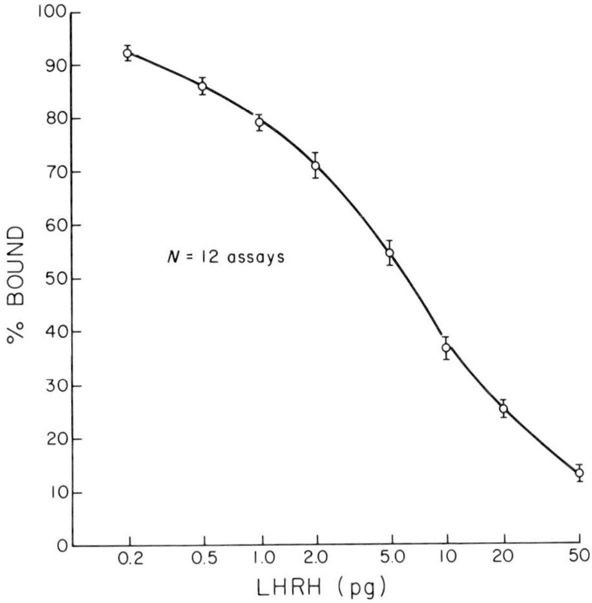

Fig. 3. Composite LHRH standard curve from 12 RIA assays (mean ± SE).

perfusate medium is being collected. Such a case has been recently reported for the estimation of *in vivo* output of endogenous biogenic amines from conscious rats by a combined PPP on-line with a high-performance liquid chromatography electrochemical detection (HPLC-EC) unit (*45*). Independently we have also adapted such a procedure (Fig. 4) to measure the output of DA and other neuroactive substances from the CN of freely behaving female and male rats (*10*.

III. FINDINGS

A. The MBH–LHRH System

A large body of experimental information indicates that the neuropeptide LHRH is the final obligatory neural signal for the maintenance of a normal secretory activity of pituitary gonadotropes (*41*). Until our first introduction of the PPC to estimate the *in vivo* output of LHRH from the nerve terminals of the ME in unrestrained, conscious rats (*42*), the *in vivo* release of this peptide was limited to measurements in hypophysial portal plasma of immobilized anesthetized animals (*7, 11, 30, 53*), in peripheral plasma (*26, 72*),

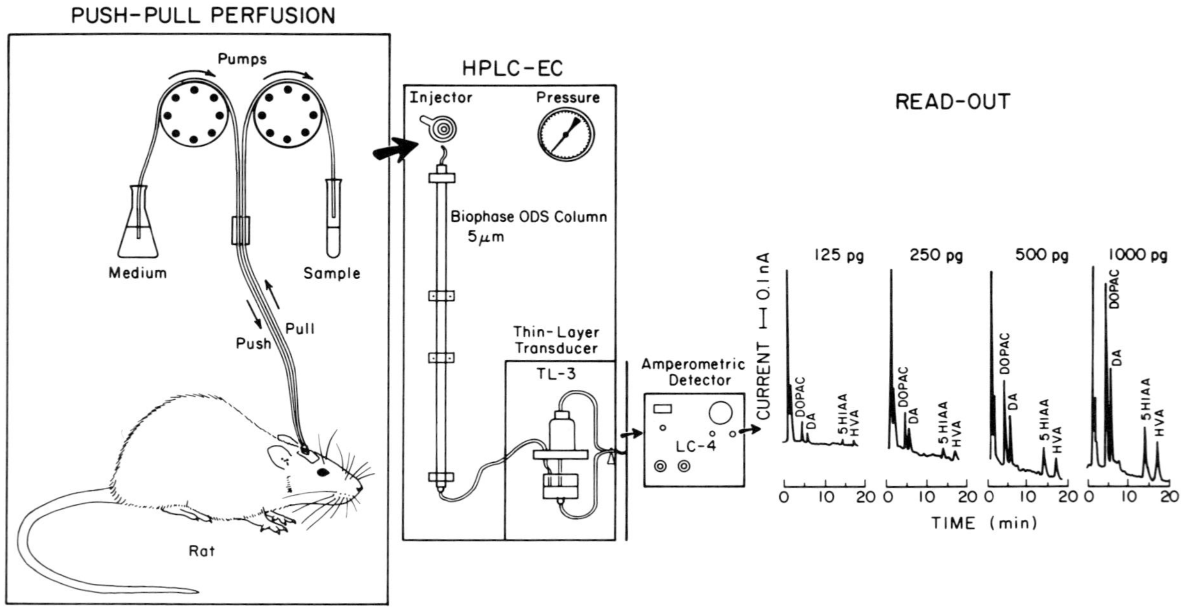

Fig. 4. PPP coupled to a Bioanalytical HPLC-EC unit to determine *in vivo* output of neurotransmitter from the caudate nucleus of conscious, unrestrained male rats. A 5-μm C-18 phase reverse column (Biophase, ODS, 25 × 1 cm) coupled with a carbon-paste (CP-O) electrode set at a potential of 0.55 V relative to the Ag/AgCl reference electrode was used to separate the different standards and generate corresponding redox currents registered in a recorder after suitable amplification. The mobile phase consists of 5.75 g citric acid, 4.1 g sodium acetate, 2.4 g sodium hydroxide, and 1.05 ml acetate acid in 1 liter of deionized and degassed water containing 0.01% merthiolate and adjusted to pH 5.4 with 5 *N* NaOH. [Reproduced from ref. (*10*) courtesy of *Neuroendocrinology*.]

or in cerebrospinal (*51*) fluid. To determine more precisely how the MBH–LHRH system operates during physiological conditions the release of LHRH must be characterized and correlated with normal physiological and behavioral events in conscious, freely behaving animals. The PPP, within their limitations, currently constitutes the method of choice to estimate the *in vivo* function of this system in the rat, given the fact that peripheral plasma or cerebrospinal fluid (CSF) LHRH determinations are questionable (*17, 18*).

In our initial studies (*42*), it was shown that the endogenous, unstimulated release of LHRH from the ME of ovariectomized (ovx) rats primed with low doses of estradiol benzoate fluctuated below and just above RIA detectability (i.e., between less than 0.2 and 1.0 pg/MBH/10 min). In contrast, the stimulated LHRH release values were as high as 3 pg/10 min when known secretagogues like progesterone (*40, 42*) or infusion through the push side of the cannula of medium containing 15 m*M* K^+ or 10^{-6} *M* PG-E_2 (Fig. 5) were used. These levels are well within the same order of magnitude as those detected in portal blood (*11, 30*) or *in vitro* determinations (*58*) considering that the values obtained with the PPP technique reflect only a fraction of total LHRH release.

After the successful application of this method to estimate the *in vivo* output of LHRH from the ME of ovx estrogen-primed rats, we abandoned this artificial endocrine condition and proceeded to examine the output of this neuropeptide during the rat estrous cycle and in response to ovariectomy (*43*). In intact female rats bearing a PPC chronically implanted in the brain with its tip aimed at the ME, 50% of the animals exhibited a 9- to 14-day period of constant diestrus, a pseudopregnancy state most probably induced by lesion of the arcuate or ventromedial nuclei. Thereafter, these animals showed normal estrous cycles despite the fact that their pre-ovulatory LH levels were only 10–30% of those observed in intact animals. In spite of the fact that the PPP is performed upon a truncated, yet operable hypothalamic–hypophysial axis, significant changes in the output of LHRH were demonstrated during the rat estrous cycle. For example, two distinct types of secretory profiles characterize the observed maximal neurosecretory activity of the MBH–LHRH system during proestrus: the so-called pulse-dominated and the surge-dominated types (see Fig. 6). In the former, a pulsatile release of LHRH with mean pulse intervals of 48 min and amplitudes fluctuating between 0.2 and 1.5 pg/12 min was the dominant feature of this LHRH secretory profile. In the surge-dominated type the LHRH release profile was characterized by abrupt manyfold increases in amplitude (2–7 pg/12 min) interspersed over undetectable or low-amplitude basal pulses. When the data for each individual rat were normalized to the largest LHRH peak, in all cases the proestrus LHRH release appeared as a biphasic secretory event.

The LHRH release was moderately or overtly elevated during the late

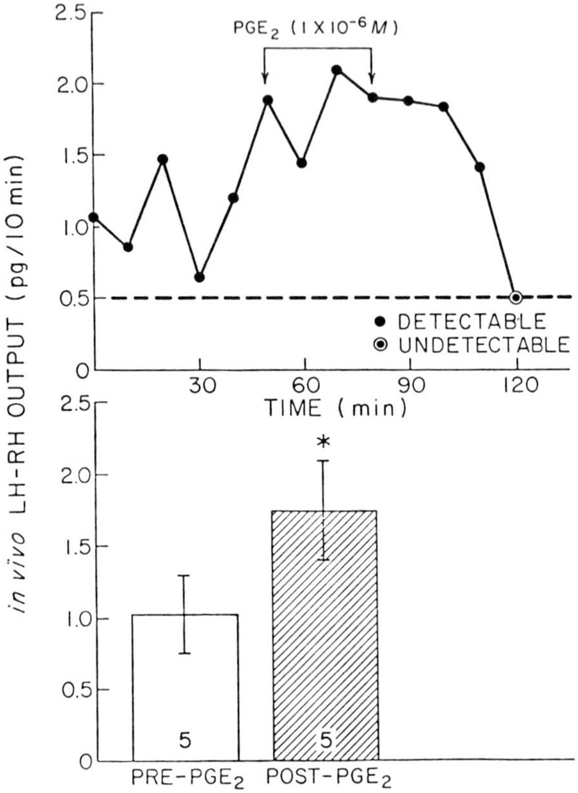

Fig. 5. Effects of PG-E_2 dissolved in medium (10^{-6} *M*) and infused locally into the ME region in *in vivo* LHRH output. In the upper figure, PG-E_2 induces a 50-min elevation of LHRH release from the MBH of an ovx rat. Bars in lower figure represent mean LHRH output during three pretreatment and three PGE_2 treatment 10-min collection intervals ($N = 5$). *$p < .05$.

afternoon hours of diestrus I, diestrus II, and proestrus but not in estrus or in long-term ovx rats, suggesting that these neurosecretory events correspond to the daily neuronal signal governing LH release, as described by Everett and Sawyer (*28*). It would appear that this neuronal signal is not expressed in long-term ovx rats or when cycling animals have been exposed 24 hr earlier to high levels of progesterone, as is the case of animals in estrus.

In long-term ovx rats the most intriguing feature of LHRH output is its consistency through the afternoon and its relative low amplitude compared to proestrus values in spite of high blood levels of pulsatile LH release. It is possible that ovarian steroids, particularly estrogen, prime the LHRH pulse generator to a maximal level of operation (acting mainly as a frequency modulatory signal). Therefore, in absence of ovarian steroids the amplitudes

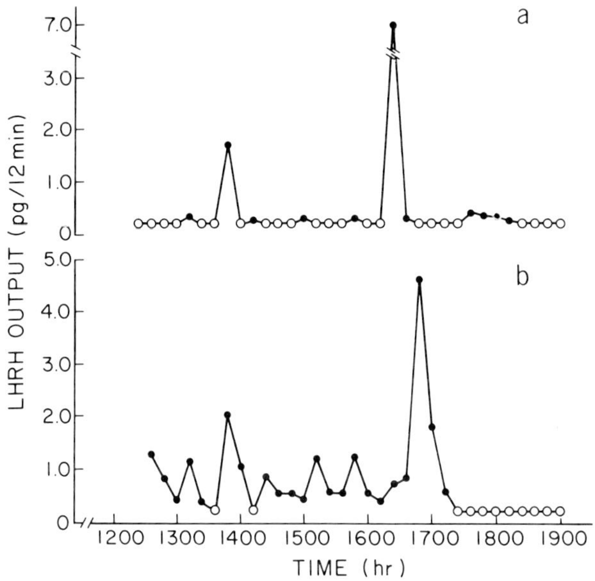

Fig. 6. LHRH release during proestrus showing "surge-dominated" (a) vs "pulse-dominated" (b) modes. In (a), two sharp peaks are evident at approximately 1400 and 1700 hr, respectively. In (b), two peaks again occur in that animal, but they appear as moderate changes in pulse amplitude over basal pulsatile release. Open circles are undetectable levels.

of the pulses are dramatically reduced which impedes frequency measurements, since most of the values are below RIA detectability. In view of these difficulties and the apparent absence of correlation between LHRH and LH determinations in long-term ovx rats, Jon Levine, in collaboration with the group of G. Jackson at our campus, attempted a first demonstration of the postulated 1:1 correlation between LHRH and LH release in the ovx, conscious, unrestrained sheep (*44*). As in rats, in ovx sheep bearing a PPC in the ME, LH levels were reduced when compared to unimplanted animals (3.5 ± 0.4 ng/ml vs 10.6 ± 1.9 ng/ml), and the frequency tended to be slightly but not significantly lower (61.9 ± 10.3 min vs 30–50 min). Nonetheless, a distinct blood pulsatile fluctuation of the hormone was still clearly observed. In this study a near perfect correlation between LH pulses and LHRH discharges (mean interpuse interval, 38.7 ± 1.5 min) was observed in the 5 animals undergoing simultaneous determinations of these two hormones. An example is depicted in Fig. 7. It should be noted that not all LHRH pulses were accompanied by corresponding LH pulses, suggesting that other factors may interfere with the final output of LH from the pituitary. Simultaneous with this study, though using a different procedure, was that depict-

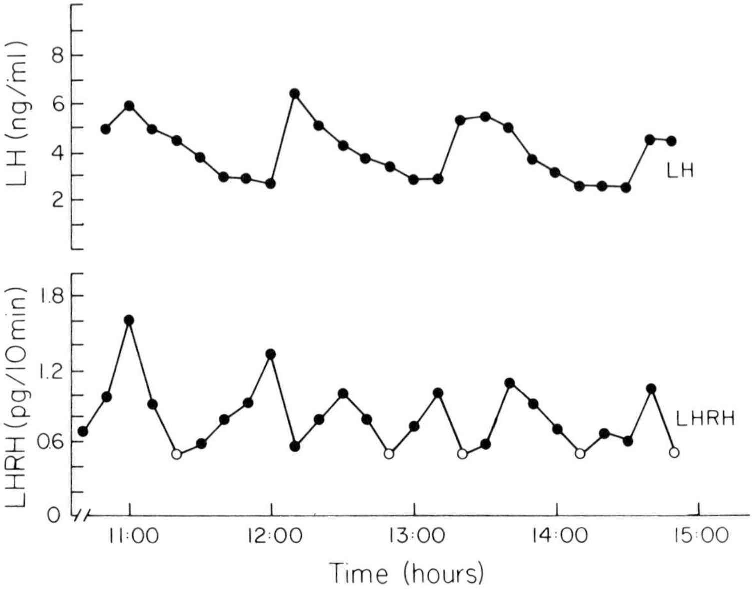

Fig. 7. Simultaneous measurements of pulsatile LHRH and LH release in an individual ovx sheep. LHRH release was estimated with the push–pull perfusion, while concomitant LH levels were determined in plasma samples. In this sheep not every LHRH pulse was accompanied or followed by an LH pulse [Reproduced from ref. (*44*). © 1982, The Endocrine Society.]

ing a similar relationship between the *in vivo* release of LH and LHRH in conscious, unrestrained ovx sheep (*13*).

Pursuing our studies in the rat and to gain a more accurate and precise temporal definition of the long-term characteristics of *in vivo* LHRH output, D. Dluzen in my laboratory implanted PPC in male rats. Figure 2 depicts the three major features that characterize the LHRH secretory profile in these animals when continuous 24-hr PPP were successfully performed. First, the release of LHRH is pulsatile as in female rats (*42, 43*) and sheep (*44*). Second, it appears to occur in bursts of increasing activity followed by silent periods, a sequence that repeats several times during the day. Third, interspersed among the basal low-amplitude pulsatile activity, which typically fluctuates between levels of detectability of the RIA and 1 pg/12 min, higher pulses [resembling typical surges of proestrus LHRH in females (*43*)] were observed in every case. The amplitude of these extremely high surges of LHRH fluctuated between 3 pg/12 min and 22 pg/12 min. As in ovx rats, long-term castrated males showed pulsatile LHRH release of low amplitude, a fact that unfortunately precludes a true estimation of frequency changes. A summary of data from 3 sham-castrated and 3 long-term castrated rats per-

TABLE I

***In Vivo* LHRH Output from the Median Eminence from Intact and Castrated Unanesthetized, Unrestrained Rats**

Condition	N	Mean LHRH release[a] (pg/12 min)	Amplitude[a] (pg)	Period[a] (min)
Sham castrated	3	0.33 (0.28–0.36)	0.47 (0.31–0.73)	83 (56–132)
Long-term castrated (> 30 days)	3	0.25 (0.22–0.26)	0.25 (0.11–0.32)	133 (62–252)

[a] Mean and range values are indicated.

fused for 8 hr is presented in Table I. The three parameters analyzed (mean release, amplitude, and period) were resolved by the use of a cycle detector program developed by Clifton and Steiner (*14*). These data indicate that in long-term castrated animals the activity of the neural LHRH apparatus markedly decreases in terms of amplitude and mean release of the neural LHRH signal. This finding suggests that a highly responsive pituitary to low-amplitude LHRH signals is presumably the primary cause for the increase in LH levels detected in castrated animals (*15, 29*). Current studies in my laboratory are addressing the question of the effect of steroid hormones on simultaneous measurements of LH and LHRH levels in gonadectomized rats.

Taken together these data indicate that the PPP technique is a powerful device to assess in conscious, freely behaving rats the *in vivo* output of this neuropeptide that represents the obligatory neural signal for a normal function of the pituitary gonadotropes. In both long-term gonadectomized male and female rats the neural LHRH apparatus operates at a low level of activity, though the frequency may be increased. In ovx sheep a good correlation exists between LHRH pulses and LH discharges. Lastly, it appears that two types of secretory LHRH activity characterize the neural LHRH apparatus in intact male and in cycling female rats: a pulse-dominated and a surge-dominated type. In the male the surge-dominated type appears to occur randomly during the day, and in the female only during proestrus in the afternoon. The significance of these findings is yet to be discovered.

B. The Nigrostriatal–Dopamine System

Previous data from our laboratory (*61*) as well as others (*12, 20, 27, 35, 36, 38, 57, 62, 73*) indicate that the nigrostriatal–dopamine (NS–DA) system may also be considered a target site for hormone action. Recently we reported that in ovx estrogen-treated rats a single injection of progesterone can initially facilitate the response of corpus striatum (CS) fragments to *in vitro* AMPH-stimulated DA release whereas 24 hr later, the CS responsiveness to AMPH markedly decreases (*21, 61*). More importantly, changes in DA concentration (*19*), turnover rate in the CS (*37*), and in *in vitro* DA release from CS fragments (6) are detected during the rat estrous cycle. Another hormone, prolactin (PRL), and not other pituitary hormones, appears to stimulate the *in vitro* release of DA from superfused CS fragments; intriguingly, the effect seems to be sex dependent since it was observed only in CS fragments from male and not from female rats (9).

To investigate the physiological significance of the effect of PRL on DA release, J. C. Chen and I decided to examine the spontaneous *in vivo* output of DA from the CN of conscious, freely behaving male rats. To this end we implanted PPC into the right and rostral part of the CN of male rats using standard stereotaxic procedures. After 2 weeks recovery the animals were perfused with a modified KRP medium, as indicated in Section II. The PPP began around 1200 and continued until 2200 hr, using a flow rate of 18 μl/min. Samples were collected continuously into plastic tubes resting on ice. To measure the output from the CN transparent 100 μl samples after 20-min collection time and without further treatment were immediately injected into the injector port of a Bioanalytical HPLC-EC unit as pictured in Fig. 4. This setting permits an immediate generation of data while the animal is being perfused and its behavior and response to different stimuli are being tested. This figure also depicts the chromatograms of four different standards diluted in perfusion medium and injected in four different concentrations. The unknown substances in the perfusate samples were identified by comparing their retention times with those of pure standards. Their concentrations were established from linear dose–response curves for each standard determined in each PPP experiment.

It was rather surprising to find from our initial experiments that the output of DA from the CN of conscious, freely behaving male rats remained rather flat and unchanged through the complete PPP session. Contrariwise, the output of 3,4-dihydroxyphenylacetic acid (DOPAC), a major nonmethoxylated metabolite of DA, showed a remarkable fourfold increase over the initial output detected in early afternoon hours (1200–1300 hr), to plateau during the evening hours (1800–2200 hr). This *in vivo* DOPAC secretory profile was a consistent finding across several animals (see Fig. 8). The outputs of 5-hydroxyindoleacetic acid (5-HIAA), a metabolite of serotonin, and a methoxylated metabolite of DA, homovanillic acid (HVA), remained also rather constant through the PPP sessions with a mean secretory output of 30 and 50 pg/min, respectively. Figures 9 and 10 document examples of the *in vivo* output of DA and DOPAC from the CN of individual rats. In each case a clear increase in *in vivo* output of DOPAC was noticed as the perfu-

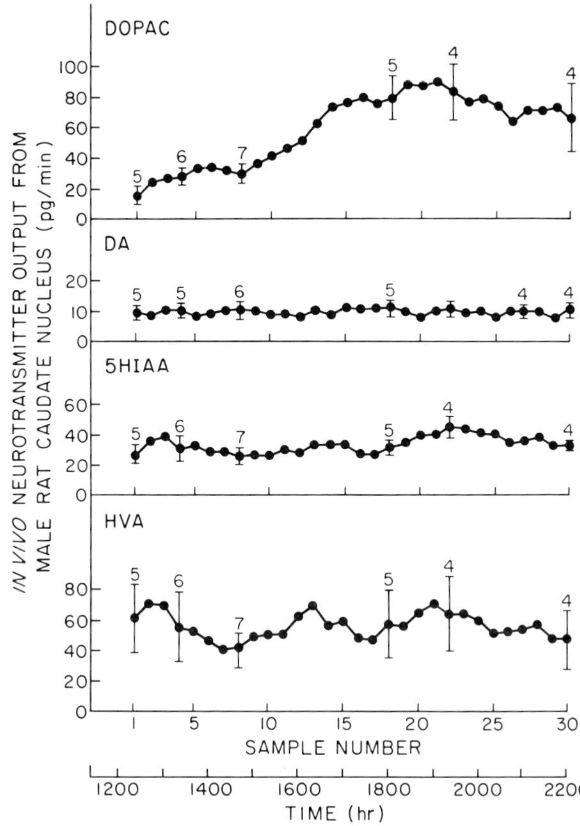

Fig. 8. Simultaneous determination of *in vivo* output (mean ± SE) of DOPAC, DA, 5-HIAA, and HVA from conscious, freely behaving male rats undergoing continuous PPP of the CN from early hours in the afternoon to late hours in the evening. Notice the selective fourfold increase in DOPAC output while the rats are being perfused from 1200–1500 to 1800–2200 hr. Lights on from 0500 to 1900 hr.

sion of the CN proceeded from early to late hours in the afternoon while the output of DA stayed unchanged.

Earlier a good correlation between stimulation of the nigrostriatal–dopamine pathway and accumulation of DOPAC in the CN was demonstrated. Conversely, lesions of the pathways resulted in decrements of DOPAC in the CN (*24, 33, 63, 71*). Up to this point it appears then that a rather selective change in nigrostriatal dopaminergic activity occurs in the male rat during the afternoon as reflected by selective increase in DOPAC output (Fig. 11).

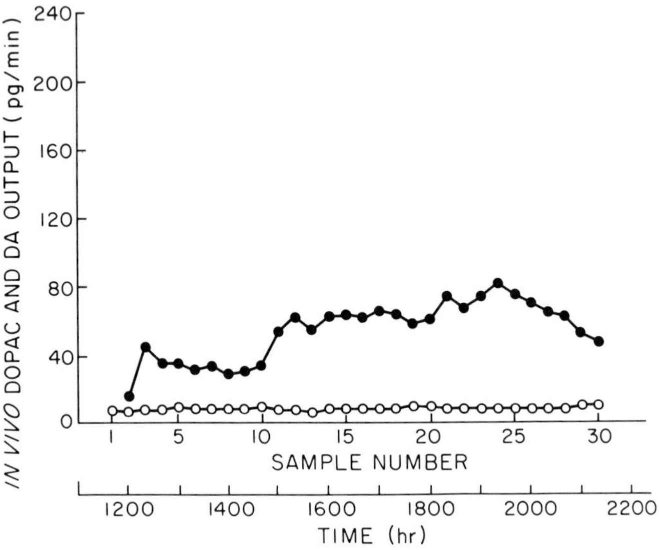

Fig. 9. *In vivo* output of DOPAC (●) and DA (○) from the CN of male rat No. 99, estimated as in Fig. 8.

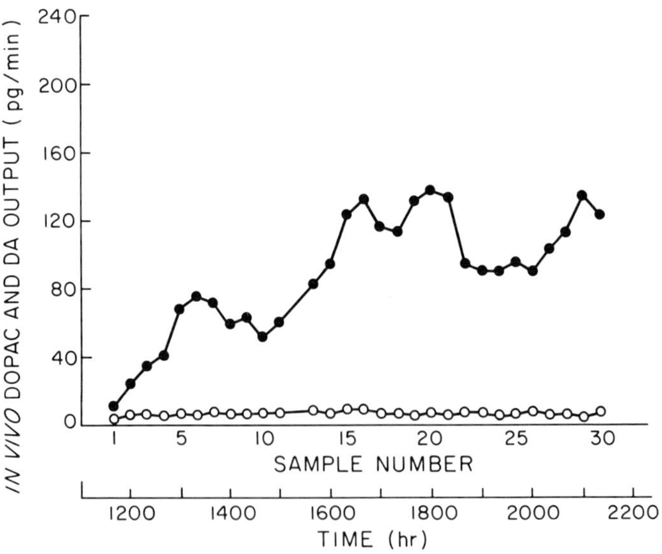

Fig. 10. *In vivo* output of DOPAC (●) and DA (○) from the CN of male rat No. 103, estimated as in Fig. 8.

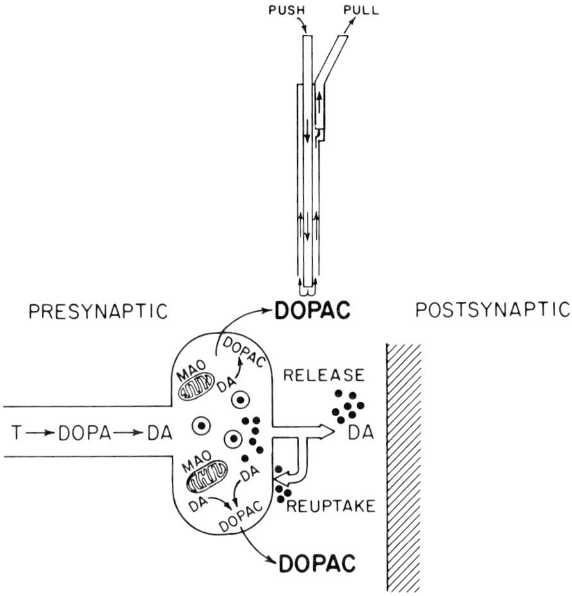

Fig. 11. Diagram indicating enzymatic oxidation of DA and conversion to DOPAC by mitochrondrial MAO in the presynaptic terminal of an NS–DA neuron.

Interestingly, plasma PRL progressively increases during the afternoon (*46, 49*), is detectable in the CSF (*54*), and is capable of inducing grooming behavior in male rats (*22, 23*). Moreover, we have previously demonstrated that PRL can directly induce DA release from male rat CS fragments superfused *in vitro* (*9*). Therefore, we decided to test the effect of a highly purified rat PRL (rPRL-I-2) preparation on the *in vivo* activity of the NS–DA system of male rats. In the preliminary result, PRL dissolved in perfusion medium at a concentration of approximately 10^{-7} *M* and infused through the push side of the cannula during a 20-min interval markedly modified the activity of the NS–DA system. As shown in Fig. 12, the first infusion of PRL coincided with the spontaneous increase in the output of DOPAC from the CN of this animal. Therefore any stimulatory effect of PRL is confounded by this spontaneous change; however, a second infusion of PRL 100 min later elicited a remarkable increase in DOPAC (close to five fold) without noticeable changes in DA levels. After the levels of this metabolite had reached normal stable values a higher dose of PRL administered 50 min later, though less effective than the previous one, still increased the output of DOPAC four fold over basal levels. No changes in DA or in the output of the other metabolites were observed. This last dose of PRL was capable of inducing yawning at a rate of 5 episodes/20 min and considerable grooming behav-

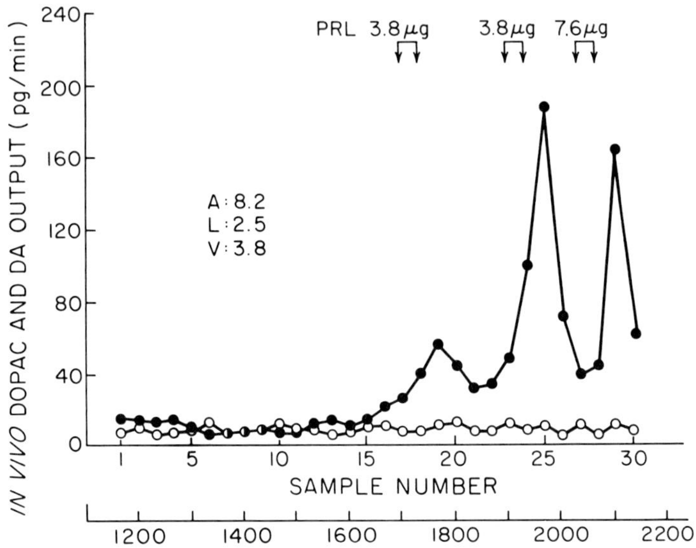

Fig. 12. In this rat, No. 76, the placement of the tip of the PPC in the CN was 8.2 mm anterior, 2.5 lateral, and 3.8 vertical (DeGroot rat atlas) from data obtained by histological control. The *in vivo* output of DOPAC (●) was rather low and started to increase rather late (about 1700 hr). Rat PRL (rPRL-I-2) was dissolved in perfusion medium (10 ng/μl) and infused for 20 min at a flow rate of 19 μl/min. The first infusion of PRL appears ineffective if one considers the spontaneous rise in the output of this metabolite of DA (○); however, the second infusion was extremely effective in stimulating the release of DOPAC. The third infusion was less effective than the second but still induced a fourfold increase in the output of DOPAC. It is worthy of mention that within this last PRL infusion time, the rat presented five episodes of yawning and considerable grooming behavior.

ior. These behavioral responses probably reflect an initial activation of the NS–DA system, since several papers have demonstrated that at least one component in the generation of these behaviors in rats is related to DA activation (*22, 23, 34, 50, 67, 68*).

Figure 13 presents a representative chromatogram of the spontaneous and selective increase in the *in vivo* output of DOPAC from the CN of rat No. 103 during the afternoon hours. Similarly, this figure documents the chromatogram of rat No. 76 showing marked changes in the DOPAC peak following PRL infusion into the CN. In both cases the appearance of an unknown substance (x) in large concentrations in the perfusates with a lower retention time than 3,4-dihydroxyphenylglycol (DOPEG) or DOPAC was also observed. Authentic DOPAC added to samples containing suspected endogenous DOPAC coeluted with the peak samples and increased proportionally the height of their elution peaks. Despite our present lack of more conclusive evidence, the relatively selected increase in the output of

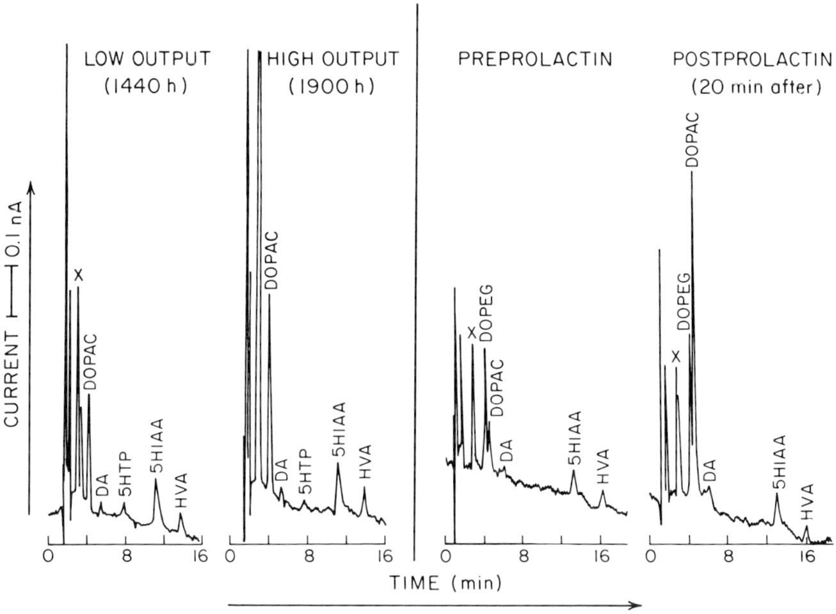

Fig. 13. Chromatograms of male rat No. 103 (left) and male No. 76 (right) describing the peak heights and retention times of identified substances in the perfusates from perfused CN of these animals. Notice also the existence of an unidentified peak (x).

DOPAC from the CN of male rats during the afternoon of the light–dark cycle may reflect changes in plasma PRL levels which then may activate the NS–DA system.

Regardless of the correctness of our speculations, this curious novel finding is a perfect example of the power of the PPP coupled to HPLC-EC to further knowledge in the study of *in vivo* output of neuroactive substances and the correlation of their changes with behavioral and physiological events that can only be investigated in conscious, freely behaving animals.

IV. PERSPECTIVES AND CONCLUSIONS

Though the application of the PPC in neuroendocrinology is of recent introduction, it has already generated valuable information and it is currently the only method available to estimate the *in vivo* output of neuropeptides from different brain loci from conscious, freely behaving animals. The mini-cannula version with compatible PPP performance is desirable in order to minimize the obligatory damage to CNS structures. A waiting period between implantation and perfusion or between perfusions appears essential to lower cannula clogging incidence.

The brain lesions produced by these cannulae do not lead to gross alterations in behavior or permanent changes in estrous cycle or ovulation in the majority of animals. The fact that PPP can be performed continuously for at least 24 hr without visible changes in gross behavior of the animals or alterating typical secretory profiles in *in vivo* output of LHRH is an index of the physiological stability of the system.

The need for new methods of assay or improvement of current methods to gain better sensitivity and capability to measure simultaneously several neuropeptides appears essential to further the application of PPP in neuroendocrinology. The application of PPP coupled to or on-line with HPLC-EC to estimate the output of neuroactive substances from the CN of conscious male rats confirms the potential of this approach, permitting useful correlations between specific behavioral outputs and *in vivo* neurosecretory events.

Lastly, the usefulness and feasibility of this technique to investigate hormone action on *in vivo* brain functions has been partially documented in this chapter for two neuronal systems: the MB–LHRH system, a classical brain target for hormone action, and the NS–DA system, a rather novel site of hormone–brain interaction.

ACKNOWLEDGMENTS

The author wishes to acknowledge the excellent collaborations of Drs. D. Dluzen and J. Levine and of the students J. C. Chen and K. Rhee who have made possible the work reported here. Also the technical help of N. Ramirez and the secretarial help of D. Meyers is greatly appreciated. This work has been supported in part by Grants HD-14625 and PCM-81-6276 to VDR.

REFERENCES

1. Arancibia, S., Epelbaum, J., Alonso, G., and Assenmacher, I. Mise en evidence d'une secretion de somatostatine (SRIF) dans le 3e ventricule cerebral chez le rat non anesthesie. *C. R. Acad. Sci. Paris* **296** (1983) 47–52.
2. Arancibia, S., Tapia-Arancibia, L., Assenmacher, I., and Astier, H. Direct evidence of short-term cold induced TRH release from the median eminence of unanesthetized rats *Neuroendocrinology* **37** (1983) 225–228.
3. Bartholini, G., Stadler, H., Ciria, M. G., and Lloyd, K. G. The use of the push–pull cannula to estimate the dynamics of acetylcholine and catecholamines within various brain areas. *Neuropharmacology* **15** (1976) 515–519.
4. Bayón, A., Shoemaker, W. J., Lugo, L., Azad, R., Long, N., Drucker-Colín, R. R., and Bloom, R. E. *In vivo* release of enkephalin from the globus pallidus. *Neurosci. Lett.* **24** (1981) 65–70.
5. Bayón, A., Solano, S., Antón, B., Castaño, I., and Diáz-Pontones, D. Push–Pull perfusion

studies on the *in vivo* release of proteins, enzymes, and the neuroactive peptides–enkephalins from the rat brain. This volume, Chapter 6.
6. Becker, J. B., and Ramirez, V. D. Sex differences in the amphetamine stimulated release of catecholamines from rat striatal tissue *in vitro*. *Brain Res.* **204** (1981) 361–372.
7. Carmel, P. W., Araki, S., and Ferin, M. Pituitary stalk portal blood collection in rhesus monkeys; evidence for pulsatile release of gonadotropin-releasing hormone (GnRH). *Endocrinology* **99** (1976) 243–248.
8. Chase, T. N., and Kopin, I. J. Stimulus-induced release of substances from olfactory bulb using the push–pull cannula. *Nature (London)* **217** (1968) 466–467.
9. Chen, Y. F., and Ramirez, V. D. Prolactin stimulates dopamine release from male but not from female rat striatal tissue superfused *in vitro*. *Endocrinology* **111** (1982) 1740–1742.
10. Chen, J. G., Rhee, K. K., Beaudry, D. M., and Ramirez, V. D. *In vivo* output of dopamine and metabolites from the rat caudate nucleus as estimated with push–pull perfusion on line with HPLC-EC in unrestrained, conscious rats: I. Chromatographic and biological validation. *Neuroendocrinology* **38** (1984) 362–370.
11. Ching, M. Correlative surges of LHRH, LH and FSH in pituitary stalk plasma and systemic plasma of rat during proestrus. Effect of anesthetic. *Neuroendocrinology* **34** (1982) 279–285.
12. Chioda, L. A., and Caggiula, A. R. Alterations in basal firing rates and autoreceptor sensitivity of dopamine neurons in the substantia nigra following acute and extended exposure to estrogen. *Eur. J. Pharmacol.* **67** (1980) 165–166.
13. Clarke, I., and Cummings, J. T. The temporal relationship between gonadotropin releasing hormone (GnRH) and luteinizing hormone (LH) secretion in ovariectomized ewes. *Endocrinology* **111** (1982) 1737–1739.
14. Clifton, D. K., and Steiner, R. A. Cyclic detection: a technique for estimating the frequency and amplitude of episodic fluctuations in blood hormones and substrate concentrations. *Endocrinology* **112** (1983) 1057–1064.
15. Cooper, K. J., Fawcett, C. P., and McCann, S. M. Augmentation of pituitary responsiveness to luteinizing hormone/follicle stimulating hormone-releasing factor (LHRF) as a result of acute ovariectomy in the four-day cyclic rat. *Endocrinology* **96** (1974) 1123–1129.
16. Cooper, K. E., Kasting, N. W., Lederis, K., and Veale, W. L. Evidence supporting a role for endogenous vasopressin in natural suppression of fever in the sheep. *J. Physiol. (London)* **295** (1979) 33–45.
17. Coppings, R. J., Malven, P. V., and Ramirez, V. D. Absence of immunoreactive luteinizing hormone-releasing hormone in ovine cerebrospinal fluid collected from the third ventricle. *Proc. Soc. Exp. Biol. Med.* **154** (1977) 219–223.
18. Cramer, O. M., and Barraclough, C. A. Failure to detect lutenizing hormone-releasing hormone in third ventricle cerebral spinal fluid under a variety of experimental conditions. *Endocrinology* **96** (1975) 913–921.
19. Crowley, W. R., O'Donohue, T. L., and Jacabowitz, D. M. Changes in catecholamine content in discrete brain nuclei during the estrous cycle of the rat. *Brain Res.* **147** (1978) 315–322.
20. DiPaolo, T., Poyet, P., and Labrie, F. Effect of prolactin and estradiol on rat striatal dopamine receptors. *Life Sci.* **31** (1982) 2921–2929.
21. Dluzen, D., and Ramirez, V. D. Bimodal effect of progesterone on *in vitro* dopamine function of the rat corpus striatum. *Neuroendocrinology* **39** (1984) 149–155.
22. Drago, F., Canonico, P. L., Bitetti, R., and Scapagnini, U. Systemic and intraventricular prolactin induces excessive grooming. *Eur. J. Pharmacol.* **65** (1980) 457–458.
23. Drago, F., Bohus, B., Canonico, D. L., and Scapagnini, U. Prolactin induces grooming in

the rat: possible involvement of nigrostriatal dopaminergic system. *Pharmacol. Biochem. Behav.* **15** (1981) 61–63.
24. Elchisak, M. A., Murrin, L. C., and Roth, R. H. Free and conjugated dihydroxyphenylacetic acid: effect of alterations in impulse flow in rat neostriatum and frontal cortex. *Psychopharmacol. Comm.* **2** (1976) 411–420.
25. Elghozi, J. L., Hanh Le Quan-Bui, K., Earnhardt, J. T., Meyer, P., and Devynck, M. A. *In vivo* dopamine release from the anterior hypothalamus of the rat. *Eur. J. Pharmacol.* **73** (1981) 199–208.
26. Elkind-Hirsch, K., Ravnikar, V., Schiff, I., Tulchinsky, D., and Ryan, K. J. Determinations of endogenous immunoreactive luteinizing hormone-releasing hormone in human plasma. *J. Clin. Endocrinol. Metab.* **54** (1982) 602–607.
27. Euvard, C., Oberlander, C., and Biossier, J. R. Antidopaminergic effects of estrogens at the striatal level. *J. Pharmacol. Exp. Ther.* **214** (1980) 179–185.
28. Everett, J. W., and Sawyer, C. H. A 24-hour periodicity in the "LH-release apparatus" of female rats, disclosed by barbiturate sedation. *Endocrinology* **47** (1950) 198–218.
29. Ferland, L., Marchetti, B., Seguin, C., Lefebvre, F. A., Reeves, J. J., and Labrie, F. Dissociated changes of pituitary luteinizing hormone-releasing hormone (LHRH) receptors and responsiveness to the neurohormone induced by 17β-estradiol and LHRH *in vivo* in the rat. *Endocrinology* **109** (1981) 87–93.
30. Fink, G., Aiyer, M., Chiappa, S., Henderson, S., Jamieson, M., Levy-Perez, V., Pickering, A., Sarkar, D., Sherwood, N., Speight, A., and Watts, A. Gonadotropin-releasing hormone. Release into hypophyseal portal blood and mechanism of action. *In* "Hormonally Active Brain Peptides," (McKerns and Pantie, eds.), 1982, pp. 397–425. Plenum, New York.
31. Gaddum, J. H. Push–pull cannulae. *J. Physiol. (London)* **155** (1961) 1–2 P.
32. Glowinski, J. *In vivo* release of transmitters in the cat basal ganglia. *Fed. Proc.* **40** (1981) 135–144.
33. Hefti, F., and Melamed, E. Dopamine release in rat striatum after administration of L-Dopa as studied with *in vivo* electrochemistry. *Brain Res.* **225** (1981) 333–346.
34. Holmgren, B., Urba-Holmgren, R., Aguilar, M., and Rodriguez, R. Sex hormone influences on yawning behavior. *Acta Neurobiol. Exp.* **40** (1980) 515–519.
35. Hruska, R. E., and Silbergeld, E. K. Increased dopamine receptor sensitivity after estrogen treatment using the rat rotation model. *Science* **208** (1980) 1466–1468.
36. Hruska, R. E., and Silbergeld, E. K. Estrogen treatment enhances dopamine receptor sensitivity in the rat striatum. *Eur. J. Pharmacol.* **61** (1980) 397–400.
37. Jori, A., and Cecchetti, G. Homovanillic acid levels in rat striatum during the oestrus cycle. *J. Endocr.* **58** (1973) 341–342.
38. Joyce, J. N., Smith, R. L., and Van Hartesveldt, C. Estradiol suppresses then enhances intracaudate dopamine-induced contralateral deviation. *Eur. J. Pharmacol.* **81** (1982) 117–122.
39. Kasting, N. W., Martin, J. B., and Arnold, M. A. Pulsatile somatostatin release from the median-eminence of the unanesthetized rat and its relationship to plasma growth hormone levels. *Endocrinology* **109** (1981) 1739–1745.
40. Kim, K., and Ramirez, V. D. *In vitro* progesterone stimulates the release of luteinizing hormone-releasing hormone from superfused hypothalamic tissue from ovariectomized estradiol-primed prepuberal rats. *Endocrinology* **111** (1982) 750–756.
41. Knobil, E. The neuroendocrine control of the menstrual cycle. *Rec. Prog. Horm. Res.* **36** (1980) 53–88.
42. Levine, J. E., and Ramirez, V. D. *In vivo* release of luteinizing hormone-releasing hormone

estimated with push–pull cannulae from the mediobasal hypothalami of ovariectomized, steroid-primed rats. *Endocrinology* **107** (1980) 1782–1790.
43. Levine, J. E., and Ramirez, V. D. Luteinizing hormone-releasing hormone release during the rat estrous cycle and after ovariectomy, as estimated with push–pull cannulae. *Endocrinology* **111** (1982) 1439–1448.
44. Levine, J. E., Pau, K. Y. F., Ramirez, V. D., and Jackson, G. L. Simultaneous measurement of luteinizing hormone-releasing hormone and luteinizing hormone release in unanesthetized, ovariectomized sheep. *Endocrinology* **111** (1982) 1449–1455.
45. Loullis, C. C., Hingtgen, J. N., Shea, P. A., and Aprison, M. H. *In vivo* determination of endogenous biogenic amines in rat brain using HPLC-EC and push–pull cannula. *Pharmacol. Biochem. Behav.* **12** (1980) 959–963.
46. Mattheij, J. A. M., and Swartz, J. J. M. Circadian variations in the plasma concentration of prolactin in the adult male rat. *J. Endocr.* **79** (1978) 85–89.
47. McLennan, H. The release of acetylcholine and of 3-hydroxytyramine from the caudate nucleus. *J. Physiol. (London)* **174** (1964) 152–161.
48. Meeker, R., and Myers, R. D. *In vivo* [^{14}C]amino acid profiles in discrete hypothalamic regions during push–pull perfusion in the unrestrained rat. *Neuroscience* **4** (1979) 495–506.
49. Mills, D. E., Buckman, M. T., and Peake, G. T. Neonatal treatment with antiserum to prolactin lowers blood pressure in rats. *Science* **217** (1982) 162–164.
50. Mogilnicka, E., and Klimek, V. Drugs affecting dopamine neurons and yawning behavior. *Pharmacol. Biochem. Behav.* **7** (1977) 303–305.
51. Morris, M., Tandy, B., Sundberg, D. K., and Knigge, K. M. Modification of brain and CSF LHRH following deafferentation. *Neuroendocrinology* **18** (1975) 131–135.
52. Myers, R. D., and Beleslin, D. B. The spontaneous release of 5-hydroxytryptamine and acetylcholine within the diencephalon of the unanesthetized rhesus monkey. *Exp. Brain Res.* **11** (1970) 539–552.
53. Neill, J. D., Patton, J. M., Dailey, R. A., Tsou, R. C., and Tindall, G. T. Luteinizing hormone-releasing hormone (LHRH) in pituitary stalk blood of rhesus monkeys. Relationship to level of LH release. *Endocrinology* **101** (1977) 430–434.
54. Nicholson, G., Greeley, S. H., Humm, J., Youngblood, W. W., and Kizer, J. S. Prolactin in cerebrospinal fluid: a probable site of prolactin antiregulation. *Brain Res.* **190** (1980) 447–458.
55. Nieoullon, A., Cheramy, A., and Glowinski, J. An adaptation of the push–pull cannula method to study the *in vivo* release of ^{3}H-dopamine synthestized from ^{3}H-tyrosine in the cat caudate nucleus: effect of various physical and pharmacological treatments. *J. Neurochem.* **28** (1977) 819–828.
56. Ondo, J., Mansky, T., and Wuttke, W. *In vivo* GABA release from the medial preoptic area of diestrous and ovariectomized rats. *Exp. Brain Res.* **46** (1982) 69–72.
57. Perkins, N. A., and Westfall, T. C. The effect of prolactin on dopamine release from rat striatum and medial basal hypothalamus. *J. Neurosci.* **3** (1978) 59–63.
58. Philippu, A. Use of push–pull cannulae to determine the release of endogenous neurotransmitters in distinct brain areas of anesthetized and freely moving animals. *In* "Measurement of Neurotransmitter Release *in Vivo*," (C. A. Marsden, ed.), 1984, pp. 3–37. Wiley, New York.
59. Ramirez, V. D. The secretory activity of peptidergic and aminergic neurons *in vitro* and *in vivo*. *In* "Neurosecretion: Molecules, Cells and Systems," (D. S. Farner and K. Lederis, eds.), 1982, pp. 153–166. Plenum, New York.
60. Ramirez, V. D. Hormones and striatal dopaminergic activity: a novel neuroendocrine

model. *In* "The Anterior Pituitary," (A. S. Bhatnagar, ed.), 1983, pp. 97–105. Raven, New York.

61. Ramirez, V. D., and Dluzen, D. Progesterone administration *in vivo* modulates *in vitro* dopamine release from the corpus striatum of ovariectomized estrogen-treated rats. *Soc. Neurosci.* abstr. 264.4 (1982) 921.
62. Robinson, T. E., and Becker, J. B. Behavioural sensitization is accompanied by an enhancement in amphetamine-stimulated dopamine release from striatal tissue *in vitro*. *Eur. J. Pharmacol.* **85** (1982) 253–254.
63. Roth, R. H., Murrin, L. C., and Walters, J. R. Central dopaminergic neurons: effects of alterations in impulse flow on the accumulation of dihydroxyphenylacetic acid. *Eur. J. Pharmacol.* **36** (1976) 163–171.
64. Ruwe, W. D., Veale, W. L., Pittman, Q. J., Kasting, N. W., and Lederis, K. Release of arginine vasopressin from the brain: correlation with physiological events. This volume, Chapter 14.
65. Szerb, J. C. Model experiments with Gaddum's push–pull cannulas. *Can. J. Physiol. Pharmacol.* **45** (1967) 613–620.
66. Ungerstedt, U. Measurement of neurotransmitter release by intracranial dialysis. *In* "Measurement of Neurotransmitter Release *in Vivo*," (C. A. Marsden, ed.), 1984, pp. 81–105. Wiley, New York.
67. Urba-Holmgren, R., Gonzalez, R. M., and Holmgren, B. Is yawning a cholinergic response? *Nature (London)* **267** (1977) 261–262.
68. Urba-Holmgren, R., Holmgren, B., and Anias, J. Pre- and post-synaptic dopaminergic receptors involved in apomorphine-induced yawning. *Acta Neurobiol. Exp.* **42** (1982) 115–125.
69. Van Der Gugten, J., and Slangen, J. L. Release of endogenous catecholamines from rat hypothalamus *in vivo* related to feeding and other behaviours. *Pharmacol. Biochem. Behav.* **7** (1977) 211–219.
70. Van Der Heyden, J. A. M., Venema, K., and Korf, J. *In vivo* release of endogenous GABA from rat substantia nigra measured by a novel method. *J. Neurochem.* **32** (1979)469–476.
71. Westerink, B. H. C., and Spaan, S. J. Estimation of the turnover of 3-metoxytyramine in the rat striatum by HPLC with electrochemical detection: implications for the sequence in the cerebral metabolism of dopamine. *J. Neurochem.* **38** (1982) 342–347.
72. Wheaton, J. E., and McCann, S. M. Luteinizing hormone-releasing hormone in peripheral plasma of normal and ovariectomized rats. *Neuroendocrinology* **20** (1976) 296–310.
73. Wood, P. L., Cheney, D. L., and Costa, E. A prolactin action on acetylcholine metabolism in striatum, hippocampus and thalamus. *J. Neurochem.* **34** (1980) 1053–1057.
74. Yaksh, T. L., and Yamamura, H. I. Factors affecting performance of the push–pull cannula in brain. *J. App. Physiol.* **37** (1974) 428–434.

16

The Efficacy of the Push–Pull Perfusion Technique in the Study of Sleep, Epilepsy, and Tremor

MARCOS VELASCO, FRANCISCO VELASCO, MARÍA TRINIDAD PACHECO, AND FRANCISCO ESTRADA-VILLANUEVA

Division of Neurophysiology
Scientific Research Department
National Medical Center
Instituto Mexicano del Seguro Social
Mexico City, Mexico

I. INTRODUCTION

In this chapter, we summarize our results on the effect of push–pull perfusion of carbachol in the mesencephalic (MRF) and pontine (PRF) re-

IN VIVO PERFUSION AND RELEASE
OF NEUROACTIVE SUBSTANCES

ISBN 0-12-083350-6

ticular formations on sleep, epilepsy, and tremor electroencephalographic (EEG) and electromyographic (EMG) patterns in cats and monkeys (*40, 46, 47, 48, 53, 54*). These experiments were made in an attempt to reproduce, by carbachol activation of MRF and PRF, the changes in cortical and spinal excitability of these normal and abnormal EEG–EMG patterns observed during spontaneous wakefulness and sleep. Although our data are still incomplete, results indicate that cholinoceptive activation of MRF produces a cortical and muscular response which resembles the one observed during spontaneous wakefulness and arousal; while activation of PRF produces a muscular response which resembles only the hypotonic component of the spontaneous paradoxical sleep.

The strategy of our experiments was initially to utilize a single cholinergic compound (carbachol) to stimulate a single structure of the central nervous system (CNS) (reticular formation) and observe its effect on a number of clinical and electrophysiological indicators of cortical and spinal excitability. We chose carbachol because it is a cholinergic compound with pharmacological stability and because there is vast evidence on the neurotransmitter nature of acetylcholine. The outstanding effects of cholinergic and anticholinergic compounds on sleep, epilepsy, and tremor have been repetitively described (see Section IV). We chose the reticular formation in view of its direct or indirect participation in wakefulness (*23*), slow wave (*19*), and paradoxical sleep (*14, 33*). We utilized the push–pull perfusion technique in view of its apparent advantages on other electrical and chemical stimulation procedures, which, according to Myers (*28*), are (1) selective activation of cholinoceptive cells at the perfusion site, (2) volumetric problems minimized after 1–2 min baseline perfusion of artificial cerebrospinal fluid (CSF), (3) control of the precise moment of initiation and termination of the chemical stimulation, and (4) determination of the dose–response curves in the same animal by controlling the time of perfusion and utilizing a constant concentration of the perfused compound in the solution and a constant perfusion velocity.

At the moment, we are in the process of improving the efficacy of the push–pull system, particularly in terms of avoiding tissue destruction by the cannula itself by preventing hydrodynamic variations of the perfused solution. The modifications proposed in the couple taps used for adjusting the various elements of the cannula system permitted us an 80% success rate for perfusions (*40, 54*). The use of a removable slot instead of a fixed concentric tip for the cannula may improve the efficacy of such a perfusion (see Chapter 6, this volume). Evidence presented here will be mainly concerned with the regional selectivity of this form of stimulation, based upon the radioactivity distribution of carbachol C-14 into the brain stem and the activation of the neuronal population adjacent to the perfusion site.

II. METHODS

A. Push–Pull Perfusions

Perfusions were made with a push–pull cannula system similar to that described by Myers (*28*), but modified in its couple taps which are used for adjusting the various elements of the system, as follows (Fig. 1, left): (1) tap for adjusting the length difference between inner and outer cannula tips, which determines the rate of inflow (optimal difference in all cats was 0.75 mm); (2) tap for adjusting the outer cannula and cylinder assembly, which determines the rate of outflow (optimal rate was individually determined in such a way that inflow and outflow rate was equal to one); (3) tap for

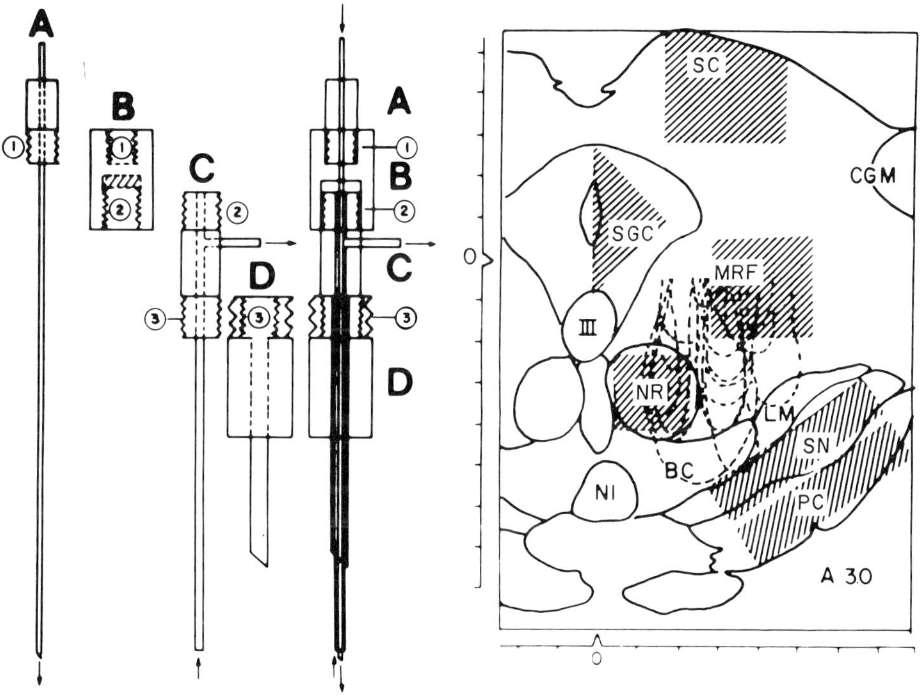

Fig. 1. Left: Diagram of the push–pull cannula system of Myers (*28*) modified in its couple taps. A, Inner cannula; B, assembly cylinder; C, outer cannula; D, cannula guide; 1–3, couple taps adjusting the various components of the system. Right: Coronal section of the cat's mesencephalon at frontal section A 3.0 (*34*) showing the site of cannula tips at the tegmental MRF (discontinuous lines) and the approximate size of the tissue biopsies taken from different brain stem structures for scintillographic determination of C-14 radioactivity (striped areas). MRF, Mesencephalic reticular formation: SGC, periaqueductal gray: SC, superior colliculus: CGM, lateral geniculate body: SN, substantia nigra: PC, cerebral peduncle: NR, red nucleus.

adjusting the length difference between cannulae and guide tips, which determine the vertical position of the cannula tip in the brain (for MRF the optimal vertical range in all cats was equal to 4.0 mm) (*40*).

The perfusion system was completed by 1-ml syringes activated by a Harvard infusion–withdrawal pump and connected to inner and outer cannulae through two 30-cm, 90-ga polyethylene catheters with a capacity of 250 μl for each catheter. The system was loaded with an aseptic, pyrogen-free artificial CSF consisting of a buffered solution (pH 7.4 and osmolarity 314.8 *M*) similar in composition to the CSF of cats (*21*).

Perfusion velocity was adjusted to 50 μl/min for a period of time from 5 to 10 min. A quantitative evaluation of intracerebral distribution of perfusates was made by marking the CSF and carbachol (1 μg/μl) with a single dose of ^{14}C-labeled glucose and ^{14}C-labeled carbachol, respectively, with a radioactivity of 2 μCi/ml. At the completion of the experiments, brains were perfused *in situ* with 10% buffered Formalin, removed, and kept for 3 days in the same solution. Subsequently, a block of 2 cm thick at the mesencephalic-pontine level was prepared by serial frozen sections of 400 μm. They were cut with the aid of a dissection microscope to obtain small biopsies of the following brain stem structures bilaterally: MRF, periaqueductal gray, superior colliculus, red nucleus, substantia nigra, lateral geniculate body, and cerebral peduncle (Fig. 1, right). Brain biopsies were collected on thin aluminum foil cups and dehydrated for 2 hr at 40°C. Then biopsies were weighed, placed in a liquid scintillation counting vials, and dissolved in hydroxyhymine (hydroxide of hyamine, 1 *M* in ethanol, Packard) for 3 days. Thereafter, a "cocktail" scintillation mixture was added and the amount of radioactivity was determined with a liquid scintillation spectrophotometer with an efficiency of 35%. The number of disintegrations per minute, per milligram dry weight was determined in each brain sample and individual corrections for quenching were made by the channel ratio method (*40, 54*).

Fig. 2. Top: Diagrams of two parasagittal sections of the cat's brain stem, lateral 1.9 and 2.9 from Berman (*4*), showing the final position of cannula (circles) and electrode (dots) tips within the pontine (FTG) and mesencephalic (FTC) reticular formations. Distance between cannula and electrode tips is indicated by diagonal lines. [Reprinted from ref. (*46*).]

Bottom: Effect of carbachol perfusion in the pontine reticular formation on adjacent pontine MUA (PRF) and in the mesencephalic reticular formation on adjacent mesencephalic MUA (MRF). A sample of baseline MUA recordings was taken during perfusion with cerebrospinal fluid (CSF), three samples during perfusion of carbachol at 2, 7, and 10 min (CARB), and one sample 10 min after perfusion (after 10′). Notice that whereas MRF perfusion produced a progressive recruitment of MUA lasting 10 min during and after perfusion, PRF perfusion produced an initial recruitment of MUA, but at 10 min there was a "suppression" response which recovered 10 min after perfusion. [Reprinted from ref. (*46*).]

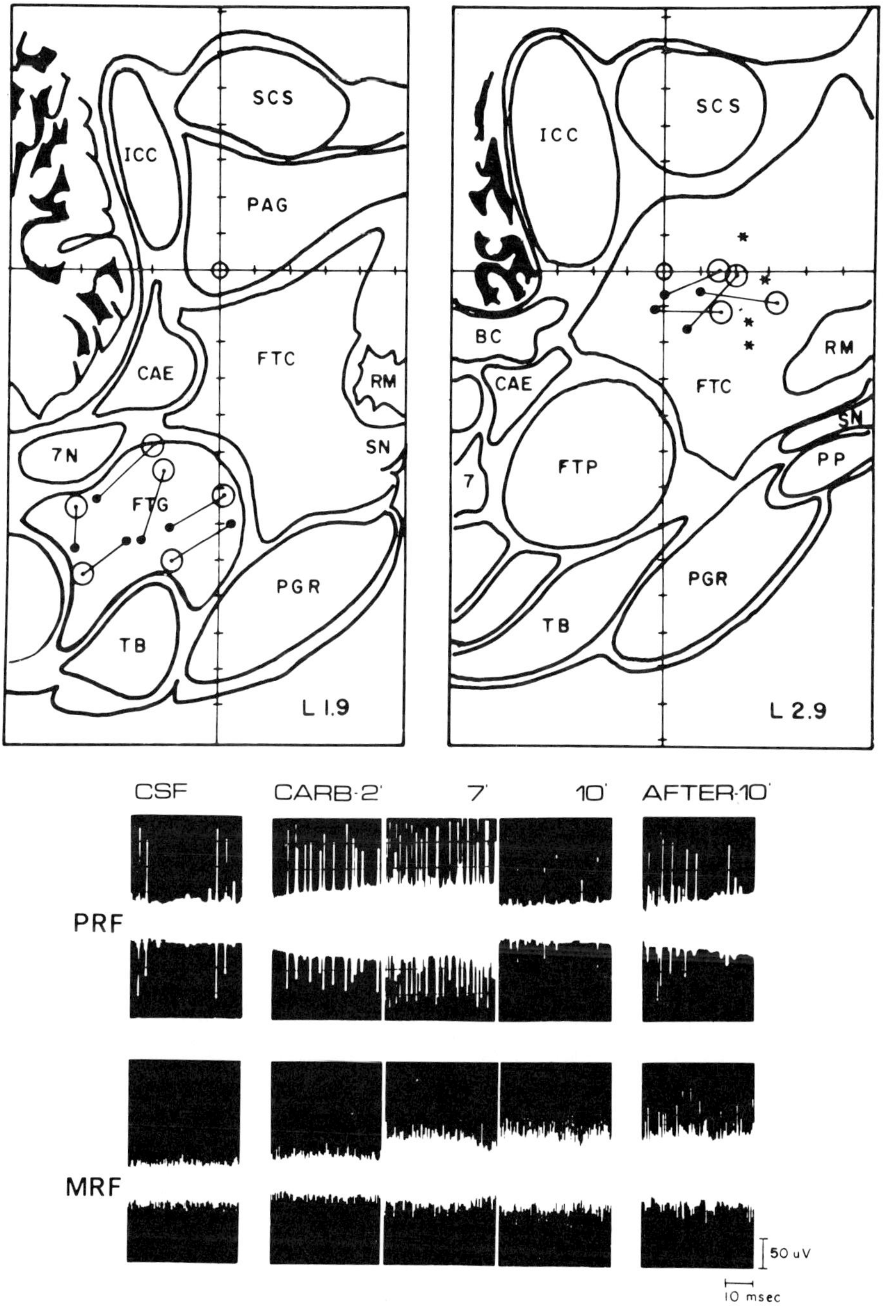
SCS
ICC
PAG
CAE
FTC
RM
SN
7N
FTG
PGR
TB
L 1.9
SCS
ICC
BC
CAE
FTC
RM
SN
PP
FTP
7
PGR
TB
L 2.9
CSF
CARB-2'
7'
10'
AFTER-10'
PRF
MRF
50 uV
10 msec

Fig. 2.

B. Adjacent Neuronal Population

Multiple-unit activity (MUA) of the reticular cells contiguous to the perfusion site was recorded through concentric, stainless-steel electrodes, insulated except at their tips (inner tip 15–30 μm, outer tip 500 μm, impedance 50 kΩ). MUA selection and integration included only those units with an amplitude of 400 and 100% larger than the noise level in PRF and MRF, respectively. The distance between the cannula tip for carbachol perfusion and the electrode tip for MUA was 1.1 ± 0.2 and 0.9 ± 0.1 mm for PRF and MRF studies, respectively. This distance was calculated after histologic verification of the final position of the cannula and electrode tips within parasagittal sections of the cat's brain stem (*46*) (Fig. 2).

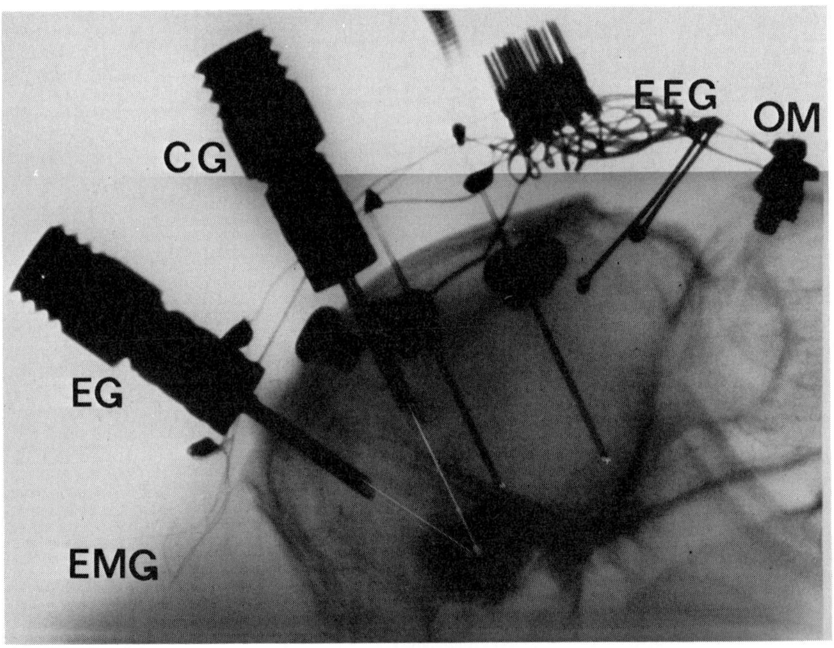

Fig. 3. Above: Lateral diagram of a cat's head showing CG, guide for push–pull perfusion system: EG, guide for MUA recording electrode: EEG, silver ball electrode for EEG recordings from the right and left motor cortices: OM, stainless-steel screws for ocular movement recordings from the outer canthus; and EMG, stainless-steel wires for EMG recordings from the neck muscles. [Reprinted from ref. (*36*).]

Right: Lateral radiogram of a monkey's head showing the complete push–pull system implanted with the cannula tips in the mesencephalic reticular formation (rf) and the cannula guide implanted in the frontal lobe for ulterior penetration of a cannula directed to the caudate nucleus (c). [Reprinted from ref. (*48*).]

C. Sleep

For sleep research, cats were implanted with two cannula guides into the cerebellum for ulterior penetration of a push–pull cannula system for perfusion of carbachol and for an electrode recording system for recording the MUA at the PRF and MRF (*46*). In addition, other electrodes for recording conventional sleep–waking parameters were also implanted (*19*), i.e., silver ball electrodes for recording EEG activity of the motor cortex, stainless-steel

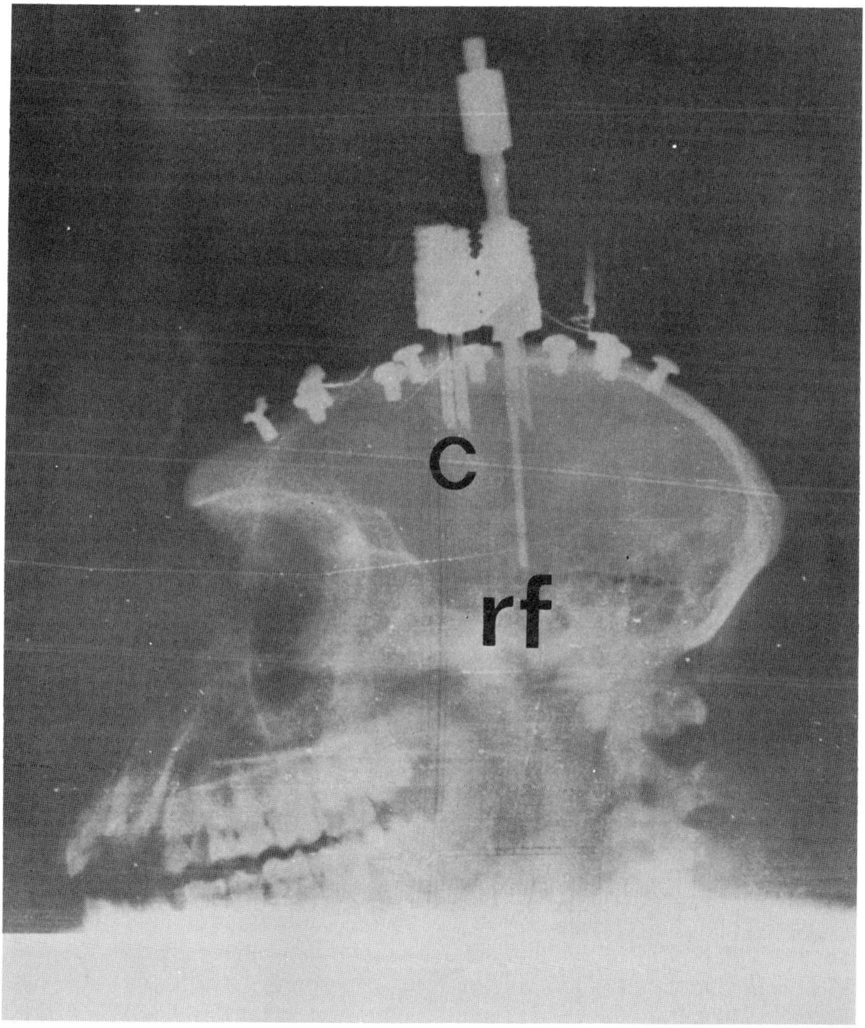

Fig. 3.

screws for recording ocular movements at the outer canthus, and wires for recording EMG activity of the neck muscles. A concentric bipolar electrode for recording MRF MUA was also implanted, in as much as it has been found to be a reliable indicator of PS in normal and epileptic cats (*11, 38*) and Parkinsonian patients (*43*). Cannula and electrode guides and other electrode connections were fixed to the skull by means of a plastic cup system with a head restraint device consisting of a leucite square with bolts extending from each side (*36*) (Fig. 3, left).

A single perfusion session in each cat (with its head attached to the stereotactic frame) was programmed 1 week after surgery as follows: (1) penetration of the perfusion cannula and MUA recording electrode; (2) 2-hr baseline recording; (3) perfusion of CSF for 2 min; (4) perfusion of carbachol for 10 min; and (5) 3-hr recovery.

D. Epilepsy

For epilepsy research, epileptogenic lesions were reproduced by single microinjections of alumina cream in the right motor cortex of cats, with the same technique and similar pathological EEG and clinical effects described elsewhere (*37, 38*). One month later and just before the development of seizures, cannula guides and electrodes were implanted. Thereafter, perfusion procedures and recording sessions were performed. Cannula guide and electrode implantation, perfusion procedures, and recording sessions were similar to those for sleep experiments.

E. Tremor

For tremor research, tremorogenic lesions were produced in the pars compacta of the substantia nigra of monkeys (*Macacus rhesus*) by means of a radiofrequency electrode. The pars compacta was identified by its typical high-voltage spikes (100–150 μV), with a 0.3- to 0.5-msec time constant, organized in 10-Hz rhythmic bursts. In the same locus, 40- to 150-μA electrical stimulation induced eyelid retraction and pupillary constriction indicating the proximity of the III cranial nerve fibers (*42*).

One week to one month later and after the development of spontaneous postural tremor, a cannula guide was implanted into the cerebellum for ulterior penetration of a cannula system, directed to the nucleus reticularis mesencephali. It was identified as a region of medium-sized cellular spikes activated by peripheral painful stimulation. In the same locus, 40- to 50-μA electrical stimulation induced an arousal response with eyes opening, pupillary dilatation, increase tremor amplitude, and EEG desynchronization (*48*). In addition, stainless-steel electrodes for EEG recordings from the motor cortex and for EMG tremor recordings from distal flexor and extensor muscles of the forelimbs were implanted (Fig. 3, right).

One week later, two consecutive perfusion sessions (10 days apart) in each monkey were programmed as follows: (1) penetration of the perfusion cannula; (2) 2-hr baseline recordings; (3) perfusion of CSF for 5 min; (4) perfusion of carbachol or atropine (1 μg/μl) for 5 min; and (5) 3-hr recovery.

Push–pull perfusion of carbachol in PRF and MRF on sleep, epilepsy, and tremor included statistics of the following parameters: number of contiguous MUA neuronal spikes, spontaneous tonic EMGMUA, EEG spikes and EMG jerks, occurrence of EEG paroxysmal discharges and EMG seizures, and amplitude and duration of the bursts of tremor.

III. FINDINGS

A. Push–Pull Perfusion

Figure 4 shows the radioactivity distribution in different brain stem structures after perfusion of ^{14}C-labeled glucose and carbachol into the MRF of "encéphale isolé" and chronically awake cats, respectively (*40, 54*). In both cases, maximal radioactivity was found in the MRF at the cannula tips (zero). The MRF radioactivity here was significantly larger than that found at other sites of MRF, located rostral and caudal to zero, and other cellular and axonal mesencephalic structures ipsi- and contralateral to the stimulated site. According to these graphs, it can be postulated that the primary behavior and electrophysiological responses are due to the activation of a circumscribed region in the MRF located at 0 ± 1.0 mm anterior–posterior from the position of the cannula tip.

B. Effect on Sleep

Perfusion of carbachol into the PRF increased the number of contiguous MUA neuronal spikes. There was a linear relationship between the number of minutes of perfusion and MUA neuronal spikes from the first to the eighth minute, followed by a plateau of maximal MUA activation from the eighth to the tenth minute and a subsequent decrease in number of MUA cellular spikes from the tenth to the eleventh minute (suppression response) when perfusion was discontinued. Concomitantly, PRF perfusion significantly decreased EMG MUA (hypotonia), but did not systematically modify MRF neuronal discharges and other electrophysiological and behavioral sleep–waking parameters (Fig. 5, PRF). Perfusion of carbachol into the MRF in-

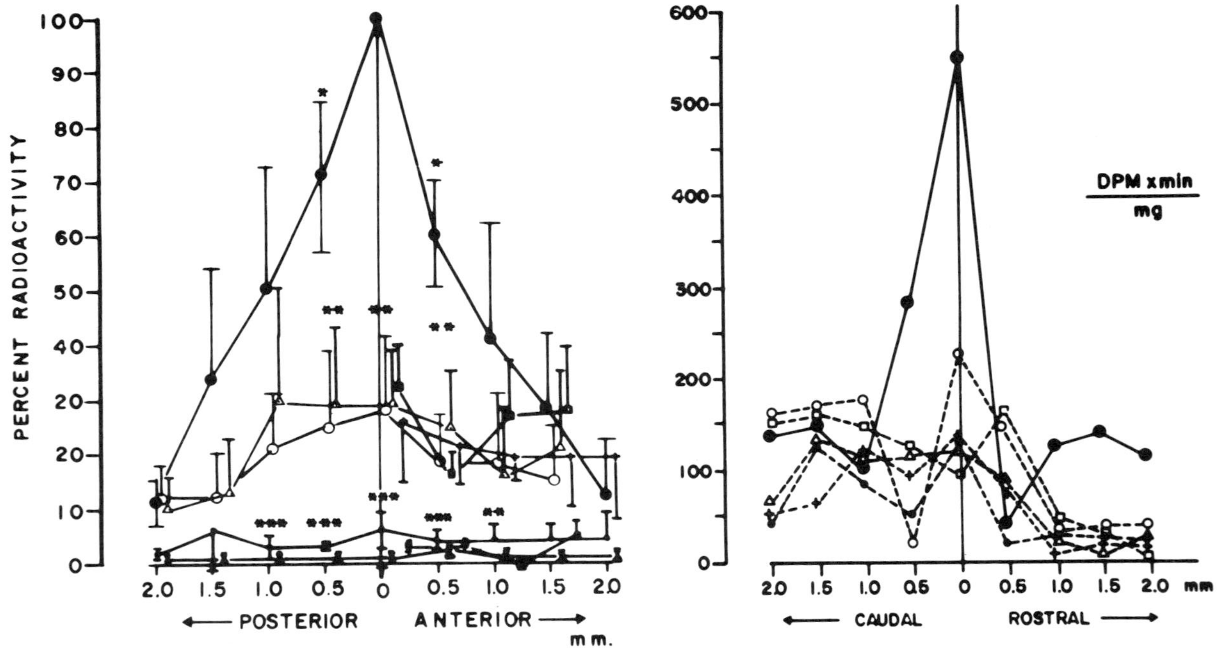

Fig. 4. Left: Distribution of radioactivity in different brain stem structures ipsi- and contralateral to the push–pull perfusion of glucose C-14 in the MRF. Ordinate: percentage radioactivity (mean ± SEM); abscissas: zero indicates the precise position of the cannula tips and millimeters posterior and anterior to zero. (*), Radioactivity in MRF at 0 level significantly ($p < .02$) larger than that of MRF at other anterior–posterior levels (filled circles); (**), Radioactivity in MRF at 0 and 0.5 anterior–posterior significantly larger ($p < .01$) than in other cellular mesencephalic structures: PAG (open circles), SC (triangles), NR (open squares), and SN (crosses); (***), radioactivity in cellular mesencephalic structures ipsilateral to the perfusion site at levels 0, 0.5, and 1.5 anterior–posterior significantly larger than that in the ipsilateral cerebral peduncle (dots) and in the average of all contralateral brain stem structures (solid squares). [Reprinted from ref. (*40*).]

Right: Radioactivity distribution in different brain stem structures ipsilateral to push–pull perfusion of carbachol C-14 into the mesencephalic reticular formation. Ordinate: absolute radioactivity (DPM × min/mg tissue); abscissas: zero indicates the precise position of perfusion and millimeters caudal and rostral to zero. MRF, filled circles: raphe, squares; periaqueductal gray, open circles; superior collicolus, triangles; lateral geniculate, crosses; and cerebral peduncle and substantia nigra, triangles. [Reprinted from ref. (*54*).]

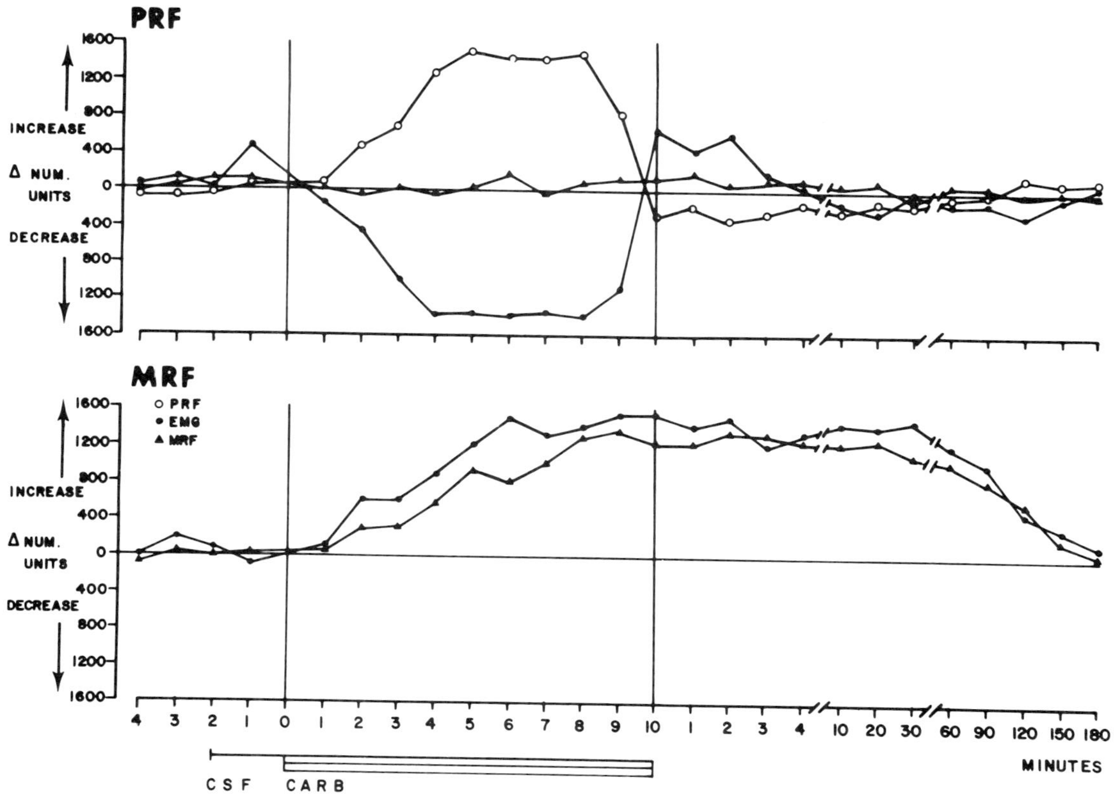

Fig. 5. Effect of carbachol perfusion into the pontine (PRF) and mesencephalic (MRF) reticular formations on contiguous MUA at pontine (circles) and mesencephalic (triangles) levels and on electromyographic MUA (dots). Mean changes in number of units per minute sequentially obtained from 4 min before to 10 min during and 180 min after carbachol perfusion. [Reprinted from ref. (*46*).]

creased the number of contiguous MUA neuronal spikes from the first to the eleventh minute when perfusion was discontinued. Concomitantly, the perfusion increased EMG MUA (hypertonia) and produced a systematic electrophysiological and behavioral arousal response, i.e., EEG desynchronization, increased number of saccadic ocular movements, opening of the eyes, contraction of nictitating membrane, pupillary dilatation, and polypnea. No systematic effects were observed after PRF perfusion while a persistent arousal response lasting 150 min was observed after MRF perfusion (Fig. 5, MRF).

C. Effect on Epilepsy

Perfusion of carbachol into the PRF produced a pure hypotonic response: decreased phasic EMG MUA (EMG activation time locked to the EEG spike) with no changes in number of EEG spikes of type B seizures.* This response lasted 80 min and was followed by an SWS-like response: a further decrease in phasic EMG MUA and an increase in the number of EEG spikes of type B seizures, which lasted 180 min after carbachol perfusion (Fig. 6, PRF).

Perfusion of carbachol into the MRF produced an arousal-like response: an increase in phasic EMG MUA and a decrease in the number of EEG spikes of type B seizures. This response lasted 80 min after perfusion and was followed by a PS-like response: a decrease in phasic EMG MUA and the number of EEG spikes of type B seizures, which lasted until 180 min after carbachol perfusion (Fig. 6, MRF).

The occurrence of type C seizures† was facilitated when impending hypotonia was present concomitant either with the SWS-like response after PRF or with the PS-like response after MRF carbachol perfusion, while such seizures were inhibited concomitant with the hypertonia produced by perfusion of carbachol into the MRF (Fig. 6, PRF and MRF, top).

*Type B seizures consist of isolated EEG spikes at the cortical epileptic focus associated to isolated EMG jerks of contralateral face, neck, and forepaw muscles. This type of seizure is due to epileptic impulses originating in the motor cortex which propagate to flexor muscles through pyramidal pathways (*50*). They continuously appear, 1–3 every second, for several days after alumina cream injection (epilepsia partialis continua) without altering sleep and waking states.

†Type C seizures consist of prolonged (1–3 min) repetitive EEG spikes (paroxysmal discharges) at the cortical epileptic focus, associated with repetitive tonic–clonic convulsions of contralateral face, neck, and limb muscles. This type of seizure is due to epileptic impulses originating outside of the motor cortex (cingulate gyrus and striatum), which propagate to extensor and flexor muscles through pyramidal and extrapyramidal pathways (bilateral pyramidal), and mesencephalic and pontine reticular formations, ipsi- and contralateral to focus and crossing fibers at the level of the raphe system (*50–52*). They spontaneously appear every 5 to 60 min after alumina cream injections (contra-adversive seizures) and immediately modify wakefulness–sleep states.

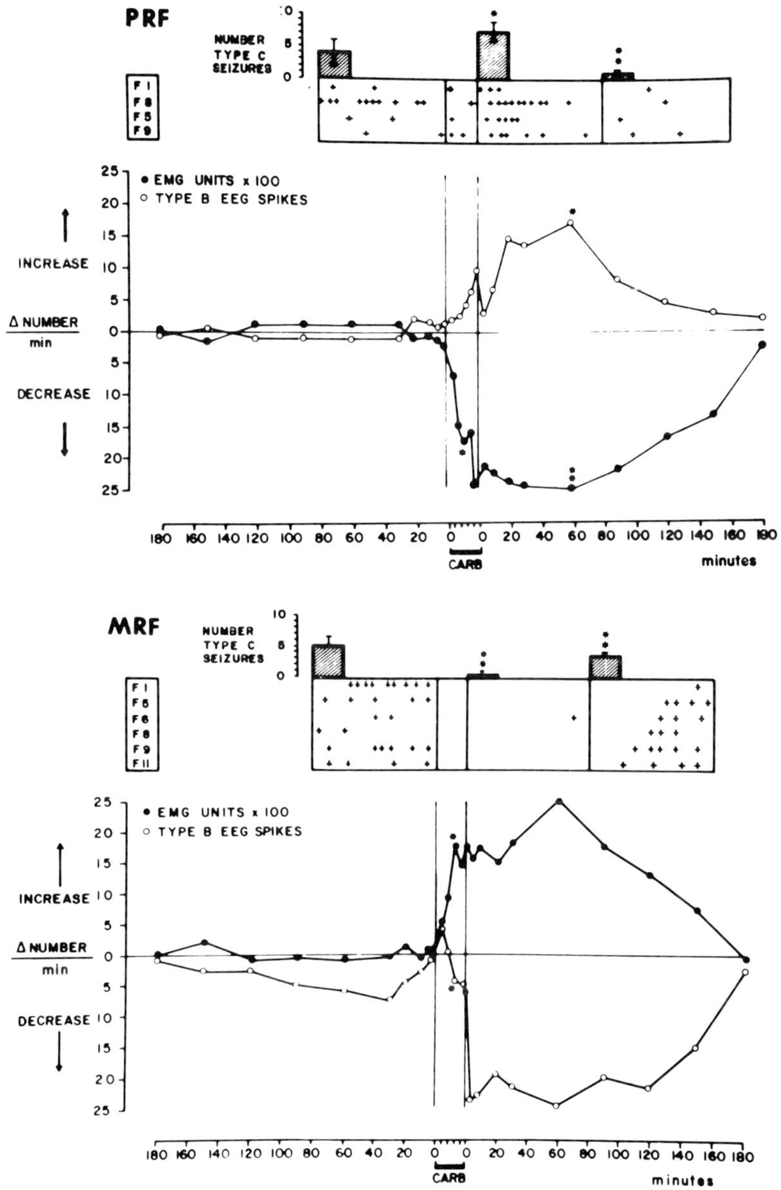

Fig. 6. Effect of carbachol perfusion into the pontine (PRF) and mesencephalic (MRF) reticular formations on contiguous type B electromyographic MUA (dots) and EEG spikes (circles) and number of type C seizures before, during, and after perfusion (crosses). Increments in number of type B electromyographic MUA units and EEG spikes per minute were calculated 5, 10, 20, 30, 60, 90, 120, 150, and 180 min before and after perfusion and every minute during perfusion (bottom graphs). Total number of type C seizures for individual cats (F1, 5, 6, 8, 9, and 11) spontaneously occurring within one period of 80 min before and two consecutive periods of 80 min each after perfusion (top graphs). Asterisks indicate significant change ($p < .05$). [Reprinted from ref. (*47*).]

D. Effect on Tremor

Perfusion of carbachol into the MRF increased duration and amplitude of spontaneous bursts of tremor at flexor and extensor muscles.* In the case of bilateral tremor, the effect was observed mainly in the extremities contralateral to the perfusion site. The effect started 0.5 min after the perfusion initiation and remitted immediately after perfusion termination. Concomitantly, there was a transient arousal response, including mild increase in spontaneous motor activity and muscular tone and EEG desynchronization.

Perfusion of atropine into the MRF produced a response opposite to that to carbachol, including decrease in contralateral tremor, motor activity, and muscular tonus with a synchronic (4–5/sec) rhythmic activity over the central region. This effect started 0.25 min after initiation and lasted 30–45 min after perfusion termination (Fig. 7). No data are available about the effect of carbachol in the PRF on tremor in monkeys.

IV. PERSPECTIVES AND DISCUSSION

A number of methodological questions about the push–pull perfusion stimulation technique have to be solved in order to interpret correctly the present results. These questions are mainly related to absolute concentration and distribution of the perfused compound into the brain stem during and after perfusion to different volumes, concentrations, and rates of perfusion. These questions are being partially solved in our laboratories by means of scintillographic determination of carbachol C-14 radioactivity at the perfusion site (*54*). Similar questions were raised by Eugene Shoener in his studies on neuronal responses to neuroactive substances administered by push–pull perfusion and are discussed in this volume (Chapter 3). In our experiments, for example, we fail to explain the nature of the "suppression" cellular response during carbachol perfusion in the PRF. Why do we have transient responses on sleep and tremor, which last for just the perfusion time in normal cats and diskinetic monkeys and are long-lasting responses in epileptic cats?

On the other hand, the use of the push–pull stimulating technique is of great interest in various areas. The pharmacological evaluation of cho-

*Experimental tremor is reliably produced by lesions in the pars compacta of the substantia nigra and suppressed in all cases by lesions in nucleus reticularis mesencephali (*42*). This kind of tremor in monkeys resembles closely that observed in Parkinsonian patients. In monkeys, it consists of rhythmic (4–5/sec) waxing and waning movements of distal flexor and extensor muscles, that are prominent at rest, increase with animals' anxiety or stress, and decrease and disappear with voluntary movements and sleep.

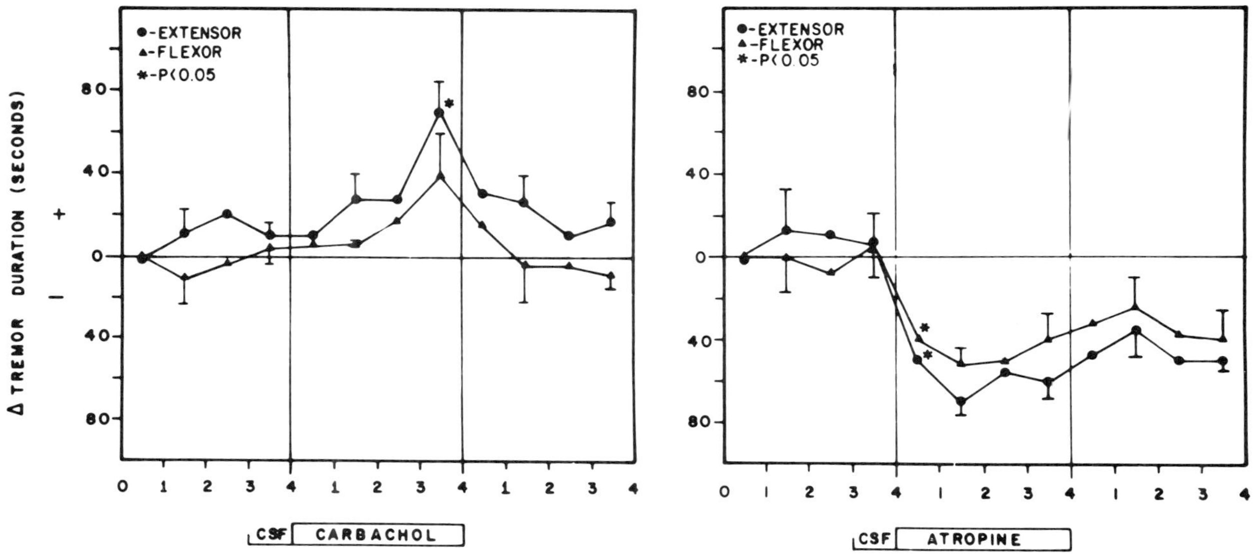

Fig. 7. Effect of carbachol (left) and atropine (right) perfusion into the mesencephalic reticular formation on tremor. Increments (mean ± SD) in duration of the tremor bursts every second for 5-sec period before, during, and after perfusion of these compounds. [Reprinted from ref. (*48*).]

linergic and anticholinergic compounds in experimental animals is promising as well as the study of other neurotransmitters or activating substances regionally perfused on sleep (*44, 45, 49, 53*), epilepsy, and tremor. In the case of the Division of Neurophysiology whose work is closely related to the Functional Neurosurgery Service at the General Hospital, S.S.A., it is urgent that a reliable technique is found which provides controllable dosages of various compounds locally delivered to several brain structures during the treatment of severe insomnia, convulsions, and extrapyramidal syndromes for which conventional medical regimes have failed.

Discussion here will be limited, however, to a cholinoceptive reticular system.

A. Sleep

With the assumption that carbachol produced its primary effect on the brain during the time elapsed between initiation and termination of a push–pull perfusion, it may be concluded that carbachol perfusion into the PRF activates a cholinoceptive system responsible for reduction of muscular tonus (*26, 30, 31, 33*). In contrast, present results do not support the idea that carbachol primary activation of PRF neurons is responsible for the activation of the whole system regulating PS, as has been proposed by George *et al.* (*12*) and Amatruda *et al.* (*2*). The idea that gigantocellular PRF neurons are related only to hypotonia but not to the other behavioral and electrophysiological parameters of PS is supported by other investigators. For example, Henley and Morrison (*13*) and Jones *et al.* (*17*) found that electrolytic lesions in this region did not modify the occurrence of PS in its normal amount, but abolished the muscular atonia. Henley and Morrison (*13*), Jones *et al.* (*18*), Mitler and Dement (*25*), and Van Dongen *et al.* (*35*) showed that activation of PRF cells in various ways generates only the atonia and not the complete pattern of PS. These findings do not necessarily invalidate the presence of the complete pattern of PS after carbachol injections or push–pull perfusion of the PRF. In fact, Vivaldi *et al.* (*56, 57*) have shown decrease latency and increase duration of sleep cycles following PRF perfusion in normal cats, and we have shown cortical and spinal indicators of complete PS after MRF perfusion in epileptic cats (*47*). These effects, however, may be due to a secondary activation of other systems outside the gigantocellular PRF field.

On the other hand, carbachol perfusion into the MRF gives rise to a primary, consistent, and complete arousal response, indicating that there is a cholinoceptive MRF system which regulates the excitability of the cerebral cortex, spinal cord, and other systems or ingredients of the wakefulness state.

B. Epilepsy

When the EEG–EMG patterns of type B and C seizures are considered electrophysiologic cortical and spinal indicators of wakefulness-sleep states, then in epileptic and in normal cats perfusion of carbachol into PRF produced a primary hypotonic response, whereas in MRF carbachol produced a primary arousal response. In addition, in epileptic cats as opposed to normals, carbachol perfusion into PRF produced a secondary SWS-like response while its perfusion in MRF produced a secondary PS-like response.

The primary and secondary effects of carbachol into PRF and MRF were in agreement with the idea of two related, although independent physiopathologic mechanisms participating in the predisposition and development of focal motor seizures, i.e., the primary hypotonic effect of carbachol into PRF was associated with a decrease in the spinal development of seizures with no concomitant changes in the cortical predisposition and development of seizures. The arousal effect of carbachol into MRF was associated with an increase in the spinal and cortical development of seizures and a decrease in their cortical predisposition.

The secondary effects of carbachol on PRF and MRF were SWS- and PS-like, and these could be dependent upon activation of other loci outside of the brain stem reticular formation.

C. Tremor

Two models of experimental tremor seem adequate to study the physiopathology of Parkinsonian tremor because they resemble the clinical and biochemical aspects of Parkinson's disease. These models are (1) lesions in the pars compacta of the substantia nigra which produce both postural tremor (*3, 5, 20*) and decrease the dopamine concentration in the striatum (*15, 32*), and (2) tremor produced by topical perfusion of cholinergic substances in the caudate nucleus which is suppressed by anticholinergic and dopaminergic substances in the same region (*6, 7, 8, 10*). Both anticholinergic compounds and dopamine are successful in controlling Parkinsonian tremor (*9, 16*). Based on these models, it has been proposed that Parkinsonian tremor results from the disruption of normal cholinergic–dopaminergic balance in the striatum. Tremor would appear after either decrease in dopamine or increase in acetylcholine in the caudate nucleus (*1, 15, 22, 24, 27, 29*). On the other hand, dorsomedial MRF lesions (*42*) and subthalamic lesions (*41*) suppress both experimental and Parkinsonian tremors, suggesting the existence of a mesencephalic ascending mechanism involved in the generation of tremor.

We have shown that carbachol perfusion in the MRF increased tremor amplitude and duration in the contralateral hand in monkeys with unilateral and bilateral tremor produced by unilateral or bilateral lesions of the pars compacta of the substantia nigra. This tremorogenic effect of carbachol was associated with a complete cortical and muscular arousal response. We believe, however, that in the monkey, cholinergic stimulation increased tremor not solely by increasing general alertness, since in the case of bilateral tremor, perfusion of carbachol and atropine in MRF modified tremor only at the contralateral hand. The fact that atropine in the MRF prevented the tremor increase produced by carbachol in the ipsilateral caudate nucleus (*48*) suggests that MRF exerts a cholinergic control on the caudate. Such a control may be directly on caudate neurons in the same way neurons in the substantia nigra control dopaminergic neurons in the striatum.

REFERENCES

1. Anden, N. E., Dahlstrom, A., Fuxe, K., and Larson, K. Functional role of the nigro-neostriatal dopamine neurons. *Acta Pharmacol. Toxicol.* (*Copenhagen*) **24** (1966) 263–274.
2. Amatruda, III, T. T., Black, D. A., McKenna, T. M., McCarly, R. W., and Hobson, J. A. Sleep cycle control and cholinergic mechanisms. Differential effects of carbachol injections at the pontine brain stem sites. *Brain Res.* **38** (1975) 501–515.
3. Battista, A. F., Nakatani, S., and Goldstein, M. The effects of L-dopa on harmaline induced tremor and on resting tremor in monkeys with tegmental lesions. *Conf. Neurol.* **32** (1969) 332–340.
4. Berman, A. L. "The Brain Stem of the Cat," 1968. Univ. of Wisconsin Press, Madison.
5. Coates, G. H. Harmine tremor after brain monoamine oxidase inhibition in the mouse. *Eur. J. Pharmacol.* **18** (1972) 284–286.
6. Connor, J. D., Rossi, G. V., and Baker, W. W. Characteristics of tremor in cats following the injection of carbachol into caudate nucleus. *Exp. Neurol.* **14** (1966) 371–382.
7. Connor, J. D., Rossi, G. V., and Baker, W. W. Analyses of the tremor induced by injections of cholinergic agents into the caudate nucleus. *Int. J. Neuropharmacol.* **5** (1966) 167–176.
8. Connor, J. D., Rossi, G. V., and Baker, W. W. Antagonism of intracaudate carbachol tremor by local injections of catecholamines. *J. Pharmacol. Exp. Ther.* **155** (1967) 545–551.
9. Cotzias, B. C., Papavasiliou, P. S., and Gelleme, R. Mofication of Parkinsonism: chronic treatment with L-dopa. *N. Eng. J. Med.* **280** (1969) 337–395.
10. Dill, R. E., Nickey, W. W., and Little, M. D. Dyskinesias in rats following chemical stimulation of the neostriatum. *Tex. Rep. Biol. Med.* **26** (1968) 102–105.
11. Drucker-Colín, R. R., Bernal-Pedroza, J. G., Díez-Mitoma, E. J., and Zamora-Quezada, J. Oscillatory changes in multiple unit activity during rapid eye movement sleep. *Exp. Neurol.* **57** (1977) 331–341.
12. George, R., Haslett, W. L., and Jenden, D. J. A cholinergic mechanism in the brain stem reticular formation: induction of paradoxical sleep. *Int. J. Neuropharmacol.* **3** (1964) 541–552.

13. Henley, K., and Morrison, A. R. A re-evaluation of the effects of lesions of the pontine tegmentum and locus coeruleus on phenomena of paradoxical sleep in the cat. *Acta Neurobiol. Exp.* **34** (1974) 215–232.
14. Hobson, J. A., McCarley, R. W., and Wyzinski, P. W. Sleep cycle oscillation: reciprocal discharge by two brain stem neuronal groups. *Science* **189** (1975) 55–58.
15. Hornykiewicz, O. Dopamine (3-hydroxytyramine) and brain function. *Pharmacol. Rev.* **18** (1966) 925–964.
16. Iivanainen, M. KR-339 in the treatment of Parkinsonian tremor. *Acta Neurol. Scand.* **50** (1974) 469–477.
17. Jones, B. E., Bobillier, P., Pin, C., and Jouvet, M. The effect of lesions of catecholamine-containing neurons upon monoamine content of the brain and EEG behavioral waking in the cat. *Brain Res.* **58** (1973) 157–177.
18. Jones, B. E., Jasper, S. T., and Halarais, A. E. Effects of locus coeruleus and the response to amphetamine in the cat. *Brain Res.* **124** (1977) 473–496.
19. Jouvet, M. Neurophysiology of the state of sleep. *Physiol. Rev.* **47** (1967) 117–177.
20. Kelly, D. M., and Naylor, R. Mechanisms of tremor induction by harmine. *Eur. J. Pharmacol.* **27** (1974) 14–24.
21. Lalley, P. M., Rossi, G. V., and Baker, W. W. Analysis of local cholinergic tremor mechanisms following selective neurochemical lesions. *Exp. Neurol.* **27** (1970) 258–275.
22. Lozoya, X., Velasco, M., Estrada, F., and Velázquez, X. Mecanismos neurohumorales que regulan los estados de sincronización cortical. *Arch. Invest. Med. (Mex.)* **3** (1972) 91–96.
23. Magoun, H. H. "The Waking Brain," Thomas, Springfield, Illinois, 1958, pp. 91–116.
24. McGeer, P. L., Boulding, J. E., Gibson, W. X., and Foukes, R. G. Drug induced extrapyramidal reaction, treatment with diphenhydramine hydrochloride and dihydroxyphenylalamine. *J. Am. Med. Assoc.* **177** (1961) 665–670.
25. Mitler, N. M., and Dement, W. E. Cataleptic-like behavior in cats after microinjections of carbachol in pontine reticular formation. *Brain Res.* **68** (1974) 335–343.
26. Morrison, A. R., and Pompeiano, O. An analysis of the supraspinal influences acting on motoneurons during sleep in the unrestrained rat. Responses on the alpha motoneurons to direct electrical stimulation during sleep. *Arch. Ital. Biol.* **103** (1965) 497–516.
27. Murphey, D. L., and Dill, R. E. Chemical stimulation of discrete brain loci as a method of producing dyskinesias in primates. *Exp. Neurol.* **34** (1972) 244–254.
28. Myers, R. D. "Handbook of Drug and Chemical Stimulation of the Brain. Behavioral, Pharmacological and Physiological Aspects," 1974, pp. 1–42. Van-Nostrand-Reinhold, New York.
29. Nashold, B. S. Cholinergic stimulation of the globus pallidus in man. *Proc. Soc. Exp. Biol. Med.* **101** (1959) 68–69.
30. Papp, M., and Bozsik, G. Comparison of the cholinesterase activity in the reticular formation of the lower brain stem of cat and rabbit. *J. Neurochem.* **13** (1966) 697–703.
31. Pavlin, R. Cholinesterase in reticular nerve cells. *J. Neurochem.* **12** (1965) 515–518.
32. Poirier, L. J., and Sourkes, T. L. Influence of the substantia nigra on the catecholamine content of the striatum. *Brain Res.* **6** (1967) 654–666.
33. Pompeiano, O., and Hoshino, K. Central control of posture: reciprocal discharge by two pontine neuronal groups leading to suppression of decerebrate rigidity. *Brain Res.* **116** (1976) 131–138.
34. Snider, R. S., and Niemer, W. T. "A Stereotaxic Atlas of the Cat Brain," 1961. University of Chicago Press, Chicago, Illinois.
35. Van Dongen, A. A. P., Broekkamp, L. E., and Cools, A. R. Atonia after carbachol microinjections near the locus coeruleus in cats. *Pharmacol. Biochem. Behav.* **8** (1978) 527–532.

36. Velasco, M. Removable plastic skull cap for chronic preparations. *Bol. Estud. Med. Biol. (Mex.)* **25** (1968) 129–134.
37. Velasco, M., Velasco, F., Estrada-Villanueva, F., and Olvera, A. Alumina cream induced focal motor epilepsy in cats. I. Lesion size and temporal course. *Epilepsy (Amsterdam)* **14** (1973) 3–14.
38. Velasco, M., Velasco, F., Cepeda, C., Almanza, X., and Estrada-Villanueva, F. Alumina cream induced focal motor epilepsy in cats. I. Wakefulness–sleep modulation of cortical paroxysmal EEG spikes. *Electroenceph. Clin. Neurophysiol.* **43** (1977) 59–66.
39. Velasco, M., Velasco, F., Cepeda, C., and Estrada-Villanueva, F. Alumina cream induced focal motor epilepsy in cats. II. Wakefulness–sleep modulation of pyramidal tract multiple unit activity. *Electroenceph. Clin. Neurophysiol.* **43** (1977) 67–73.
40. Velasco, M., Velasco, F., Lozoya, X., Estrada-Villanueva, F., and Gallegos, A. J. Effect of crossed-perfusion of homologous loci of the mesencephalic reticular formation on electrical synchronization of acute "encéphale isolé" cats. *Exp. Neurol.* **59** (1978) 16–29.
41. Velasco, F., and Velasco, M. A reticulo-thalamic system mediating propioceptive attention and tremor in man. *Neurosurgery* **4** (1979) 30–36.
42. Velasco, F., Velasco, M., Romo, R., and Maldonado, H. Production and suppression of tremor by mesencephalic tegmental lesions in monkeys. *Exp. Neurol.* **64** (1979) 516–527.
43. Velasco, F., Velasco, M., Cepeda, C., and Muñoz, H. Wakefulness–sleep modulation of thalamic multiple unit activity and EEG in man. *Electroenceph. Clin. Neurophysiol.* **47** (1979) 597–606.
44. Velasco, M., Velasco, F., and Romo, R. Specific and nonspecific multiple unit activities during pentylene-tetrazol seizures. I. Animals with "encéphale isolé." *Electroenceph. Clin. Neurophysiol.* **49** (1980) 600–607.
45. Velasco, M., Velasco, F., and Romo, R. Specific and nonspecific multiple unit activities during pentylene-tetrazol seizures in animals with pretrigeminal brain stem transections. *Exp. Neurol.* **74** (1981) 1–10.
46. Velasco, M., Velasco, F., Romo, R., and Estrada-Villanueva, F. Carbachol push–pull perfusion in the reticular formation: effect on the contiguous multiple unit activity and other sleep–waking parameters in the cat. *Exp. Neurol.* **72** (1981) 318–331.
47. Velasco, M., Velasco, F., Romo, R., and Martínez, A. Effect of carbachol push–pull perfusion in the reticular formation on alumina cream induced focal motor seizures in cats. *Exp. Neurol.* **72** (1981) 332–345.
48. Velasco, F., Velasco, M., and Romo, R. Effect of carbachol and atropine perfusions in the mesencephalic tegmentum and caudate nucleus on experimental tremor in monkeys. *Exp. Neurol.* **78** (1982) 450–460.
49. Velasco, F., Velasco, M., and Romo, R. Specific and nonspecific multiple unit activities during pentylene-tetrazol seizures in animals with mesencephalic transections. *Electroenceph. Clin. Neurophysiol.* **53** (1982) 289–297.
50. Velasco, M., and Velasco, F. Pyramidal and extrapyramidal propagation of alumina cream induced focal motor seizures in cats. *In* "Epilepsy and Motor Systems," (E. J. Speckman and C. E. Elger eds.), 1983, pp. 238–249. Urban & Schwarzenberg, Munich.
51. Velasco, M., Velasco, F., Cepeda, C., Martínez, A., and Estrada-Villanueva, F. Alumina cream induced focal motor epilepsy in cats. IV. Peduncular and midline tegmental lesions. *Electroenceph. Clin. Neurophysiol.* **56** (1983) 63–73.
52. Velasco, M., Velasco, F., Romo, R., and Martínez, A. Effect of sagittal transections of the brain stem tegmentum on alumina cream induced focal motor seizures in cat. *Exp. Neurol.* **81** (1983) 226–239.
53. Velasco, F., Velasco, M., and Pacheco, M. T. Generalized seizures produced by push–

pull perfusion of pentylenete-trazol in the reticular formation. *Electroenceph. Clin. Neurophysiol.* (in press) (1983).

54. Velasco, M., Velasco, F., Pacheco, M. T., and Gallegos, A. J. Radioactivity distribution in the brain stem after push–pull perfusion of carbachol C-14 into the mesencephalic reticular formation. *Exp. Neurol.* (in preparation) (1983).
55. Velasco, M., Velasco, F., Márquez-Rubio, I., and Estrada-Villanueva, F. Alumina cream induced focal motor seizures in cats. V. Ablations of the cerebral cortex. *Electroenceph. Clin. Neurophysiol.* (in press) (1983).
56. Vivaldi, E., McCarley, R. W., and Hobson, J. A. Evocation of desynchronized sleep signs by carbachol filled micropipettes in the pontine brain stem. *In* "Sleep Research, UCLA" (M. H. Chase *et al.*, eds.), 1979, p. 88.
57. Vivaldi, E., McCarley, R. W., and Hobson, J. A. Evocation of stereo-typed PGO waves by placing carbachol (filled) micropipettes in the pontine tegmentum. *In* "Sleep Research, UCLA," (M. H. Chase *et al.*, eds.), 1979, p. 89.

17

The Use of Push–Pull Perfusion Techniques for Measuring the Efflux of [^{3}H]Dopamine in the Striatum of the Conscious Rat

GREGORY E. MARTIN* AND
DEAN R. HAUBRICH†

Department of Pharmacology
Merck Sharp & Dohme Research Laboratories
West Point, Pennsylvania

*Present address: McNeil Pharmaceutical, Department of Biological Research, Spring House, Pennsylvania 19477.
†Present address: Sterling-Winthrop Research Institute, Rensselaer, New York 12144.

ISBN 0-12-083350-6

I. INTRODUCTION

A. Rationale for Push–Pull Perfusion

The use of the push–pull perfusion technique is actually the latest refinement in a methodology that launched the study of neuropharmacology. Using isolated but innervated frog hearts, Loewi (*15*) was the first to demonstrate stimulation-induced release of a neuroactive substance, later determined to be acetylcholine, into perfusate collected from cardiac tissue during nerve stimulation. Perfusing innervated tissue *in situ* via a push–pull cannula, be it via concentric (*11*) or side-by-side collection tubes (*9*), represents an enormous stride forward as a tool for examining dynamic alterations in the biochemical sequelae of neural activity in the behaving animal. The intracerebral release of neuroactive substances mediating thermoregulation (*21*), food intake (*31*), and sleep (*10*) has been demonstrated in conscious animals using push–pull cannula in crossed-perfusion studies somewhat analogous in design to Loewi's original experiments in the isolated heart. The major premise of the push–pull method is that the perfusate will absorb a sampling of the transmitter substances released in the vicinity of the perfusion, making it possible to examine changes in transmitter release during behavior or after drug administration. The dramatic evocation of integrated physiologic responses in animals given donor perfusate in the aforementioned cross-perfusion studies validates this basic supposition. Although the push–pull perfusion may cause some traumatization of tissue (*3*), the technique has a unique advantage over methods in which an animal must be sacrificed, its nervous tissue removed, and levels of transmitter measured so that inferences may be drawn about transmitter release. The push–pull method is unique in that it allows repeated control experiments to be performed at the same anatomical site in the same animal. Furthermore, dynamic alterations in transmitter fluxes can be examined *in vivo* and correlated with behavior. The significance of this is obvious for the behavioral pharmacologist concerned with the biochemical events underlying behavior. In this chapter, the efflux of ^{3}H-labeled dopamine (DA) into push–pull perfusate collected within the striatum of the rat is studied in two different experimental paradigms.

B. Influence of Nigral GABA on Dopamine Neurons and Behavior

In the first experiment, the push–pull perfusion technique was the most direct method of answering a puzzling question which had arisen from our experiments with the GABA agonist muscimol. To place in perspective the importance of the push–pull method in resolving this experimental issue, a short history of the question is required. There were very few *in vivo* models for GABAergic activity in the mid-1970s. On the other hand, GABA was known to be present in large quantities within the substantia nigra (*2, 25*). Furthermore, GABA was thought to act within the substantia nigra to inhibit the firing of dopamine (DA) neurons which project via the nigrostriatal tract to the striatum (*1, 27*). The elegant studies of Ungerstedt (*30*) on these dopaminergic neurons and their role in the locomotor behavior of the rat suggested that the unilateral infusion of a GABAergic agent within the substantia nigra should, via inhibition of the dopaminergic neurons on that side of the brain, cause the activity of DA neurons in the opposite striatum to predominate, resulting in a rotational response, viz., directed ipsilateral to the side of the microinjection. The presence and magnitude of such a turning response might provide a feasible *in vivo* screen for putative GABA agonists.

Upon infusion into the substantia nigra, muscimol or other GABAergic agents were indeed found to produce rotation, but the rotation was directed contralateral to the infusion site. The turning was opposite to the predicted direction, a finding made simultaneously in several laboratories (*17, 18, 24, 26, 29*). Although the results produced an *in vivo* screen for GABA agonists, the chain of events producing the contralateral turning was unclear. According to Ungerstedt's theory (*30*), dopamine release in the striatum on the side of the muscimol injection should mediate the contralateral turning. Therefore, one was forced to assume that either the infused GABA was not inhibiting the DA neurons in the substantia nigra, or, alternatively, that DA release within the striatum was not mediating the turning. In fact, if Ungerstedt's theory were true, the intranigrally infused GABA should somehow be promoting DA release within the ipsilateral striatum. Presumably the only scheme by which this could occur is via GABAergic inhibition of an interneuron tonically inhibiting DA nerve cells within the substantia nigra.

To resolve this question, the push–pull method was employed in conscious animals in which GABAergic agonists were perfused within the substantia nigra. In these animals, rotation was observed as [^{3}H]DA efflux from the ipsilateral striatum was ascertained. Two push–pull cannula assemblies were utilized, one to apply the GABA agonist within the substantia nigra and one to perfuse ^{3}H-labeled tyrosine through the striatum. The push–pull method was the only apropos method for looking at the dynamic alteration in [^{3}H]DA release in the conscious behaving animal.

C. Effect of a Novel Compound, MK-801, on Striatal [^{3}H]Dopamine Efflux

The second experiment is an example of what push–pull perfusion can reveal about the dynamics of a drug interacting with striatal tissue. In this experiment, MK-801, a novel agent with apparent sympathomimetic activity (*7*), was perfused directly within the striatum. MK-801 is very potent in producing ipsilateral turning in 6-OHDA lesioned rats. Ipsilateral turning is generally evoked by agents, i.e., amphetamine and amfonelic acid, which cause the release of DA. The effect of MK-801 on [^{3}H]DA efflux was ascertained and compared with standard sympathomimetic compounds also known to evoke ipsilaterally directed turning in the lesioned rat.

In the first experiment, a complex question about neuropharmacological and anatomical interconnections is explored and in the second, the events underlying a specific drug action are examined.

II. METHODS

A. Species and Tissue Sites

There is one serious drawback to the use of push–pull cannulae, namely, the cannula assembly invariably produces tissue damage either during the perfusion itself (*28*) or simply via its insertion into tissue. The push–pull cannula utilized in these experiments is a concentric assembly essentially the same as described by Myers (*20*) (see Fig. 1). The outer pull tube is fashioned from 23-ga thin-wall stainless-steel tubing which has an outside diameter of 0.6 mm. When utilizing the rat, therefore, one must be wary of which anatomical structure one wishes to perfuse. Clearly, anatomical structures whose circumference is $\leq$ 0.6 mm would be difficult to study for two reasons. First of all, the entire region may be obliterated by insertion of the cannula assembly, and even if the cannula could be lowered so that only the perfusing medium impinged on the tissue, there would be some question as to whether the perfusate were collected exclusively from the tissue in question or also from bordering anatomical structures. As a result and of necessity, most push–pull studies in the rat are performed in anatomical regions of adequate size. Since the striatum is a rather large mass of tissue, it can survive the insertion of the push–pull cannula. Hence, as can be seen by examining other chapter titles in this book, the striatum has become the anatomical region which has been utilized the most in push–pull perfusion studies in the rat. If one were interested in studying a smaller central nervous system (CNS) structure, the use of a larger animal would be required.

B. Unanesthetized vs Free-Moving Animals

The potential for measuring dynamic alterations in transmitter fluxes within the brain of the conscious and behaving animal is one of the most exciting aspects of push–pull methodology. Performing a perfusion within the CNS of a freely moving animal, however, does require additional practical con-

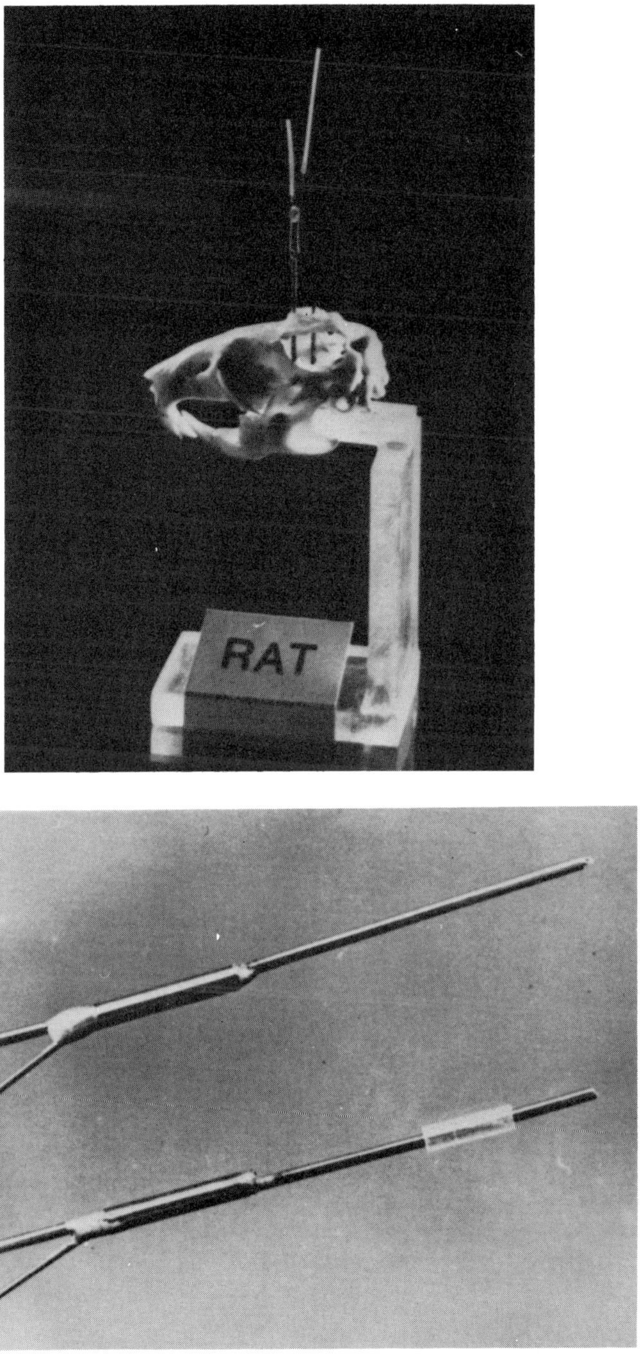

Fig. 1. A picture of the push–pull cannula assembly lowered into the skull of a rat. The lower panel is a close-up photo of the push–pull assembly. A polyethylene shim can be seen on the lower cannula which is used to adjust the cannulae to different perfusion depths.

siderations. Whether or not the animal should be anesthetized may depend on the questions that the experimenter is posing. Of the two experiments discussed here, the results issuing from the first are greatly enhanced by the simultaneous observation of behavior and [^{3}H]DA efflux, whereas the second experiment is not as concerned with the behavior but more with the biochemical sequalae of direct drug application to brain tissue. Both experiments, however, were carried out in the unanesthetized rat. The first question that comes to mind when using an anesthetized preparation is what effect will the anesthetic agent have on the dynamics of release of the transmitter or other bioactive substance being examined. The appropriate control experiments must be done before results from an anesthetized animal can be properly interpreted. The use of a free-moving rat usually requires the prior implantation of a guide cannula or the push–pull assembly. Hence, it is not as convenient as merely lowering a push–pull assembly into an anesthetized rat held in a stereotaxic device. In our laboratory, a guide cannula is implanted so that it terminates 3 to 4 mm above the intended perfusion site 4–7 days prior to the first perfusion. Although the implantation of a guide cannula does require additional work, it does circumvent a problem that is encountered when a cannulae is lowered into tissue just prior to perfusing. The recovery time following the implantation of the guide permits the brain tissue to heal around the cannula. Subsequently, upon insertion of the perfusion cannula, perfusing media does not escape up the sides of the cannula onto the surface of the cortex as we have observed to occur in acute preparations.

In a classic experiment on the dynamics of the push–pull perfusion, Yaksh and Yamamura (32) reported that the rat must be immobilized and the push–pull cannula held in place throughout an experiment since removing and replacing the cannula produced alterations in recovery of ^{14}C-labeled urea of 2.0- to 40.0-fold. In our experiments, the animal was free-moving which may have resulted in shifts in the orientation of the push–pull cannula *in situ*. In addition, the cannula assembly was removed, flushed, and then replaced at 15-min intervals throughout the experiment. In our control experiments, however, the baseline was stable enough (see figs. 5 and 13) that it seems these factors did not appreciably increase the variability of the recovery of [^{3}H]DA.

C. Assaying Push–Pull Perfusion Effluent

Radioactive labeling of endogenous stores of transmitter provides the experimenter with a very sensitive method of observing the activity of that transmitter. What method should be used to label the endogenous stores? In examining [^{3}H]DA efflux in our laboratory, two methods have been tried.

In the first method, a bolus injection of either ^{3}H- or ^{14}C-labeled DA was microinjected into the perfusion site via an injector needle cut to the same length as the push–pull cannula. After a period of from 30 min to 1 hr, serial perfusions of the labeled site were carried out and control efflux of radioactivity due to labeled DA was plotted against time to derive a washout curve. This method was subsequently abandoned for two reasons. First, one could not be sure that the injected [^{3}H]DA was being taken up exclusively into DA cells. The [^{3}H]DA could be taken up into glial, serotonergic, or noradrenergic cells. Alternatively, it might be sitting in the extracellular fluid as a residue of the bolus injection. This latter fear was raised by the fact that the washout curve had a very steep negative slope, with about 98% of the recovered radioactivity contained in the first two serial perfusions. The second reason was the shape of the radioactivity washout curve which varied greatly from animal to animal. There was no reliably reproducible plateau portion of the washout curve, making interanimal comparisons difficult.

The second method, adopted from the work of Nieoullon *et al.* (*23*) who used the push–pull method in the cat, was preferable for two reasons. In this system, a high concentration of [^{3}H]tyrosine [50 μCi/ml cerebrospinal fluid (CSF] was perfused through striatal tissue. [^{3}H]DA was then assayed in samples of the recovered push–pull effluent. Since [^{3}H]DA was measured in the effluent, one must assume it has undergone transformation from [^{3}H]tyrosine to [^{3}H]DA within a dopaminergic neuron. Hence, it is safer to assume that the [^{3}H]tyrosine was taken up and released by a DA neuron, and has not merely resided in the extracellular fluid or been released via a noncatecholaminergic neuron. Second, a stable baseline level of [^{3}H]DA recovered in control perfusates was also established rapidly which made inter- and intra-animal comparisons easier. The precise timing of the pharmacological or behavioral stimulation was therefore not as crucial as it was following the bolus injection. In some of our experiments, a 45-min perfusion of [^{3}H]tyrosine (30 μl/min, containing 50 μCi/ml of [^{3}H]tyrosine) was performed before the actual experiment was begun. This procedure, however, failed to increase the baseline levels of [^{3}H]DA collected in subsequent perfusates, so it was abandoned.

D. Methods Used to Examine Striatal [^{3}H]Dopamine Release during Intranigral Perfusion of GABA Agonists

Male Sprague–Dawley rats weighing 400–600 g were used. With the head held level, a 20-ga thin-wall guide cannula was stereotaxically implanted (coordinates in parentheses) above the striatum (stereotaxic coordinates, anterior–posterior (AP), −0.2 mm from bregma, L 2.2 and V − 3.2 mm from skull) and another above the ipsilateral substantia nigra (SN) (AP 3.1, L 2.0, V

−1 from skull). At least 1 week following surgery, a push–pull cannula (*20*), specially modified for the rat and pictured in Fig. 1, was lowered into the striatum and an artificial CSF (*19*) containing 50 μCi/ml of [^{3}H]tyrosine (40–50 μCi/mmol, NEN) was perfused at a rate of 30 μl/min. The experiment consisted of eight serial perfusions of the striatum, each 15 min in duration. To minimize possible tissue damage due to a suction lesion, the flow of the perfusion was constantly monitored by watching the progress of a small air bubble, about 2 mm in length, down the effluent tube. The effluent PE tubing

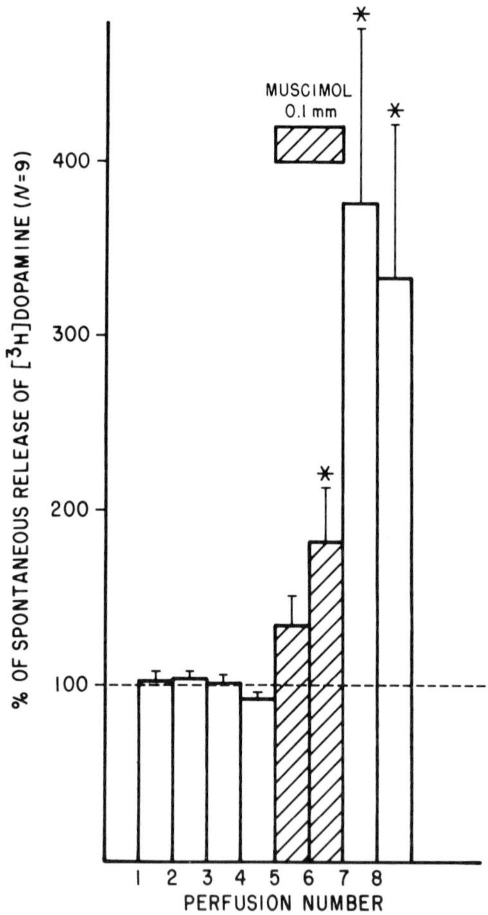

Fig. 2. The percentage of spontaneous release of [^{3}H]dopamine obtained in serial perfusions of the striatum. Muscimol (0.1 m*M*) was perfused simultaneously through the substantia nigra during the perfusions indicated by the cross-hatching. In this and in figures to follow, the asterisks denote a significant difference from the values derived for the CSF control group (see Fig. 5) ($p < .05$, t test).

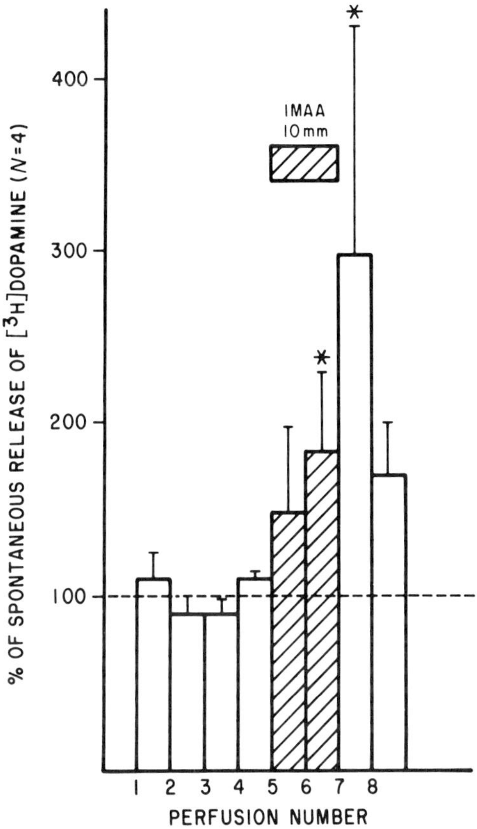

Fig. 3. Striatal [^{3}H]dopamine efflux in the rat. A 10 m*M* solution of IMAA was perfused through the ipsilateral SN during the perfusions denoted by the cross-hatching.

(PE-50) was calibrated in 30-μl volumes so that the rate of perfusion could be constantly monitored. If an outflow bubble failed to progress at a rate of 30 μl/min, the perfusion was immediately stopped. At the end of each 15-min perfusion, the push–pull assembly was removed from the guide cannula. The PE-50 outflow tubing was removed from the system and the effluent quickly expelled into a chilled test tube containing cold DA carrier and an antioxidant. A fresh length of PE-50 tubing filled with CSF except for the 2-mm bubble was quickly fastened to the pull side of the push–pull cannula which was then reinserted in the striatum for the next perfusion. The perfusions were conducted using a Harvard apparatus withdrawal infusion pump with a variable speed motor. The perfusing medium was loaded in the infusion pumps in 5-ml plastic syringes. During the fifth and sixth perfusion of striatal tissue, a second push–pull cannula was lowered into the ipsilateral substan-

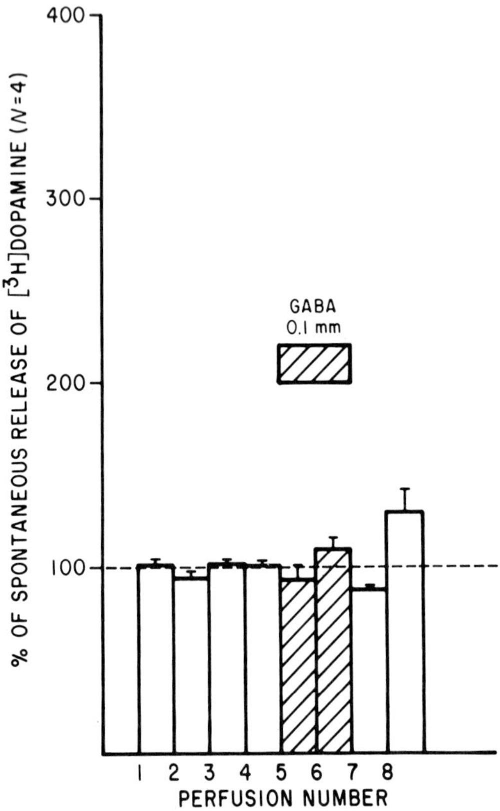

Fig. 4. Striatal [^{3}H]dopamine efflux in the rat. A 0.1 m*M* solution of GABA (cross-hatching) was perfused intranigrally during striatal perfusions 5 and 6.

tia nigra. Through this cannula, either the CSF vehicle solution, muscimol (0.1 m*M*), imidazole acetic acid (IMAA, 10 m*M*), or GABA (0.1 m*M*) was perfused at a rate of 30 μl/min. A 400-μl aliquot of each striatal perfusate was assayed for [^{3}H]DA content using the ion-exchange method of Neff *et al.* (22). The behavior of the rat, viz., circling, was also noted but not quantified throughout the experiment.

The mean amount of [^{3}H]DA in the four striatal perfusates preceding the intranigral perfusions was used as a control value indicative of spontaneous release of [^{3}H]DA. [^{3}H]DA in each perfusate was then expressed as a percentage of this spontaneous release value. [^{3}H]DA levels in striatal effluent collected during the nigral perfusion of the GABA agonists was compared with that collected during CSF perfusions of the substantia nigra in a control group using a *t* test. The grouped data only included data from experiments in which the perfusion sites had been localized via examination of histological material to the striatum and substantia nigra. The stereotaxic atlas of König and Klippel (*14*) was used to verify the perfusion sites.

Data are not shown for perfusions of IMAA in concentrations of 0.1 and 1.0 m*M*, nor for muscimol perfused in a concentration of 0.01 m*M*, since these perfusions failed to elicit either turning or [^{3}H]DA release.

E. [^{3}H]Dopamine Release during Direct Intrastriatal Perfusion of Sympathomimetics

A single guide cannula was stereotaxically implanted above the striatum (for coordinates see Section II,D). In these experiments, three intrastriatal

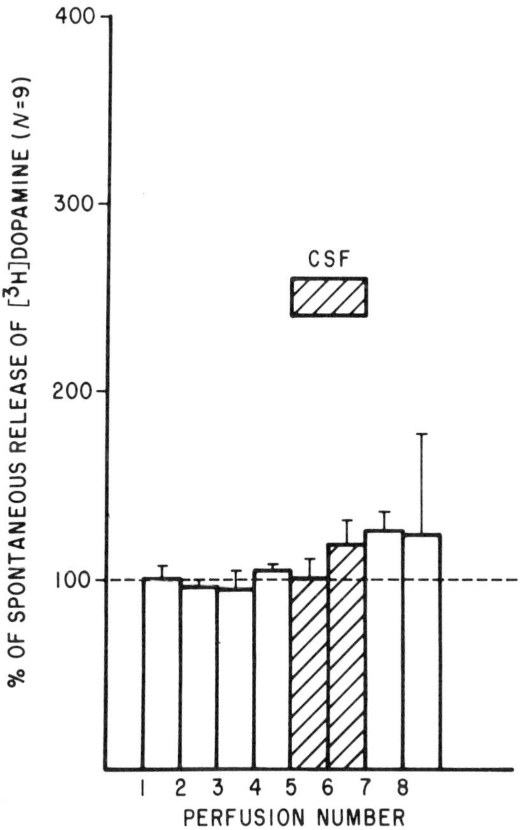

Fig. 5. Striatal [^{3}H]dopamine efflux in the rat. A CSF vehicle solution (cross-hatching) was perfused intranigrally during striatal perfusions 5 and 6.

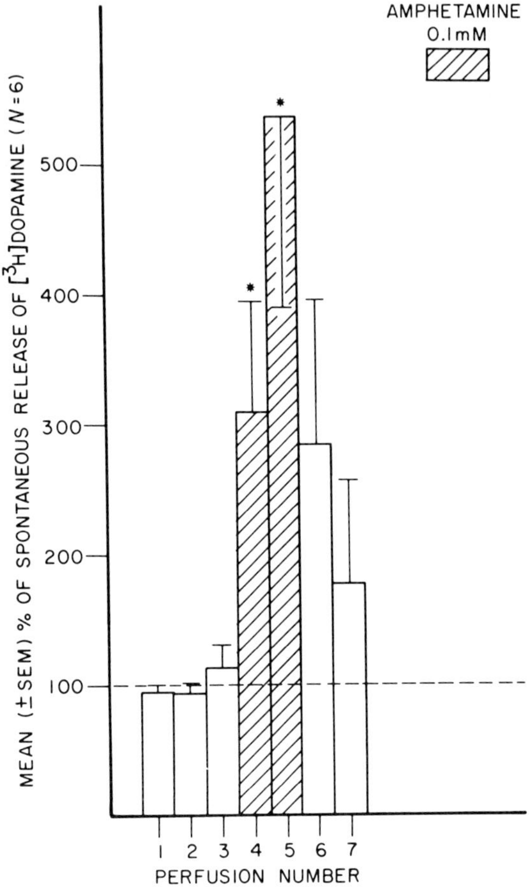

Fig. 6. Efflux of striatal [^{3}H]dopamine during the direct intrastriatal perfusion of 0.1 m*M* amphetamine (cross-hatching) (perfusions 4 and 5).

control perfusions of [^{3}H]tyrosine (30 μl/min) preceded two perfusions of 0.1 m*M* solutions of either amphetamine, amfonelic acid, methylphenidate, nomifensine, apomorphine, (±)-5-methyl-10,11-dihydro-5*H*-dibenzo[*a,d*]-cyclohepten-5,10-imine, or its (+) isomer (MK-801) which were in turn followed by two additional control perfusions of CSF contained [^{3}H]tyrosine. There also was a series of control experiments in which CSF alone was perfused in seven serial perfusions. Artificial CSF containing 50 μCi/ml of [^{3}H]tyrosine was the vehicle for all perfusions. The assays and statistical analyses were identical to those in the first experiment. These animals were also observed for overt behavioral reactions during the perfusion.

III. FINDINGS

A. [³H]Dopamine Efflux into Striatal Perfusates during the Intranigral Perfusion of GABA Agonists

The intranigral perfusion of muscimol produced contraversive turning which varied in time to onset from 30 sec to 8 min into the first intranigral perfusion. A significant efflux of [³H]DA into the push–pull effluent was not seen until the second perfusion of muscimol, but it did persist through the

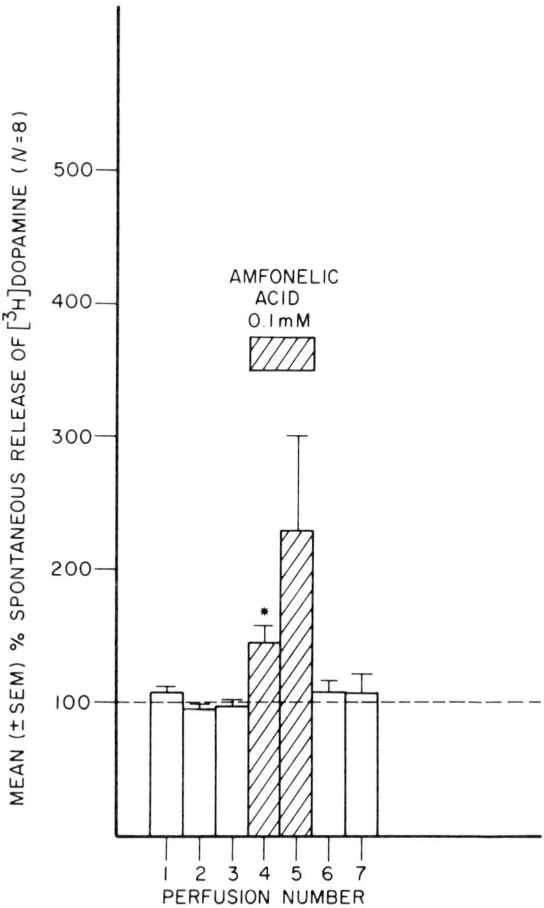

Fig. 7. Efflux of striatal [³H]dopamine during the direct intrastriatal perfusion of 0.1 mM amfonelic acid (cross-hatching) (perfusions 4 and 5).

seventh and eighth striatal perfusions, as shown in Fig. 2. The intranigral perfusion of IMAA also produced contraversive turning and a significant increase in [^{3}H]DA levels detected in striatal perfusate. As shown in Fig. 3, IMAA induced [^{3}H]DA release in a pattern similar to that seen following muscimol. Neither the amount of turning, nor the magnitude of the IMAA-induced increase in [^{3}H]DA in the perfusate were as great as following muscimol despite the 100-fold greater concentration of IMAA in the nigral perfusate.

GABA (0.1 m*M*) failed to elicit either turning or a significant increase in [^{3}H]DA efflux into the striatum, as shown in Fig. 4. The pattern of recovery for [^{3}H]DA during the intranigral perfusion of GABA was similar to that seen

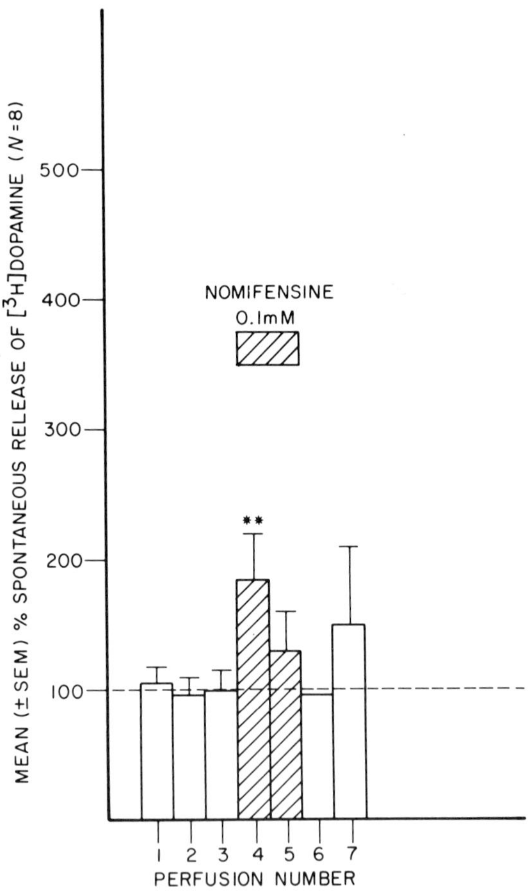

Fig. 8. Efflux of [^{3}H]dopamine during the direct intrastriatal perfusion of 0.1 m*M* nomifensine (cross-hatching) (perfusions 4 and 5).

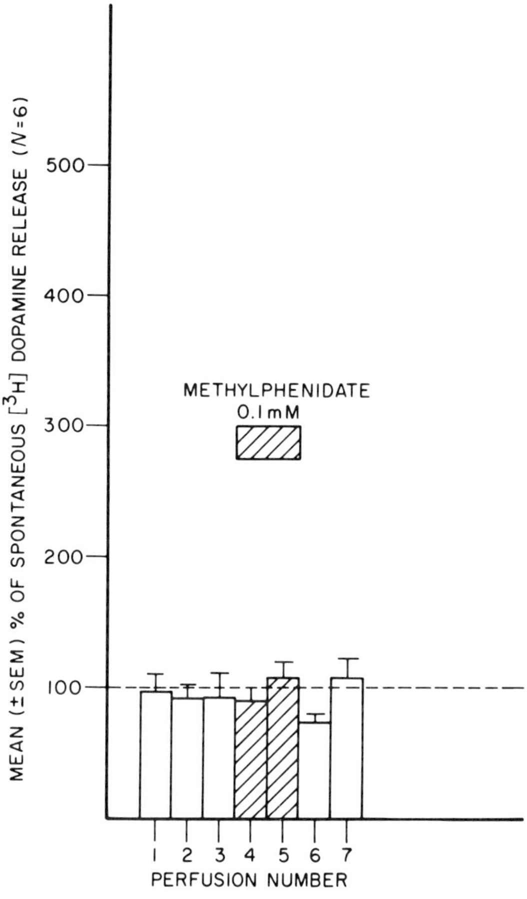

Fig. 9. Efflux of [^{3}H]dopamine during the direct intrastriatal perfusion of 0.1 m*M* methylphenidate (cross-hatching) (perfusions 4 and 5).

for the intranigral perfusion of the CSF vehicle (Fig. 5). The lack of activity of GABA is not surprising since it is much less potent than muscimol or IMAA in producing contraversive turning when given into the SN.

B. [^{3}H]Dopamine Efflux during Intrastriatal Perfusion of Sympathomimetics

The direct intrastriatal perfusion of amphetamine produced a greater than fivefold increase in the efflux of [^{3}H]DA into the push–pull perfusate (Fig. 6). Behaviorally, the intrastriatal perfusion of amphetamine produced a mild form of stereotypy which consisted mainly of sniffing but not turning. Amfonelic acid also produced a significant increase in [^{3}H]DA recovered in the perfusate causing a doubling of the amount recovered, as shown in Fig. 7. The DA uptake inhibitor, nomifensine (Fig. 8), was somewhat less potent than either amphetamine or amfonelic acid but did produce a significant increase in [^{3}H]DA recovery.

Methylphenidate, on the other hand, failed to evoke a significant efflux of [^{3}H]DA from the striatum (Fig. 9). Similarly, the direct application of either MK-801 or its racemic parent failed to produce a significant efflux of [^{3}H]DA into the perfusing medium (Figs. 10 and 11). The direct-acting DA agonist, apomorphine, also failed to significantly alter the basal efflux of [^{3}H]DA (Fig. 12) from the pattern of release observed in control animals (Fig. 13).

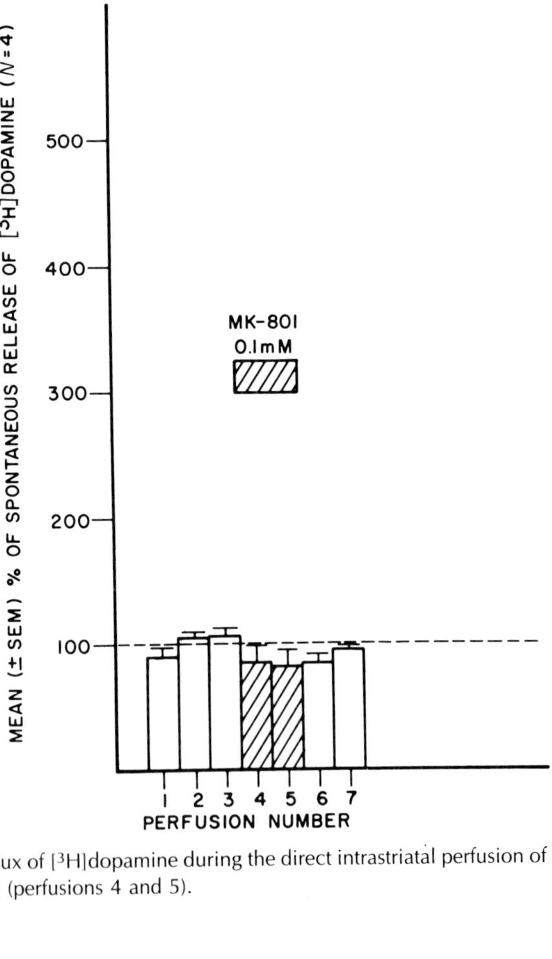

Fig. 10. Efflux of [^{3}H]dopamine during the direct intrastriatal perfusion of 0.1 m*M* MK-801 (cross-hatching) (perfusions 4 and 5).

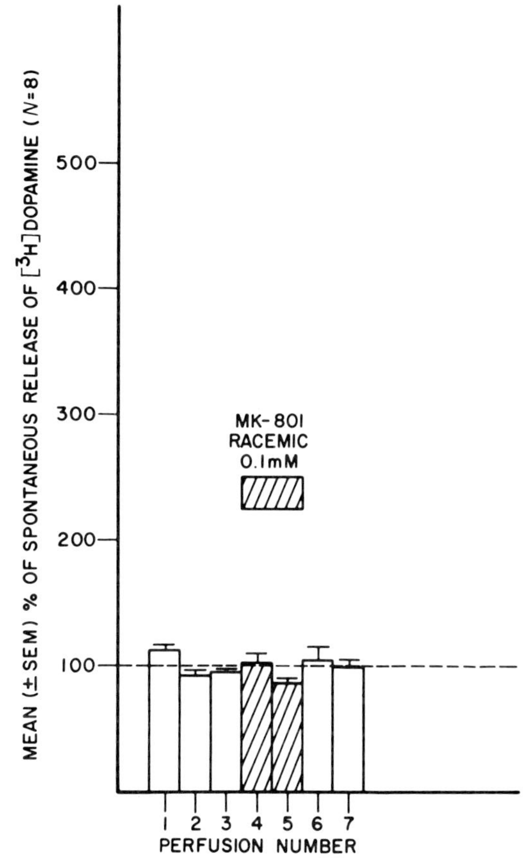

Fig. 11. Efflux of [^{3}H]dopamine during the direct intrastriatal perfusion of 0.1 m*M* racemic MK-801 (cross-hatching) (perfusions 4 and 5).

IV. DISCUSSION AND PERSPECTIVES

Through use of push–pull cannulae, the resolution of a complex question is provided in the first set of experiments. The turning elicited by the intranigral infusion of a GABA agonist, reported by several authors (*17, 18, 24, 26, 29*), is indeed accompanied by the release of [^{3}H]DA, newly synthesized from [^{3}H]tyrosine, within the ipsilateral striatum. The finding preserves the integrity of Ungerstedt's heuristic framework for explaining the neurochemical events mediating this turning (*30*). The present experiments, however, do not resolve the issue of how the GABA agonist produces the

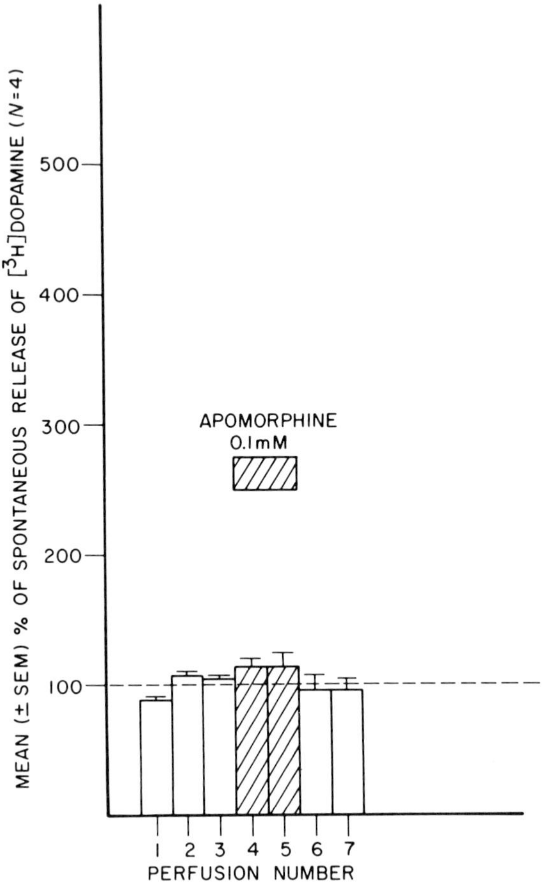

Fig. 12. Efflux of [^{3}H]dopamine during the direct intrastriatal perfusion of 0.1 m*M* apomorphine (cross-hatching) (perfusions 4 and 5).

apparent striatal release of [^{3}H]DA. The data are in agreement with those reported in the immobilized cat by Chéramy and co-workers (4–6) who have clearly shown in the anesthetized cat that the intranigral infusion of GABA agonists increases the release of [^{3}H]DA into the ipsilateral striatum. GABA may produce this apparent excitatory effect on DA neurons via inhibition of the inhibitory action of an interneuron within the substantia nigra. The precise neuronal circuitry involved, however, remains to be fully elucidated.

In the series of experiments in which compounds were perfused directly through striatal tissue, the push–pull perfusion method was used in an attempt to delineate the profile of activity of a novel sympathomimetic drug,

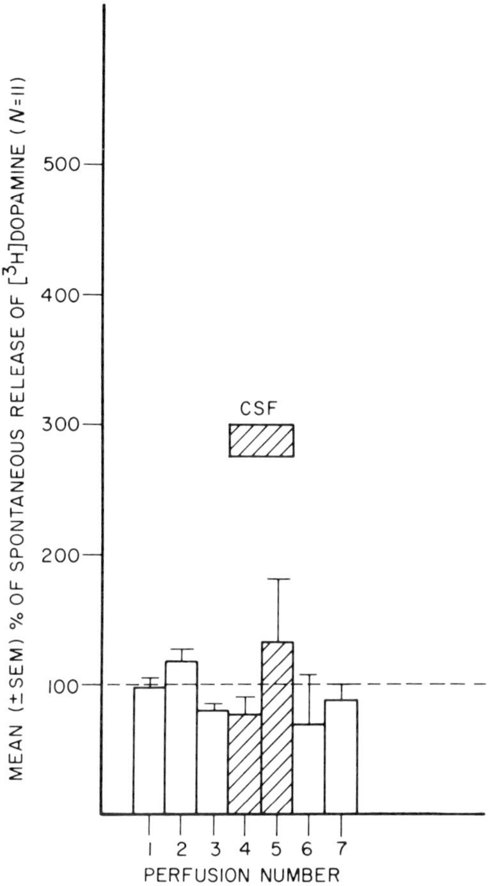

Fig. 13. Efflux of [³H]dopamine into seven serial 15-min (30 μl/min) perfusions of the striatum with a solution of artificial CSF (cross-hatching) containing 50 μCi/ml of [³H]tyrosine.

MK-801. This agent, which is more potent than amphetamine in producing turning in 6-OHDA-lesioned rats (*7*), surprisingly failed to elicit the release of [³H]DA into striatal perfusates. Amfonelic acid, which releases DA from nerve endings (*16*), and nomifensine, which blocks reuptake of DA (*12*), both produced an increased efflux of [³H]DA from the striatum. MK-801 is clearly more methylphenidate-like in this test, as has been reported in other *in vivo* test systems (*7, 8*), insofar as it failed to increase the level of [³H]DA recovered in the perfusate. These results do not preclude the possibility that MK-801 releases [³H]DA following parenteral administration. MK-801 may undergo preliminary metabolism in the bloodstream to an active agent, which then produces the release of DA. Alternatively, MK-801 may act on cell bodies in the substantia nigra to evoke DA release in the striatum. These questions form the basis of additional experiments. It is interesting to note that none of the sympathomimetic agents elicited contraversive turning when perfused intrastriatally. This may be due to the fact that either a sufficient number of striatal cells were not bathed by the perfusing solution to result in a behavioral response, or that the concomitant stimulation of the nucleus accumbens may also be required to produce the turning response (*13*).

The push–pull perfusion technique was utilized to answer two different questions in these experiments. The effect of a locally applied drug on release of [^{3}H]DA from neural tissue was examined as well as the dynamics of striatal [^{3}H]DA release during drug stimulation at a distant site. When utilized with the proper caution and control experiments, the push–pull technique provides a powerful method for monitoring changes in transmitter release. With the advent of new and more sensitive assays for measuring the efflux of endogenous substances, the technique promises to be even more useful in unraveling the function of specific cerebral structures and the mechanisms of action of drugs on the central nervous system.

REFERENCES

1. Anden, N.-E., and Stock, G. Inhibitory effect of gamma-hydroxybutyric acid and gamma-aminobutyric acid on the dopamine cells in the substantia nigra. *Naunyn-Schmiedeberg's Arch. Pharmacol.* **279** (1973) 89–92.
2. Balcom, G. J., Lenox, R. H., and Meyerhoff, J. L. Regional γ-aminobutyric acid levels in rat brain determined after microwave fixation. *J. Neurochem.* **24** (1975) 609–613.
3. Chase, T. N., and Kopin, I. J. Stimulus induced release of substances from olfactory bulb using the push–pull cannula. *Nature (London)* **217** (1968) 466–467.
4. Chéramy, A., Nieoullon, A., and Glowinski, J. Stimulating effects of γ-hydroxybutyrate on dopamine release from the caudate nucleus and the substantia nigra of the cat. *J. Pharmac. Exp. Therap.* **203** (1977) 283–293.
5. Chéramy, A., Nieoullon, A., and Glowinski, J. GABAergic processes involved in the control of dopamine release from nigrostriatal dopaminergic neurons in the cat. *Eur. J. Pharm.* **48** (1978) 281–295.
6. Chéramy, A., Nieoullon, A., and Glowinski, J. *In vivo* changes in dopamine release in cat caudate nucleus and substantia nigra induced by nigral application of various drugs including GABAergic agonists and antagonists. *In* "Interactions between Putative Neurotransmitters in the Brain," 1978, pp. 175–190. Raven, New York.
7. Clineschmidt, B. V., Martin, G. E., Bunting, P. R., and Papp, N. L. Central sympathomimetic activity of (+)-5-methyl-10,11-dihydro-5*H*-dibenzo[*a,d*]cyclohepten-5,10-imine (MK-801), a substance with potent anticonvulsant, central sympathomimetic, and apparent anxiolytic properties. *Drug Dev. Res.* **2** (1982) 135–145.
8. Clineschmidt, B. V., Martin, G. E., and Bunting, P. Anticonvulsant activity of (+)-5-methyl-10,11-dihydro-5*H*-dibenzo[*a,d*]cyclohepten-5,10-imine (MK-801), a substance

with potent anticonvulsant, central sympathomimetic, and apparent anxiolytic properties. *Drug Dev. Res.* 2 (1982) 123–134.
9. Delgado, J. M. R. Electrodes for extracellular recording and stimulation. *In* "Physical Techniques in Biological Research," Vol. V, 1964, pp. 88–143. Academic Press, New York.
10. Drucker-Colín, R. R. Crossed perfusion of a sleep inducing brain tissue substance in conscious cats, *Brain Res.* **56** (1973) 123–134.
11. Gaddum, J. H. Push–pull cannulae. *J. Physiol. (London)* **155** (1961) 1–2P.
12. Hoffman, I. Pharmacology of nomifensine. *Int. Pharmacopsychiat.* (Suppl 1) **17** (1982) 4–20.
13. Kelly, P. H., and Moore, K. E. Dopamine concentrations in the rat brain following injections into the substantia nigra of baclofen, γ-aminobutyric acid. γ-hydroxybutyric acid, apomorphine and amphetamine. *Neuropharmacology* **17** (1978) 169–174.
14. König, J. F. R., and Klippel, R. A. *In* "The Rat Brain," 1963. Williams & Wilkins, Baltimore, Maryland.
15. Loewi, O. Uker humorale ubertragbarbeit der herznervenwerkung. *Pflugers Arch.* **89** (1921) 239–242.
16. McMillen, B. A., and Shore, P. A. Amfonelic acid, a non-amphetamine stimulant, has marked effects on brain dopamine metabolism but not noradrenaline metabolism: association with differences in neuronal storage systems. *J. Pharm. Pharmac.* **30** (1978) 464–466.
17. Martin, G. E., Bacino, C. B., and Papp, N. L. Contraversive circling induced in the rat by the intranigral microinjection of muscimol. *Soc. Neurosci. Abst.* **3** (1977) 41.
18. Martin, G. E., Bacino, C. B., and Papp, N. L. Contralateral turning evoked by the intranigral microinjection of muscimol and other GABA agonists. *Brain Res.* **155** (1978) 297–312.
19. Myers, R. D. General laboratory procedures. *Meth. Psychobiol.* **1** (1971) 27–67.
20. Myers, R. D. Methods for perfusing different structures of the brain. *Meth. Psychobiol.* **2** (1972) 169–211.
21. Myers, R. D., and Sharpe, L. G. Temperature in the monkey: transmitter factors released from the brain during thermoregulation. *Science* **161** (1968) 572–573.
22. Neff, N. H., Spano, P. F., Groppetti, A., Wang, C. T., and Costa, E. A simple procedure for calculating the synthesis rate of norepinephrine, dopamine and serotonin in rat brain. *J. Pharmacol. Exp. Therap.* **176** (1971) 701–710.
23. Nieoullon, A., Chéramy, A., and Glowinski, J. An adaptation of the push–pull cannula method to study the *in vivo* release of [^{3}H]dopamine synthesized from [^{3}H]tyrosine in the cat caudate nucleus: effects of various physical and pharmacological treatments. *J. Neurochem.* **28** (1977) 819–828.
24. Oberlander, C., Dumont, C., and Boissier, J. R. Rotational behaviour after unilateral intranigral injection of muscimol in rats. *Eur. J. Pharm.* **43** (1977) 389–390.
25. Okada, Y., Nitsch-Hassler, C., Kim, J. S., Bak, I. J., and Hassler, R. Role of γ-aminobutyric acid (GABA) in the extrapyramidal motor system. 1. Regional distribution of GABA in rabbit, rat, guinea pig and baboon CNS. *Exp. Brain Res.* **13** (1971) 514–518.
26. Olpe, H.-R., Schellenberg, H., and Koella, W. P. Rotational behavior induced in rats by intranigral application of GABA-related drugs and GABA antagonists. *Eur. J. Pharmacol.* **45** (1977) 291–294.
27. Precht, W., and Yoshida, M. Blockade of caudate-evoked inhibition of neurons in the substantia nigra by picrotoxin. *Brain Res.* **32** (1971) 229–233.
28. Redgrave, P. A modified push–pull system for the localized perfusion of brain tissue. *Pharm. Biochem. Behav.* **6** (1977) 471–474.
29. Scheel-Krüger, J., Arnt, J., and Magelund, G. Behavioural stimulation induced by mus-

cimol, and other GABA agonists injected into the substantia nigra. *Neurosci. Lett.* **4** (1977) 351–356.
30. Ungerstedt, U. Striatal dopamine release after amphetamine or nerve degeneration revealed by rotational behaviour. *Acta Phys. Scand. Suppl.* **367** (1971) 49–68.
31. Yaksh, T. L., and Myers, R. D. Neurohumoral substances released from hypothalamus of the monkey during hunger and satiety. *Am. J. Physiol.* **222** (1972) 503–515.
32. Yaksh, T. L., and Yamamura, H. I. Factors affecting performance of the push–pull cannula in brain. *J. App. Physiol.* **37** (1974) 428–434.

Index

V